AF364434

# Novel Drug Delivery Systems

# Novel Drug Delivery Systems

DK Tripathi

Amit Alexander

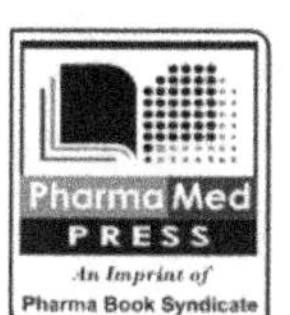

**PharmaMed Press**
*An imprint of Pharma Book Syndicate*

**A unit of BSP Books Pvt. Ltd.**
4-4-309/316, Giriraj Lane,
Sultan Bazar, Hyderabad - 500 095.

*Published by*

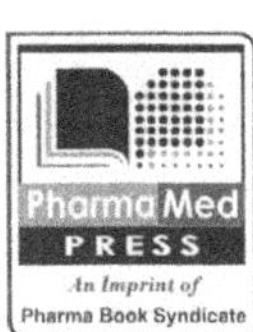

# PharmaMed Press

*An imprint of Pharma Book Syndicate*
**A unit of BSP Books Pvt. Ltd.**

4-4-309/316, Giriraj Lane, Sultan Bazar, Hyderabad - 500 095.
Phone: 040-23445600, 23445688; Fax: 91+40-23445611
E-mail: info@pharmamedpress.com
www.pharmamedpress.com/pharmamedpress.net

**ISBN: 978-93-89354-18-8**

# PREFACE

The driving force behind writing this book is to inculcate the fundamentals of the Novel Drug Delivery Systems (NDDS) into the students. The chapters in the book cover the majority of NDDS required for the students to strengthen their research domain. The adherence of the content is following the standard syllabus of the Pharmacy Council of India (PCI), New Delhi. The book comprises of Eleven chapters describing different prospects of novel drug delivery system. The first chapter elaborates the basic principle and design of the controlled drug delivery system along with the properties of drug and polymers suitable for the development of CDDS. The second chapter explains the types, properties, and application of various polymers in CDDS explicitly. Moving ahead, the chapter three deals with the microencapsulation process, its advantages, disadvantages, and application as a novel drug carrier system.

Further, chapter four explains mucosal drug delivery system, the concept of bioadhesion, mucoadhesive polymers, transmucosal permeability and formulation consideration of different mucoadhesive formulations specifically the buccal drug delivery system. The next chapter illustrates the implantable drug delivery devices, the concept of implants and different types of osmotic pumps. After that, chapter six elucidates the transdermal drug delivery system, drug permeation through the skin, use of permeation enhancers, components of transdermal drug delivery devices and its formulation approaches.

Moreover, chapter seven enlightens gastro-retentive drug delivery system. More emphasis has been paid on the novel approaches of gastro retention including the floating tablets, inflatables, high-density system, and gastro adhesive system. The next chapter, chapter eight deals with nasopulmonary drug delivery system. It explains the essential features, concept, and designing of the inhaler, nasal sprays, nebulizer, and other naso-pulmonary devices. Afterward, chapter nine explains the basic concept and approaches of targeted drug delivery system along with the properties and applications of a different nano-carrier system including liposome, niosome, nanoparticles, monoclonal antibodies and many more.

Further, chapter ten elucidates the ocular drug delivery system, intra-ocular barriers, formulation parameters of occusert and other ophthalmic formulations. Thereafter, the last chapter describes the intrauterine drug delivery system different types of IUDs, its application and limitations. Overall, in the book, we tried to cover all the critical areas of NDDS according to the PCI scheme.

The entire writing was done with a clear intention to target the UG and PG students' competencies of learning the NDDS. The contents of the chapters are kept complete and straightforward with maximum use of original illustrations and diagrams to make the content clearer, and easy to understand.

However, we will be grateful to have your comments on the content of the book for future improvement and revision of the book. Your contribution in this regard will be highly appreciated.

*-Authors*

# ACKNOWLEDGEMENT

I must express my sincere thanks to the Management of Santosh Rungta Group of Institutions, Bhilai. In particular, I am grateful to Sri Santosh Rungta ji, the mentor of the mentors, for providing the facilities and encouragement for completion of this book. I am also thankful to Dr. Saurav Rungta, Director (Tech) and Mr. Sonal Rungta, Director (F & A) for their inspiration and cooperation.

I am heartily thankful to Mrs. Bimala, my wife for her cooperation without which it would not be possible for me to complete the work.

I am also thankful to Dr. Amit Alexander, who has worked with me and has written five chapters. Dr. Alexander happens to be one of my colleagues.

I express my thanks to my colleagues Dr. Ajazuddin and others for their cooperation.

*DK Tripathi*

# ABOUT THE AUTHORS

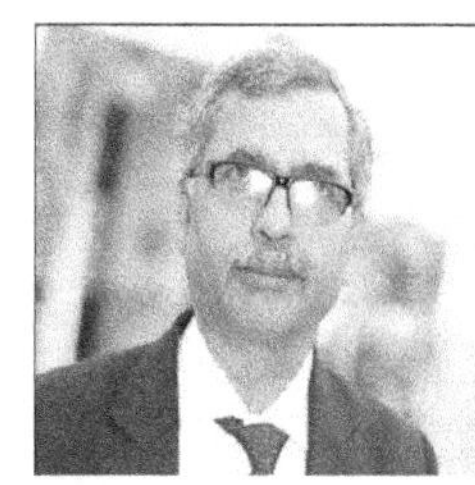

**Dr. DK Tripathi** has been working in the profession of Pharmacy since 1974, about forty five years. He has completed his Bachelor, Master's and PhD degree from Jadavpur University, Kolkata. His specialization is Pharmaceutics, he has worked in various departments such as Quality Control, Production, and in R&D of different pharmaceutical industries in different capacities during a period of more than two decades.

Since he has been working in academic institutions for more than twenty one years, he understands the needs of the students and where the students lack. Dr. Tripathi has authored five books – Introduction to Pharmaceutics (Theory & Practice), Pharmaceutics (Basic Principles & Formulations), Industrial Pharmacy (A Comprehensive Approach) and Elementary Pharmaceutical Calculations, Career Opportunity in Pharmacy. Each of the books has gained readers' acceptance; since in each book there is a touch of industrial approach which is desired.

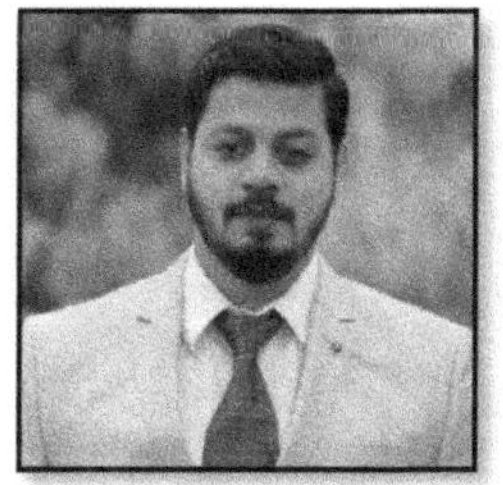

**Dr. Amit Alexander** is working as an **Associate Professor** in the Department of Pharmaceutics at Rungta College of Pharmaceutical Sciences and Research (RCPSR), Bhilai, Chhattisgarh, India. He received the Doctorate Degree from the University Institute of Pharmacy, Pt. Ravishankar Shukla University, Raipur, Chhattisgarh, India in 2015. **Dr. Alexander** has an overall teaching experience of 11 years and 8 Years of Research Experience. He is also serving as a **Review Editor** in Frontier in Biomaterial Journal. He is also serving as a **Reviewer** in various reputed Journals like Biomacromolecules (ACS Publication); Journal of Neuroscience method (Elsevier); Material Science and Engineering (Elsevier); Neurochemistry International reviews (Elsevier); and Journal of Cellular Physiology (Wiley Online), etc. He is also contributing his scientific writing in various labs of different countries like the USA, GREECE, EGYPT, and TEHRAN. He won the title of "**Young Scientist**" (2013), recipient of **P. D. Sethi** Best Research Paper award (2013); recipient of the outstanding faculty of the year award (2016) by G.D.R., Educational society, etc. Dr. Alexander is frequently contributing as a **Grant Evaluator** in Government Funding Agencies like Science and Engineering Research Board (SERB), New Delhi, India and associated with various esteemed international journals as well.

# CONTENTS



## CHAPTER 1   CONTROLLED DRUG DELIVERY SYSTEMS



## CHAPTER 2  POLYMERS

## CHAPTER 3  MICROENCAPSULATION



## CHAPTER 4  MUCOSAL DRUG DELIVERY SYSTEM

# CHAPTER 5 IMPLANTABLE DRUG DELIVERY SYSTEMS

# CHAPTER 6 TRANSDERMAL DRUG DELIVERY SYSTEMS

## CHAPTER 7   GASTRORETENTIVE DRUG DELIVERY SYSTEMS



## CHAPTER 8   NASOPULMONARY DRUG DELIVERY SYSTEM

# CHAPTER 9  NANOTECHNOLOGY AND ITS CONCEPTS

# CHAPTER 10  OCULAR DRUG DELIVERY SYSTEMS

## CHAPTER 11  INTRAUTERINE DRUG DELIVERY SYSTEMS

# CHAPTER 1

# Controlled Drug Delivery Systems

*Introduction, terminology/definitions and rationale, advantages, disadvantages, selection of drug candidates Approaches to design-controlled release formulations based on diffusion, dissolution and ion exchange principles, Physicochemical and biological properties of drugs relevant to controlled release formulations*

## Introduction

Drugs are administered through various routes such as oral, topical, parenteral, etc. Among all these routes, the oral route is the most common, convenient and popular. There are various reasons for such popularity. The most important and common reasons for their popularity are the convenience of administration, easy to carry and the ease of preparation on an industrial scale. About 80% of the dosage forms sold in the market are tablet dosage form. These dosage forms have been used since long, but these are found to have the following limitations.

1. The frequency of administration in a day, 'dosage regimen' is high.
2. It is difficult to monitor the daily-dose; in many cases, it is not exactly maintained.
3. There is a greater chance of missing dose.
4. Non-specific administration
5. The careful calculation is required to prevent overdosing; it is difficult to calculate the exact dose for a child or elderly patient who should not receive the adult dose.
6. The drug goes to non-target cells and can cause damage; orally administered drug must reach circulatory bloodstream every time and pass through the liver. Thus, the drug is available in the sites which are not affected.
7. Low concentrations can be ineffective. After oral administration fraction of the dose may not be absorbed, a fraction of dose is metabolized; hence, the amount of drug must be sufficient to elicit its therapeutic action.

8.    High concentrations can be toxic, causing side effects or damage to organs.

9.    Consumption of more drug than necessity.

After oral administration of a drug, the concentration of the drug increases gradually with time (absorption phase) as shown in **Fig. 1.1**.

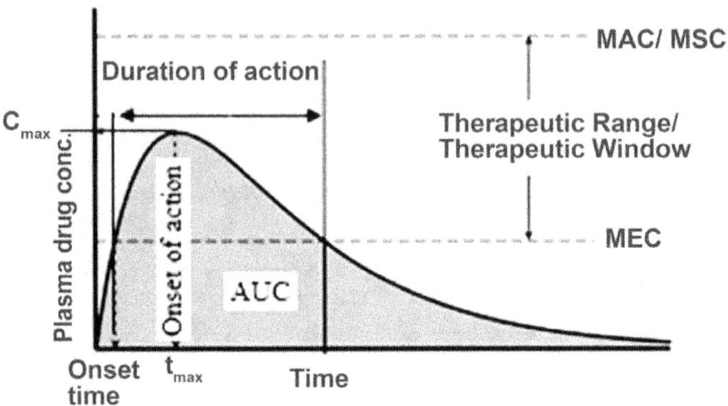


**Fig. 1.1:** Bioavailability profile of drug after oral administration. The curve plotted between plasma drug concentration vs. time, showing all the pharmacokinetic parameters, where; MEC- minimum effective concentration; MSC- maximum safe concentration; AUC- area under curve; $C_{max}$- maximum drug concentration and $t_{max}$- maximum time.

During this phase, absorption >> elimination. Therapeutic action starts when the concentration of the drug reaches the minimum effective concentration (MEC); the ascending portion of the curve. Once the concentration reaches to peak level, the descending phase starts (elimination phase); the metabolism and elimination phase predominates. During this phase elimination >> absorption. The therapeutic effect is observeduntil the concentration remains above the MEC. The period during which the concentration of the drug remains above the MEC is

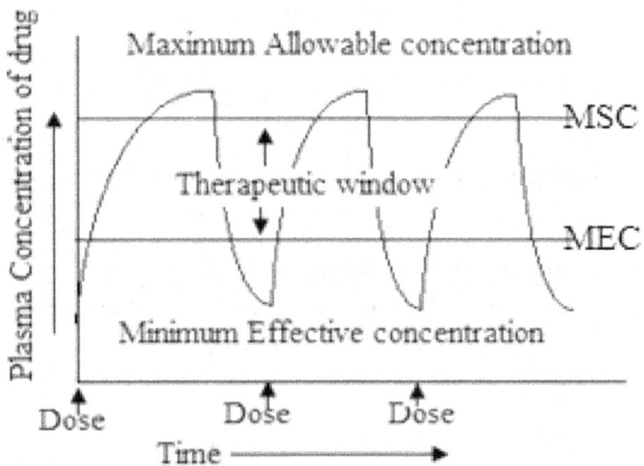


**Fig. 1.2:** Fluctuation in plasma concentration of drug following conventional dosage forms

called *duration of action*. After the concentration falls below the MEC, a second dose is required to achieve continuous therapeutic action of the drug; this is shown in **Fig. 1.2**.

## Terminology/Definitions

A.  **Immediate release dosage forms:** The conventional dosage forms belong to this class. The dosage form releases the drug present in it after administration to achieve rapid and complete systemic absorption. After absorption of the drug from the dosage form, plasma concentration of the drug starts decreasing according to its pharmacokinetic profile. Finally, the concentration falls below the minimum therapeutic concentration (MEC) and therapeutic activity ceases. The period at which the drug concentration remains within the therapeutic window is called the *duration of action* and the time at which the maximum concentration is attained is called the *onset of action*. To maintain a steady state concentration, the next dose is administered. Thus, a conventional dosage form shows 'see-saw' or 'peak and valley' pattern of drug concentration in plasma and tissue compartments (**Fig 2**). Depending on the drug kinetics such as the rate of absorption, distribution, elimination and dosing intervals, the magnitudes of these fluctuations varies.

B.  **Modified release dosage form:** The dosage forms, in which the rate of release of the drug and the time at which the release of the drug would take place are different from conventional type, are called modified release dosage form. An enteric coated tablet can be considered as a common example of a modified release dosage form. For example, erythromycin gets decomposed in the stomach; hence it is formulated as an enteric coated tablet. The multi-layered tablet is a further advancement of the modified release delivery systems.

C.  **Site-specific targeting:** These systems refer to targeting the release of a drug straight to a particular biological location. In this case, the target is adjacent to or in the diseased organ or tissue.

D.  **Receptor targeting:** These systems refer to targeting a specific biological receptor. In this case, the target is the specific receptor for a drug within an organ or tissue. Site-specific targeting and receptor targeting systems satisfy the spatial aspect of drug delivery and are also considered to be sustained drug delivery systems.

E.  **Delayed release dosage form:** When a dosage form does not release the drug immediately after administration like immediate release or conventional dosage form but releases the drug in portions at a predetermined time or at times, it is called delayed release dosage form. However, in some cases, a portion of the drug may be released immediately after administration.

F.  **Extended-release dosage form:** If a dosage form reduces the frequency of dose at least by two-fold as compared to the frequency of administration of immediate release or conventional dosage form, the dosage form is said to be the extended release dosage form. Sustained-release, controlled-release, or long-acting dosage forms belong to this class.

G. **Sustained release dosage form:** The drug release from sustained release dosage form exhibit a predetermined rate in order to maintain an approximately constant drug concentration in the body over a prolonged period. The rate of release of drug follows first-order kinetics. Usually, the drug content of one dose of SR dosage form is more than that of its conventional or immediate release dosage form.

H. **Prolonged action dosage form:** In this type of dosage form the drug is released at a rate relatively slower rate, but for a long period; so that, the therapeutic action of the drug remains for an extended period. In this type of dosage form, one dose of the drug is released immediately after administration and later on, the second dose is released.

## Rationale of Controlled Drug Delivery

Therefore, extensive researches have been conducted to reduce the frequency of administration. The outcome is the development of controlled or sustained release drug delivery system. Controlled delivery of the drug is possible by combining a polymer with the drug or active agent; so that, the release of the drug can take place at the right time, at a predetermined rate and the right place. In this system, the release of drug can bepre-designed. Thus, controlled release dosage forms have gradually gained acceptance of the medical practitioner and popularity among the patients.

Compared to conventional dosage forms such delivery systems offer numerous advantages including improved efficacy, reduced toxicity, and improved patient compliance and convenience. All controlled release systems are developed to improve the therapeutic effectiveness of the drug.

According to the patent history, the earliest patent on SR dosage form was filed by Israel Lipowskiin 1938, who coated the pellets/particles. The basic objective of this therapy is to maintain a steady state therapeutic concentration of drug in blood or tissue for an extended period, as shown in **Fig. 1.3**. The controlled or sustained release dosage form can be defined as; *The dosage forms that release a drug at a predetermined rate so that a constant drug concentration is maintained for a specific period with a minimum side effect.* A single dose of such dosage form is used for extending the therapeutic action. The dose size is more than a single conventional dose, but the total daily dose is reduced.

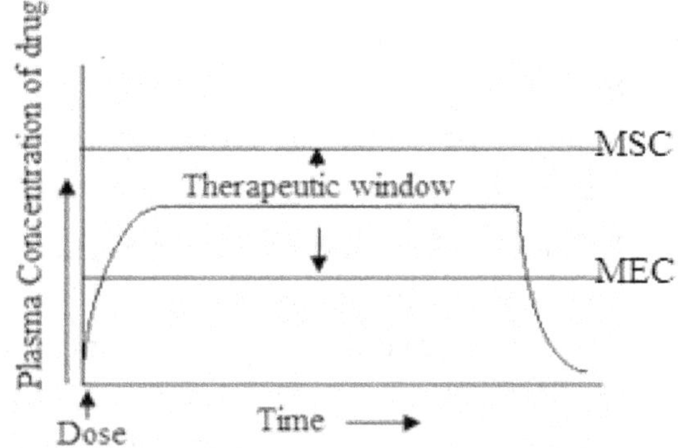


Fig. 1.3: No fluctuation in plasma concentration of drug following controlled release dosage form

The primary reason for controlled drug delivery is to alter the pharmacokinetic and pharmacodynamic properties of the drug substance. This is possible by using a novel drug delivery system or by modifying the molecular structure and physiological parameters. A properly designed dosage form should provide the drug action for a prolonged period. The key objective of controlled drug delivery is to confirm safety and to improve the efficiency of drugs as well as patient compliance. This is achieved by better control of plasma drug levels and frequency of dosing. For conventional dosage forms, only the dose (D) and dosing interval (C) can vary for each drug. For every drug, there is a definite therapeutic window. Below the MEC, the therapeutic effect of the drug is ineffective, and above MSC toxic side effects are elicited. The therapeutic index is defined as the ratio of the median lethal dose ($LD_{50}$) to the median effective dose ($ED_{50}$). The rationale of controlled release dosage form can be summarized as below:

- To provide a location-specific action within the GIT.
- To avoid an undesirable local action within the GIT.
- To provide a programmed delivery pattern.
- To increase the rate and extent of absorption/bioavailability.
- To extend the duration of action of the drug.

## General Advantages

The release of the active ingredient (drug) may be constant over a long period; it may be cyclic. The environment or other external events may trigger it. Controlled release drug delivery systems provide one or more of the following advantages.

- Maintenance of drug level within the desired range
- Delivery of 'difficult' drugs: the slow release of water-soluble drugs, and/orfast release of poorly soluble drugs
- Reduces dosing frequency
- Eliminates over or underdosing
- Prevention or reduction of side effects
- Reduction in total health care cost
- Improved efficacy in the treatment
- Reduction in adverse side effects and improvement in tolerability
- Improved patient compliance
- Employ less amount of total drug
- Minimizes or eliminates local or systemic side effects
- Minimal drug accumulation on chronic usage
- Cures or controls the condition more promptly
- Reduces the fluctuation in drug level

- Improves the bioavailability of some drugs
- Makes use of special effects

## Disadvantages

Various disadvantages of the controlled drug delivery systems are mentioned below:

- Likely to be costly
- Unpredictable and often provide poor *in-vitro – in-vivo correlations*
- May cause dose dumping, if the release design is failed
- Provides less scope for dosage adjustment
- May increase the first pass clearance
- Poor systemic availability in some cases
- Effective drug release period is influenced and limited by the gastric residence time

### Clinical Advantages of Control Release Dosage Forms

- Reduction in frequency of drug administration
- Improved patient compliance
- Reduction in drug level fluctuation in blood
- Reduction in total drug usage, when compared with conventional therapy
- Reduction in drug accumulation with chronic therapy
- Reduction in drug toxicity (local/systemic)
- Stabilization of medical condition (because of more uniform drug levels)
- Improvement in bioavailability of some drugs because of spatial control
- Economical to the health care providers and the patient

### Commercial / Industrial Advantages

- Illustration of innovative/technological leadership
- Product life-cycle extension
- Product differentiation
- Market expansion
- Patent extension

### Major Limitations

- Delay in the onset of action
- The possibility of dose dumping in the case of a poor formulation strategy
- Increased potential for first-pass metabolism
- Greater dependence on the gastric residence time of the dosage form
- The possibility of less accurate dose adjustment in some cases
- Cost per unit dose is higher when compared with conventional doses
- All drugs are not suitable for formulating into ER dosage form

## Selection of Drug Candidates

All the drugs cannot be formulated as their controlled release dosage forms. A drug must have the following characteristics for the formulation of controlled release dosage forms.

- Very short elimination half-life
- Very long elimination half-life
- Narrow therapeutic index
- Rate of absorption
- Mechanism of absorption
- First pass effect

**Factor Influencing the Design and Performance of Controlled Drug Delivery System**

1. Biopharmaceutic characteristics of the drug
   - The molecular weight of the drug
   - The aqueous solubility of the drug
   - Apparent partition coefficient
   - Drug pKa and ionization physiological pH
   - Drug stability
   - Mechanism and site of absorption
   - Route of administration.
2. Pharmacokinetic characteristics of the drug
   - Absorption rate
   - Elimination half-life
   - Rate of metabolism
   - Dosage form index
3. Pharmacodynamic characteristic of the drug
   - Therapeutic range
   - Therapeutic index
   - Plasma–concentration-response relationship

The fabrication of the formulation depends on the physicochemical properties of the drug and on the pharmacokinetic behavior of the drug. In conventional dosage form, the rate-limiting step in drug's bioavailability is usually absorption through the bio-membrane; where as in controlled drug delivery system the rate-limiting step is the release of drug from the dosage form.

## Approaches to Design Controlled-release Formulations

Primarily there are two approaches or concepts to design and prepare controlled/sustained release dosage form:

(a) Modification of the drug molecule, and   (b) Modification of the dosage form.

There are hundreds of commercial products based on controlled release technologies. Only a few show distinct mechanisms of controlled drug release. Oral controlled-release formulations are designed mainly based on physical mechanisms. The chemical degradation, enzymatic degradation, and prodrug approach are less. **Table 1.1** presents different classes of marketed products based on controlled release mechanisms. All controlled-release formulations are designedby one mechanism or combination of a few mechanisms.

**Table 1.1:** Marketed formulations of drugs with the technology used

| S.No. | Drug | Branded Formulation | Technology |
|---|---|---|---|
| 1 | Bupropion | WellbutrinWL | Diffusion controlled-release |
| 2 | Zolpidem tartarate | Ambien CR | Matrix system (Tablet) |
| 3 | Chlorpheniramine Polistirex and Hydrocodone Polistirex | TussionexPennkinetic ER suspension | Ion-exchange system |
| 4 | Chlorpheniramine Maleate Glipizide | Efidac 24® Glucotrol XL® | Osmosis-based system Elementary osmotic pump Push-pull osmotic system |
| 5 | Propranolol HCl | Inderal ® LA | pH independent formulation |
| 6 | Levodopa and Benserazide | Modapar | Altered density formulation |

The modified-release dosage form can be categorized into the following;

- Delayed release
- Extended-release
- Sustained release
- Controlled release
- Timed release
- Prolonged release

Broadly the modified release dosage form can be classified as below **(Fig. 1.4),**

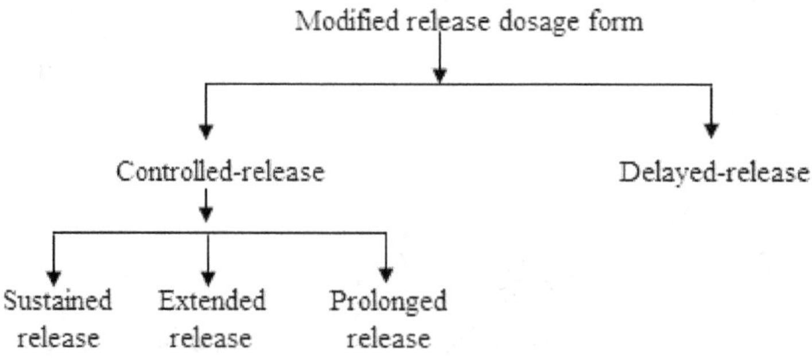


**Fig. 1.4:** Classification of modified release dosage form.

Based on the mechanism of drug-release and carrier used, the modified-release dosage form can be classified into the following six categories;

1.  Diffusion sustained system
    (a)  Reservoir type          (b)  Matrix type
2.  Dissolution sustained the system.
    (a)  Reservoir type          (b)  Matrix type
3.  Methods using Ion-exchange
4.  Methods using osmotic pressure
5.  pH-independent formulations
6.  Altered-density formulations

## Dissolution Controlled-release

The simple preparation of this category is sustained-release oral products, where dissolution is the rate-limiting step. When the rate of dissolution of a drug is high, the drug is mixed with a carrier having a slow rate of dissolution, and a tablet is prepared to sustain or control the release of the drug.

When the dissolution process is diffusion layer controlled, the rate of diffusion of the drug from the solid surface to the bulk solution through an unstirred liquid film is the rate-limiting step. Insuch case, the dissolution process at steady-state would be described by Noyes-Whitney equation,

$$\frac{dC}{dt} = K_D A(C_s - C) \qquad \qquad .....(1.1)$$

Where,          $\dfrac{dC}{dt}$ = Dissolution rate.

$K_D$ = Dissolution rate constant.

$C_s$ = Saturation solubility of drug, and

$C$ = The concentration of drug in bulk of the solution.

There are two ways to prepare dissolution-controlled preparations:

- Dissolution-controlled encapsulated/coated system
- Dissolution-controlled matrix system

- **Dissolution-controlled encapsulation:** In this method, the particles or granules of the drug are coated individually with slowly dissolving coating material (**Fig. 1.5**). The coated particles are compressed into a tablet directly; such as space tabs or Spansules.

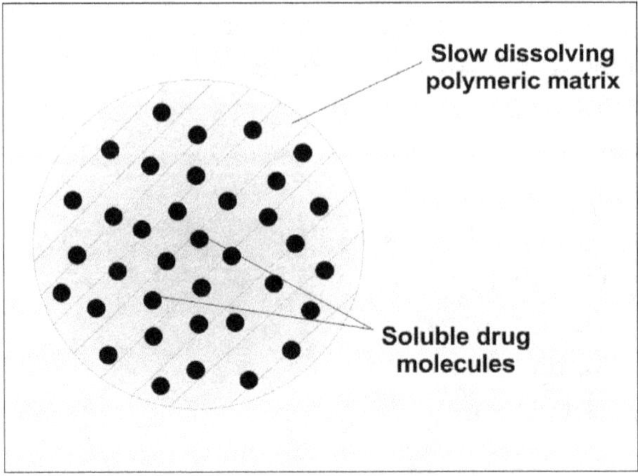



**Fig 1.5:** Schematic diagram of the drug release from the reservoir system by dissolution of polymeric matrix.

### Erosion-controlled systems

Erosion-controlled drug delivery systems are alternatively called *stimuli-induced systems*. These systems are activated by an external stimulus, such as pH, temperature, enzymes or osmotic pressure and release the drug. Drug release occurs depending on the mechanism of erosion surface or bulk. If the pH of the environment is not favorable for dissolution of the dosage form, the drug release will not occur (pH sensitive dosage form). Polymers are commonly used for coating of the pH-sensitive systems. Usually acrylates (methacrylic acid copolymers) and cellulose esters (cellulose acetate phthalate) are used for coating; however, these can also be used to make matrix systems (**Fig. 1.6**).

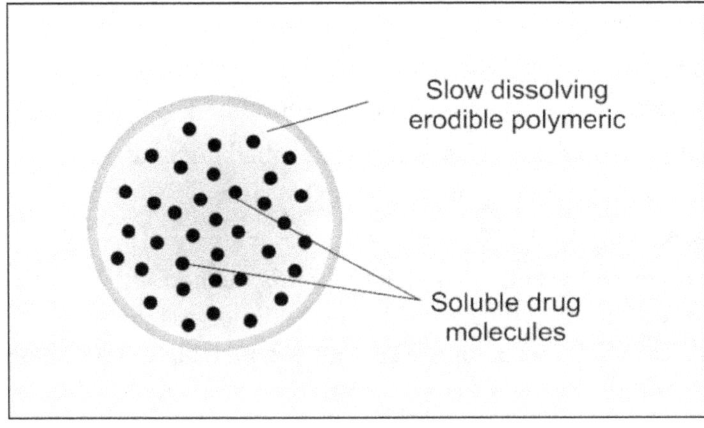



**Fig. 1.6:** Schematic representation of an erosion controlled system

### Dissolution-controlled matrix

In this method, the drug is mixed with a slowly dissolving carrier to prepare a matrix material, which is then compressed. The rate of bioavailability of the drug is controlled by the rate of penetration of the dissolution fluid into the matrix. The penetration of the medium is controlled by the porosity of the tablet matrix, the presence of hydrophilic material, the wettability of the tablet, and the particle surface.

Poorly water-soluble drugs (BCS class II and IV) inherently show sustained release. In the case of water-soluble drugs, a water-insoluble carrier is incorporated in the formulation to reduce the rate of dissolution of the drug particles, which are pre-coated with this type of materials; such as polyethylene glycol. In this type of formulation disintegrating agent may not be used to help delayed release.

### Hybrid systems

These are a combination of the robustness of matrix systems with the constant-release kinetics of reservoir systems. The drug is incorporated (entrapped) into a release-controlled matrix, and the matrix is then coated with a polymer. High molecular weight compounds can also be incorporated. The advantages of this system are many folds –

- Cost-effectiveness,
- Easy to manufacture, and
- Can be prepared by conventional processes and equipment.

### Diffusion-controlled release

These systems may be of two types:

1. Diffusion-controlled encapsulation, and
2. Osmotic pressure is rate limiting.

### Diffusion controlled encapsulation

In diffusion-controlled formulations, drug molecules diffuse through a polymer membrane or a polymer matrix and are released. Depending on whether a polymer membrane surrounds a drug or distributed within the polymer matrix, diffusion-controlled formulations can be divided into categories:

- Reservoir system, and
- Monolithic systems.

In nonporous reservoir systems, drug molecules diffuse through the polymer membrane; but in microporous reservoir systems, the drug molecules are released by diffusion through micropores. The micropores are usually filled with either water or oil.

In addition to nonporous and microporous systems, diffusion-controlled monolithic systems can be further classified by the concentration of the loaded drug. In the monolithic system, the drug is loaded by soaking a polymer matrix in a drug solution. The concentration of drug inside the matrix cannot be higher than the solubility of the drug; if the partition coefficient of a drug is 1. If the drug loading is higher than the drug's solubility, the monolithic system is called monolithic dispersion.

Fick's law gives the flux of the drug J (in amount/area - time), across a membrane in the direction of decreasing concentration.

$$J = - D \, dc/dx$$

Where, D = diffusion coefficient in area/ time,

dc/dx = change of concentration 'c' with distance 'x'

A release rate of the drug characterizes diffusion systems is dependent on its diffusion through inert water insoluble membrane barrier. There are two types of diffusion devices.

**(a)** **Reservoir Type:** In the system, a water-insoluble polymeric material encloses a core of drug, which controls release rate.

The drug will partition into the membrane and exchange with the fluid surrounding the particle or tablet. The additional drug will enter the polymer, diffuse to the periphery and exchange with the surrounding media.

The polymers commonly used in such devices are Ethyl cellulose and Poly-vinyl acetate. The rate of drug released (dm/dt) can be calculated using the following equation

$$\frac{dm}{dt} = ADK \frac{\Delta c}{l}$$

Where, A = Area,

D = Diffusion coefficient,

K = Partition coefficient of the drug between the drug

core and the membrane,

$\ell$ = Diffusion path length and

$\Delta$C = Concentration difference across the membrane.

**Advantage**
- Zero-order delivery is possible with this method,
- Release rates variable with polymer type.

**Disadvantages**
- The system must be physically removed from implant sites.
- Difficult to deliver high molecular weight compound,
- Generally increased cost per dosage unit,
- Potential toxicity may occur if the system fails.

**(b)** **Matrix Type:** A solid drug powder is homogeneously dispersed within a rate controlling medium, an insoluble matrix. The waxes such as beeswax, carnauba wax, hydrogenated castor oil, etc. are used to prepare the matrix. These waxes control drug dissolution by controlling the rate of dissolution in fluid and subsequent penetration into the matrix. The medium alters the porosity of the tablet, decreases its wettability or dissolves at a slower rate. The drug release from such matrices follows the first order kinetics. The wax-the embedded drug is generally prepared by dispersing the drug in molten wax and solidifying and granulating the same. The rate of drug release is subject to the rate of drug-diffusion, not on the rate of dissolution of the drug.

**Advantages**

- Production of this system is more accessible than reservoir or encapsulated devices,
- High molecular weight compounds can be delivered.


**Disadvantages**

- Cannot provide zero order release,
- Removal of the remaining matrix is necessary for the implanted system.

**Osmosis-Based Formulations:** Osmosis is the movement of a solvent (water) from its higher concentration to its lower concentration through a semipermeable membrane. While diffusion is the movement of solute from its higher concentration to lower concentration.This principle of osmosis has been used for the development of zero-order release drug delivery systems.

These systems are made-up by encapsulating an osmotic drug core (**Fig 1.7**) comprising an osmotically active drug (or a blend of an osmotically inactive drug with an osmotically active salt such as NaCl, **Fig 1.8A**) within a semi-permeable membrane made from biocompatible polymers, such as cellulose acetate. Once a difference (gradient) in osmotic pressures is created, the drug (solute) is continuously pumped out of tablet through small delivery orifice present in tablet coating. This continues for a prolonged period, about 24hrs. This type of drug system provides drug solutes continuously at a zero-order rate and release of the drug is independent of the environment of the gastrointestinal tract but depends on the osmotic pressure of the release medium. However, the manufacturing process is complicated. Basic osmotic systems can deliver only water-soluble drugs. Water-insoluble drugs can be delivered by "push-pull" osmotic systems (**Fig 1.8B**). There is a non-swelling solubilizing agent that enhances the solubility of insoluble drugs and a non-swelling agent that enhances the contact-surface area of the drug substances with the incoming aqueous liquid when it is dispersed throughout the composition. Different polymer membranes have different water vapor transmission value. The semipermeable membrane should be selected based on the nature of the application.

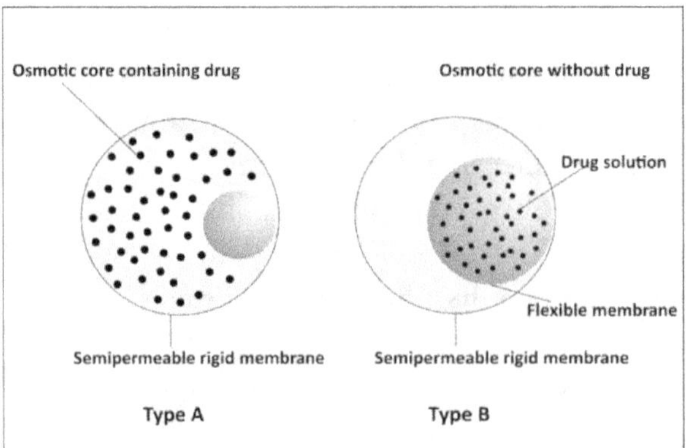



**Fig. 1.7:** Schematic representation of drug encapsulation in Osmotic system; Type A: Drug present in the osmotic core and Type B: Osmotic core without drug and the drug is present inside a flexible membrane.

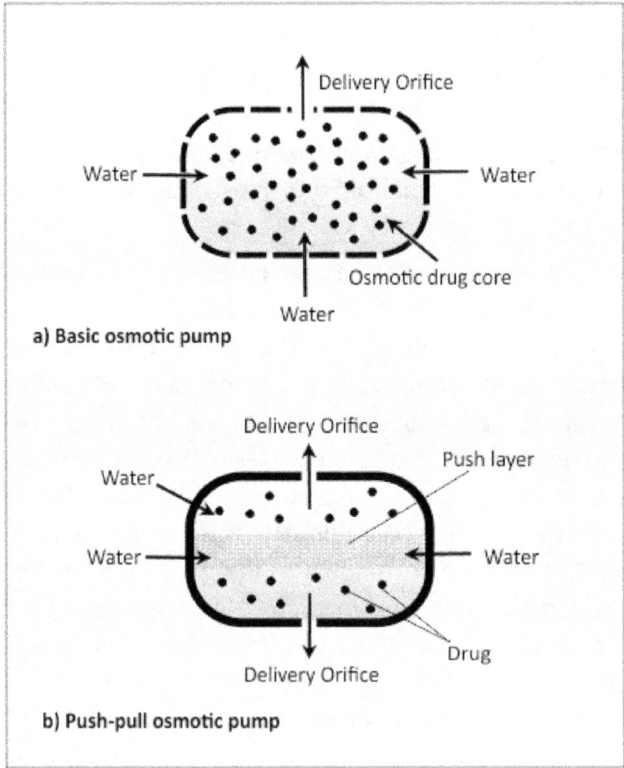



**Fig. 1.8:** Schematic representation of different types of osmotic pumps; (a) represents the basic osmotic pump and (b) represents the Push-pull osmotic pump.

## Based on Ion exchange Principles

Ion exchange resins are also used to control the release of drugs. The water-insoluble polymeric materials containing ionic groups are used as resins. Through electrostatic interaction, the drug molecules attach onto the oppositely charged ionic groups of the resin. The drug molecules can be exchanged with other ions having the same charge and accordingly, the drug molecules are released from the ion-exchange resin. This principle is used to prepare the controlled-release dosage form of anionic or ionizable drug. The method of preparation is simple:

    (a) The ionized drug is absorbed onto the ion-exchange resin granules; for example, codeine base (drug) is absorbed onto amberlite (resin).

    (b) The resins are filtered from the alcoholic medium,

    (c) The filtered drug-resin complex granules are coated with a water permeable polymer, such as a modified copolymer of polyacrylic and methacrylic ester, by spray drying method.

The drug is released by replacing with appropriately charged ions in the GIT, and then the drug diffuses out of the resin. The release of the drug depends on;

    (a) the strength and type of ionic environment (pH, electrolyte conc.) and

    (b) the properties of the resin.

The rate of diffusion is controlled by:

    (a) the area of diffusion,

    (b) diffusion path length, and

    (c) the rigidity of resin.

$$Resin^+\text{-}Drug^- + X^- \longrightarrow Resin^-\text{-} X^- + Drug^-$$

**Advantage**

- It offers a protective mechanism by temporarily changing the substrate.
- Suitable for the drugs which are highly susceptible to degradation by enzymatic processes.

**Limitation**

- The release rate is proportional to the concentration of the ions present in the proximity of the granules in the site of administration.
- The rate release varies with diet, water intake, and intestinal contents.

**Processes used to prepare controlled-release formulations**

Based on the mechanism of drug-release such as dissolution, diffusion, and osmosis, the oral controlled- release (CR) formulations are developed. Accordingly, the approaches/technology used to develop CR formulations can be roughly divided into three types: (A) matrix tablets, (B) multi-particulates, and (C) osmotic tablets; although different processes can be used in a particular formulation approach.

**(A) Matrix Tablets:** Both hydrophilic CR systems and lipophilic CR systems can be present in Matrix tablets. From hydrophilic systems, the drug is released through both diffusion and dissolution (i.e., matrix erosion), and from lipophilic systems, the drug-release takes place only through diffusion mechanism.

In general, the processes such as direct compression, roller compaction, wet granulation, fluid bed granulation, foam granulation, and melt extrusion granulation have been used to prepare both types of matrix tablets.

The selection of a process for the preparation of matrix tablets is similar to that used for immediate release tablets. The major factors influencing the process selection are;

- Drug loading,
- Flowability, and
- Compatibility.

For moisture-sensitive drugs, both wet granulation and fluid bed granulation would not be suitable. The melt extrusion granulation would not be suitable for thermally unstable drugs. For different processes, generally, the maximal drug loading follows approximately in the order of melt extrusion granulation>wet granulation >roller compaction ≈ fluid bed granulation> direct compression.

**(B) Multi-particulates:** Multi-particulate CR systems constitute both drug layered beads and microspheres. Fluid bed coating has been found very useful in preparing different multi-particulate CR systems. The process uses three different spraying methods – top spray, bottom spray (Wurster process), and tangential spray. Commonly the top spray method is used for fluid bed granulation; in some cases, for particle coating also. For the coating of particles/beads, the bottom spray(Wurster) coating is usually followed.

For the preparation of the multi-particulate CR systems, Wurster coating has been found very useful for layering of the drug on nonpareils as well as functional coating. Similar film quality can be achieved by the tangential spray (rotary) method as is obtained by Wurster coating. However, it is more difficult to scale up the technology. Besides fluid bed granulation, many other processes have been used to prepare microspheres or beads, such as;

- Extrusion and spheronization,
- Hot-melt extrusion granulation,
- Spray congealing, and
- Roller compaction.

For making pellets Extrusion–spheronization (palletization process) is usually used. The pellets can be used for the preparation of both immediate and controlled release formulation. If a solution of calcium chloride is added to sodium alginate solution, insoluble calcium alginate precipitates out, and the beads are formed. These beads have been widely used for preparing controlled release formulation. The beads can be collected by filtering and drying, or by one-step spray drying.

**(C) Osmotic Tablets:** The method of preparation of osmotic tablets can be roughly divided into three operations:

1. formation of drug layer and/or sweller layer,
2. formation of a membrane(s), and
3. making of microscopic hole(s) for drug release.

The drug layer and the sweller layer can be made by using the traditional method of granulation to prepare granules. To prepare an elementary osmotic pump, monolayer tablets can be compressed easily. For the 'pull-push' osmotic pump, that is, both drug layer and sweller layer need to be compressed into bilayer tablets. After membrane(s) has been coated onto the core tablets, holes for releasing drug from membrane are normally created by laser drilling technique. In Merck osmotic delivery system, high concentrations of porosigens are incorporated inside cellulose acetate, which generates holes for drug release.

## Physicochemical Properties of Drugs Suitable for Controlled Release Formulations

For designing a controlled drug delivery system, the following physicochemical properties of drugs must be considered:

1. **The molecular weight of the drug:** Drugs of lower the molecular weight, more accurately, of lower molecular size, are absorbed faster and more completely. Through passive diffusion, about 95% of the drugs are absorbed. Diffusivity is well-defined as the ability of a substance (drug) to diffuse through the membrane. It is inversely related to the molecular size. Thus, drugs with large molecular weight rather large molecular size are not ideally suitable for oral controlled release systems.

2. **The diffusion coefficient and molecular size:** After reaching the systemic circulation, the drug needs to diffuse (1) through rate-controlling polymeric membranes or matrix (in case of extended-release or matrix system), and through (2) different biological membranes. The capacity of a drug to diffuse through these membranes is called diffusibility or diffusion coefficient (D). Diffusibility of the drug depends on its molecular size or molecular weight. The diffusivity of a drug through a polymer can be interrelated with its molecular size or weight as follows;

$$\log D = -S_v \log V + k_v = -S_M \log M + k_m \qquad .....(1.1)$$

Where V is the molecular volume, M is the molecular weight; $S_v$, $S_M$, $k_v$, and $k_m$ are constants. Thus, the value of D depends on the size and shape of the drug. Usually, drugs having a molecular weight within 150 to 400 Da (Dalton) possess diffusivity of $10^{-6}$ $-10^{-9}$ cm$^2$/sec through flexible polymers. The drugs having molecular weight more than 500 Da have very small diffusivity such as $10^{-12}$cm$^2$/sec. It is challenging to measure such a low diffusivity. High molecular weight drugs usually show very slow release kinetics in extended release dosage form; if the mechanism of drug release is diffusion control.

3. **The aqueous solubility of the drug:** For oral controlled release dosage form, the drug should have excellent aqueous solubility and are independent of pH; such drugs are good candidates. The solubility of the drug is a factor for selection of the mechanism to be employed for preparing CRDDS. For example, the diffusional systems are not appropriate for poorly soluble drugs. Absorption of poorly soluble drugs is dissolution rate-limited; hence, control release device does not control the absorption process. So, they are poor candidates.

Solubility refers to the concentration of solute in a saturated solution. In other words, solubility can be expressed as the amount of solute remaining in a solution containing a given volume of solvent with some undissolved solute in equilibrium– saturated solution. Solubility is a thermodynamic property of solute. The amount of drug absorbed into systemic circulation is a function of the amount of the drug present in anunionized form in a solution of G.I fluid. This is the intrinsic solubility of the drug and permeation of drug under such condition is called intrinsic permeability.

Before absorption, the drug must go into a solution of GI fluid and then partitions into the absorbing membrane. Thus, absorption of a drug is related to its partitioning between the lipid layer and an aqueous phase, and the rate of dissolution is related to its aqueous solubility. The Noyes-Whitney equation can express the relation between the rate of dissolution and aqueous solubility as below;

$$\frac{dC}{dt} = k_D.A.C_S \text{ (under sink condition)} \qquad .....(1.2)$$

Where, $\frac{dC}{dt}$ is the rate of dissolution, $k_D$ is the dissolution rate constant, A is the total surface area of the drug particle, and $C_S$ is the saturation solubility of the drug. Thus, drugs which are soluble in water are generally absorbed adequately when administered orally. On the other hand, poorly soluble drugs have low dissolution rates, and their bioavailability becomes a problem when administered orally.

Since most drugs are either weak acids or weak bases, their aqueous solubility greatly influenced by the pH of dissolution medium. The aqueous solubility of a weak acid can be expressed as;

$$S_t = S_u \left( 1 + \frac{K_a}{[H^+]} \right) \qquad .....(1.3)$$

Where $S_t$ is the total solubility (both ionized and nonionized forms) of the weak acid, $S_u$ is the solubility of the unionized form, $K_a$ is the dissociation constant of the acid, and $[H^+]$ is the hydrogen ion concentration of the medium. Similarly, the aqueous solubility of weakly basic drugs can be expressed as;

$$S_t = S_u\left(1 + \frac{[H^+]}{K_a}\right) \qquad .....(1.4)$$

Where, $S_t$ is the total solubility (both conjugate acid and free base forms) of the weak base, $S_u$ is the solubility of the free-base form, $K_a$ is the dissociation constant of the conjugate acid, and $[H^+]$ is the hydrogen ion concentration of the medium.

The equations 3 and 4 indicate that the pH of the medium can influence the total solubility of a weakly acidic or weakly basic drug having a given pKa.

According to the pH-partition hypothesis, the unionized form of a weakly acidic drug present in the stomach (pH $\approx$ 1–2) will be absorbed very well. Similarly, weakly basic drugs predominantly remain unionized in the small intestine (pH $\approx$ 5–7) and will be excellently absorbed; but these drugs remain in ionized form in the stomach resulting poor absorption.

Therefore, the above discussion can be summarized as: *for better absorption in GI tract (oral route) the drug must have an adequate aqueous solubility, must be released from the dosage form at a required rate, and be available as unionized form at the site of its absorption.*

The ratio of equation 2 and 3 indicates the driving force, R for absorption based on the pH gradient. Then,

$$R = \frac{\left(1 + 10^{pHb} - p^{K_a}\right)}{\left(1 + 10^{pHg} - p^{K_a}\right)} \qquad .....(1.5)$$

When, pHb = 7.4 (pH of blood), pHg = 2 (pH of gastric fluid), and if the pKa value of the drug is 3.4 then the value of R becomes $10^{3.8}$. It indicates that the drug would be absorbed in the stomach. Similarly, by using the pH value of intestinal fluid, the value of R can be calculated, and the potential site of absorption can be speculated.

The effect of three major factors -solubility, dissolution, and intestinal permeability on oral drug absorption can be measured with the help of biopharmaceutical classification (BCS) system. According to BCS, the drugs are of 4 classes:

Class I: high solubility-high permeability,

Class II:  low solubility-high permeability,

Class III: high solubility-low permeability,

Class IV:  low solubility-low permeability.

High solubility means the largest dose of a drug is dissolved in 200 – 250 ml of water over a pH range from 1 to 8 and when the extent of absorption is more than 90% the drug is said to be highly permeable. Accordingly, the drugs of class III and IV are not suitable for SR/CR formulation. Usually, the drugs whose solubility is less than 0.1mg even up to 10mg per ml are challenging to be formulated as SR/CR dosage form.

4. **Apparent partition coefficient:** Larger the apparent partition coefficient of a drug ($K_{o/w}$), greater its lipophilicity and hence, greater would be its rate and extent of absorption. These types of drugs even cross the highly selective blood-brain barrier. This parameter is also significant in deciding the release rate of a drug from a lipophilic matrix or device.

   Both permeation of a drug across the biological membrane and diffusion through the rate controlling membrane or matrix depend on the partition coefficient of the drug. After administration and before elimination from the body the drug is supposed to diffuse through various biological membranes. These membranes perform primarily as a lipid-like barrier. The apparent oil/water partition coefficient of a drug is considered as a measure of its membrane permeability. The apparent oil/water partition coefficient, K is defined as;

$$K = \frac{\text{The concentration of drug in oil}}{\text{The concentration of drug in water}} = \frac{C_o}{C_w} \qquad .....(1.6)$$

   Where, Co represents the equilibrium concentration of all forms of the drug in an organic phase, usually in n-octanol, and Cw represents the equilibrium concentration of all forms of the drug in the aqueous phase. Drugs having a high value of K are readily soluble in oil and partition easily into membranes. *Hansch correlation* describes the parabolic relationship between the logarithm of the ability of a drug to be absorbed and the logarithm of its partition coefficient. This relationship expresses that the activity of a drug is a function of the ability to cross the membranes and interact with the receptor. There should be an optimum partition coefficient for required permeability. When the value of partition coefficient is more than the optimumvalue, the aqueous solubility of a drug is reduced, and the lipid solubility is increased; under this circumstance of once the drug enters into lipid membrane cannot diffuse out of the lipid membrane. Usually, the optimum value of K is 1000 when measured using the n-octanol/water system. Drugs having partition coefficient value more than or less than the optimum values are not suitable candidates for making extended-release formulation.

5. **Drug pKa and ionization at physiological pH:** The pKa value can indicate the strength of an acid or a base. Thus, at a particular pH, the charge on a drug molecule can be determined through its pKa value. Drug molecules are therapeutically active only in their unionized form and in this form the drug can easily penetrate the lipoidal membrane.

   The amount of drug that remains in unionized form is a function of its dissociation constant and pH of the fluid at the site of absorption. Thus, the drug which remains in ionized form at its absorption site is not suitable for SR/CR dosage form.

   For optimum passive absorption, the drugs should be non-ionised at the site for an extent of 0.1–5%. Drugs, such as hexamethonium, exist largely in ionized forms are poor candidates for controlled delivery systems.

6. **Drug stability:** Drugs which are unstable in the GI environment are not suitable candidates for controlled release systems. Drugs which are unstable in gastric pH can be designed for release in the intestine with limited or no release in stomach

and drugs which are unstable in intestinal pH (alkaline pH) can be designed for release in the stomach with limited or no release in the intestine.

Some amount of the drug administered orally may be lost in the GI tract due to acid hydrolysis and metabolism in the liver. Omeprazole, pantoprazole, lansoprazole, rifampicin, erythromycin, riboflavin, etc. are the most common examples of acid-susceptible drugs; i.e., these are unstable in the stomach. While captopril, ranitidine, etc. are not stable in the intestine; (alkaline media). Hence, the stability of the drug in the GI tract is an essential factor. The relative bioavailability of a drug which is unstable in the stomach can be improved significantly by making a slowly releasing or controlled releasing formulation. However, it would be most beneficial when the formulation can control the release of the drug only in the intestine.

Similarly, there are drugs which are unstable in the intestine. Their stability can be increased significantly by making a sustained/controlled release formulation which can slowly release the drug in the stomach only. Hence, the drugs which have stability problem in any region of the gastrointestinal tract can be formulated as sustained/controlled/extended release formulation; but the release characteristics must be decided based on absorption site where the drugs are most stable. The desired physicochemical properties of a drug are summarized in the **Table 1.2.**

**Table 1.2:** Physicochemical properties of drug

| Physicochemical properties | Desired value |
| --- | --- |
| Molecular weight/size | < 1000 Daltons |
| Solubility | > 0.1g/lt at pH 1 to 7.8 |
| Apparent Partition coefficient | High |
| Absorption mechanism | Diffusion control |
| General absorbability | Throughout entire GI tract |
| Drug release | Should not depend on enzyme and pH |

7. **Mechanism and site of absorption:** Drugs which are absorbed by carrier-mediated transport procedure or through a window are not entirely suitable candidates for the development of controlled release systems, such as Vitamin B.

8. **Route of administration:** Oral and parenteral routes are the most preferred for controlled release, this is followed by transdermal.

   (i) *Oral route*: The drug should have the following properties to be a successful candidate

   - It must get absorbed through the entire length of GIT.
   - The main limitation is transit time (mean of 14 hours), which can be extended for 12-24 hours.

- Dose as high as 1000mg can be given through this route.

**(ii)** ***Intramuscular/subcutaneous route:*** This route is preferred because

- The action is to be prolonged for 24 hours to 12 months.
- A small amount of drug is administered (2mL/2gm).
- Factors important are solubility of the drug in surrounding tissue, molecular weight, partition coefficient and pKa of the drug.

**(iii)** ***Transdermal route:*** This route is selected for drugs which show extensive first-pass metabolism upon oral administration or drugs with a low dose. Important factors to be considered are:

- The partition coefficient of drugs,
- Contact area,
- Skin condition,
- Skin permeability of drug,
- Skin perfusion rate, etc.

# Biological Properties of Drugs Suitable for Controlled Release Formulations

## Pharmacokinetic Properties of a Drug

**(a)    Dose and Release rate:**

To achieve a sustained or extended action, the concentration of the drug is to be maintained within the therapeutic window for a long period. For this, it is essential to provide a therapeutic concentration immediately after administration;

so that the absorption pool of drug is maintained. Using a conventional or immediate release dosage form this can be done. This can be illustrated schematically as follows;

$$\text{Dosage form} \xrightarrow[\text{Drug release}]{kr} \text{Absorption pool} \xrightarrow[\text{Absorption}]{ka} \text{Site of action} \xrightarrow[\text{Elimination}]{ke}$$

Where, kr, ka, and ke are release rate constant, absorption rate constant, and overall elimination rate constant respectively. Absorption pool indicates the amount of drug present at the site of absorption. When the drug is released immediately as in case of the conventional dosage form, kr>>> ka. Thus, the absorption of the drug becomes the rate-limiting step for the drug to reach its site of action. On the other hand, for a dosage form which does not release the drug immediately, kr<<< ka and release of drug at the site of absorption become the rate-limiting step for the drug to reach its site of action.

$$\text{Dosage form} \xrightarrow[\text{Drug release}]{kr} \text{Site of action} \xrightarrow[\text{Elimination}]{ke}$$

The three-step process is reduced to the two-step process. This indicates that once the drug is released from the dosage it is immediately absorbed, and it reaches its site of action. Thus, to design or develop a sustained/extended release dosage form attention should be paid towards altering the rate of release (*alteration of the* kr). While designing or developing an SR/CR dosage form, it is theoretically expected that the plasma concentration of the drug should remain at a constant level. In fact, practically it is complicated and, in most cases, not necessary also to maintain the constant level. The concentration of the drug should remain within the therapeutic window throughout the period. Ideally, an extended release dosage form should release the drug at the desired site and at a rate as per the need of the body. Many attempts have been, and no commercial product is available that fulfills this requirement. Since there is no feedback information about the rate at which a drug should be infused into the body to maintain the steady-state blood concentration; the drug may be administered at a rate equivalent to the rate of elimination from the body.This means that the drug should be administered at a constant rate over a period without considering the amount of drug remaining in the dosage form. Thus, the drug would be released from the dosage form following zero-order kinetics;

$$K_r^o = k_e C_d V_d = \text{Rate of administration} = \text{Rate of elimination} \qquad .....(1.7)$$

Where, $K_r^o$ is the zero-order rate constant for the drug release (amount/time), $k_e$ is the first, order rate constant for theoverall elimination of the drug from the body (time$^{-1}$), $C_d$ is the desired drug concentration in plasma (amount/volume), and $V_d$ is the apparent volume of distribution of the drug in the body (volume).

The equation 7 may be used to calculate the amount of drug to be released per unit time for maintaining a constant plasma drug concentration. This may be used in the simple case where elimination of the drug from the body follows first order kinetics.

- ***Use of Zero order release technique***

  There are many drugs whose elimination is a complex process and disposition of drugs is influenced by several factors. These influence the release kinetics of the dosage form for maintaining constant drug level in the body. Although theoretically zero order release kinetics is desired for sustaining or extending the action, in some cases non-zero order release has been found to be equally clinically useful. However, there are intra- and inter-subject variations. Depending on the degree of such variations the clinical performance of some drugs may vary. In some cases, due to this intra- and inter-subject variations average change in drug concentration in tissues does not show a significant change in the clinical performance of the drug. As a result, the difference between the clinical effects of constant plasma drug level and of non-constant plasma drug level becomes insignificant.

The purpose of SR/CR dosage form is to provide an immediate effect and to extend this effect for a more extended period. Hence, there are two parts of SR/CR dosage form – immediate or initial dose (Di) and sustaining or maintenance dose (Dm). The sum of these doses makes the total dose, W.

$$W = Di + Dm \qquad .....(1.8)$$

When the maintenance dose releases the drug by zero order process for a definite period, the total dose may be calculated as;

$$W = Di + K_r^o T_d \qquad .....(1.9)$$

Where, $T_d$ is the total time required for the extended release of drug from one dose. If the maintenance dose starts releasing the drug along with the initial dose (when t = 0), the total amount of drug released shall be more than the amount released from the initial dose. In such case, a correction is necessary to account for the extra amount (amount released from maintenance dose, $K_r^o T_p$) and the equation is rewritten as;

$$W = Di + K_r^o T_d - K_r^o T_p \qquad .....(1.10)$$

Where, $T_p$ is the time required for attaining peak drug level, $C_{max}$. In fact, the maintenance dose starts releasing the drug after the time, $T_p$. This is an ideal situation; making the maintenance in such a way that it releases the drug following zero-order kinetics is the simplest way to achieve this.

- ***Use of First order release technique***

  A constant drug level can be maintained by formulating the initial dose and maintenance dose which releases the drug by first order process. Total dose for such a system can be calculated as;

$$W = Di + \left(\frac{k_e C_d}{k_r}\right) V_d \qquad ....(1.11)$$

Where, $k_e$, $C_d$, and $V_d$ carry the same meaning as described earlier; $k_r$ is the first order release rate constant.

Now, in this case also if the maintenance dose releases the drug along with the initial dose (when t = 0), a correction factor needs to be included as indicated below;

$$W = Di + \left(\frac{k_e C_d}{k_r}\right) V_d - Dm.k_e.T_p \qquad .....(1.12)$$

The conventional dose of a drug provides some information of the amount of drug required to be present in an extended release dosage unit. This has been mentioned earlier that both dose-size and half-life of drugs are essential characteristics of a drug to become suitable for SR/CR dosage form **(Table 1.3)**.

**Table 1.3:** Pharmacokinetic properties of the drug

| Pharmacokinetic properties | Desired value |
|---|---|
| Absolute bioavailability | > 75% |
| Intrinsic rate of absorption | Greater than the release rate |
| Elimination half-life | 0.5 to 8 hr |
| Elimination rate constant | As necessary for the design |
| The apparent volume of distribution, $V_d$ | Should not be large |
| Minimum effective concentration, MEC | Should not be high; if both MEC and $V_d$ are less, the dose size of SR/CR dosage form will be small. |
| Toxic concentration | Toxic concentration or maximum safe concentration should be large; i.e., wider therapeutic window can provide safety of the dosage form. |

## (b) Absorption rate

A drug which is fabricated into a controlled release system should be absorbed efficiently. The rate-limiting step is the rate of drug release. A drug which is slowly absorbed is a poor candidate for such dosage forms; since continuous release will result in a pool of unabsorbed drug. If a drug is absorbed by active transport, or transport is limited to a specific region ofthe intestine, sustained-release preparations may be disadvantageous to absorption; hence should be avoided.

For an extended release dosage form, the rate, extent, and uniformity of absorption of the drug are important factors to be considered. When the formulation is prepared for oral route, these are most critical; because for smooth and regular absorption from GI tract the release of the drug must be very less than the rate of absorption, i.e., $k_r<<<k_a$.

If the transit time of a drug in the gastrointestinal tract is assumed to be within 9 – 12 hours, the maximum absorption half-life would be 3 – 4 hours. Then the minimum absorption rate constant, Ka would be 0.17 – 0.23/hr for about 80 – 95% absorption during 9 – 12 hours.

When a drug is very slowly absorbed ($K_a<< 0.17$), the first order release rate constant, $k_r$Would be less than 0.17/hr and the drug is considered to be very poorly bioavailable in many patients. Such poorly bioavailable drug is not suitable for formulating extended release dosage form. Because for extended release dosage form $k_a>>>k_r$.

The absorptive surfaces of the gastrointestinal tract vary. If the absorption of a drug is erratic in the GI tract, e.g., iron, dicoumarol; it becomes difficult to design an extended/controlled release dosage.

Drugs which are not suitable for formulating sustained/controlled/extended release dosage form can be categorized into four types by biological factors;

> Drugs which are absorbed by active transport system; e.g., Methotrexate, pyridoxine, riboflavin, nicotinamide, enalapril, methyl-dopa, 5-fluorouracil, 5-bromouracil, etc.

> Drugs which are absorbed through amino acid transporter in the intestine; e.g., cephalosporin, baclofen, gabapentin, methyl-dopa, levodopa, etc.

> Drugs which are absorbed through oligo peptide transporters; e.g., cephalexin, cefadroxil, cefixime, captopril, lisinopril, etc.

> Drugs used for local therapeutic effect in the stomach; e.g., antacids, 5-fluorouracil, misoprostol, anti-helicobacter pylori agents, etc.

The normal pH range and enzyme present in different areas of gastrointestinal tract mentioned in **Table 1.4**;

**Table 1.4:** The pH range and Enzyme present in different region of GIT.

| Part of GIT | pH range | Enzymes present |
|---|---|---|
| Mouth | 7.4 | Amylase |
| Stomach | 0.8 - 5.0 | Pepsin, lactase |
| Small intestine | 5.0 - 6.5 | Lactase, Bile, Protease, Amylase, Lipase |
| Colon | 6.0 - 8.0 | |

- *Absorption window*

  The term 'absorption window' refers to the area or range of areas of the gastrointestinal tract where the drug is absorbed beyond which there is no/negligible absorption. Different regions of the gastrointestinal tract have different pH; accordingly, solubility and stability of some drugs vary from region to region due to change in pH and enzymatic degradation. For the formulation of a controlled/extended release dosage form, the rate, extent, and uniformity of absorption of a drug are essential factors. In a controlled or extended release system the release of the drug is the rate limiting step for absorption. Once the drug crosses the absorption window, it is almost wasted. Thus, absorption window is one more limiting factor for bioavailability of orally administered drugs. It can appear as a major constraint in developing SR/CR dosage form. Drugs show site absorption in the GI tract is metformin, acyclovir, captopril, ranitidine, levodopa, furosemide, sulphonamides, salbutamol, cephalosporins, tetracycline, verapamil, thiamine, quinolines, etc.

**Table 1.5:** Apparent volume of distribution of different drugs.

| S. no. | Drug | Apparent volume of distribution (L) |
|---|---|---|
| 1. | Amiodarone | 4620 |
| 2. | Azithromycin | 2170 |
| 3. | Chloroquine | 12950 |
| 4. | Doxepin | 1400 |
| 5. | Digoxin | 500 |
| 6. | Flurazepam | 1540 |
| 7. | Haloperidol | 1400 |

- ***Distribution***

  In overall elimination kinetics, the distribution of a drug in vascular and extravascular spaces in the body is an important factor to be considered. The distribution characteristic of a drug is expressed using its apparent volume of distribution and ratio of drug in tissues to the drug in plasma (T/P). The larger volume of distribution means the more considerable amount of drug is bound to the tissues and drug present blood is relatively less. The drug present in circulating blood is exposed to hepatic or renal clearance. That is if the apparent volume of distribution of a drug is less most of the drug is in blood and is exposed to renal or hepatic clearance.

  Some drugs such as chloroquine are widely bound to extravascular tissues. Their apparent volumes of distributions are more significant than the real volume of distributions, and their elimination half-lives are reduced. In such cases, the drugs go away from the body slowly provided their rate of elimination be limited by the rate of release from tissue binding sites. If the amount of drug released from the tissues is within the therapeutic range, therapeutic action of the drugs becomes sustained. The **Table 1.5** shows some drugs whose apparent volume of distribution is more than the real volume of distribution.

  Use of apparent volume of distribution to assess drug present in the body may sometimes create ambiguity. To avoid this ambiguity the ratio T/P may be used for this purpose. If the amount of drug present in the blood (P) is known, the amount of the drug present in the peripheral compartment (T) and hence, T/P can be calculated as;

  $$T/P = k_{12}(k_{21} - \beta) \qquad \qquad .....(1.13)$$

  Where $\beta$ represents the slow disposition rate constant of the drug. T/P indicates the relative distribution of the drug in peripheral and central compartments, while $V_d$ indicates the apparent distribution of the drug in the body. Some use the $V_{dss}$, the volume of distribution at the steady state level in place of $V_d$; but it does not yield any conclusion. However, the values of T/P and of $V_{dss}$ can be correlated, and some interpretations can be made (**Table 1.6**).

**Table 1.6:** Relation of T/P ratio, total body clearance and disposition characteristics

| T/P ratio | Total body clearance | Disposition characteristics |
|---|---|---|
| High | High | Weak tissue binding |
| High | Low | Strong tissue/protein binding |
| Low | Low | Strong protein binding |
| Low | High | Weak plasma protein binding |

- *Metabolism*

  Metabolism is a process which converts the drug in the body. Through metabolism either an inactive molecule is converted into therapeutically active metabolite or a therapeutically active molecule is converted into an inactive metabolite. When the process of metabolism is complex, it becomes difficult to design an SR/CR dosage form particularly if the metabolite is an active molecule. There are two situations related to metabolism which affect the design of SR/CR dosage form significantly.

  1. A drug will be considered a poor candidate for SR/CR formulation if it induces or inhibits synthesis of the enzyme when it is administered for an extended period (chronic administration).

     (i)  Drugs which induce enzymes are primidone, phenytoin, griseofulvin, rifampicin, barbiturates, meprobamate, cyclophosphamide, etc.

     (ii) Drugs which inhibit enzymes are erythromycin, Fluconazole, ketoconazole, isoniazid, cimetidine, Amiodarone, MAO-inhibitors, 4-aminosalicylic acid, allopurinol, coumarins, etc.

  2. A drug will be considered a poor candidate for SR/CR formulation, if there is a varying concentration of it in the blood either due to tissue/intestinal metabolism or due to hepatic metabolism (first pass effect). Other reasons are: most of the process can be saturated, depending on the dose the amount or fraction of the drug would be lost, and due to this loss, the bioavailability of the drug may reduce appreciably. An appreciable reduction in bioavailability will result particularly when the drug is released slowly as in case of SR/CR dosage form.

     Drugs which are metabolized in the intestine are chlorpromazine, clonazepam, hydralazine, levodopa, salicylamide, isoproterenol, etc.

- *Elimination half-life*

  Time is taken for the amount of a drug in the body (plasma concentration) to be reduced by 50% 0f its initial concentration is called elimination half-life. The half-life elimination can be determined by using clearance (Cl) and volume of distribution ($V_d$).

$$t_{\frac{1}{2}} = 0.693 V_d / Cl \qquad \qquad .....(1.14)$$

  According to the eqn. 14 the elimination half-life increases when the volume of distribution, $V_d$ is increased or when clearance, Cl is decreased. When the volume of distribution is high, the drug remains distributed more in tissues than in blood. Similarly, if the volume of distribution is less the drug is present more in the blood and less in tissues. The drug is subjected to elimination. The effect of clearance and volume of distribution on the elimination of some drugs has been presented in the **Table 1.7**.

**Table 1.7:** The effect of drug clearance and volume of distribution on elimination half-life.

| Drug | Clearance (L/hr) | Volume of Distribution (L) | Elimination half-life (hr) |
|---|---|---|---|
| Morphine | 63 | 280 | 3.0 |
| Haloperidol | 46 | 1400 | 20.0 |
| Chloroquine | 45 | 12950 | 200 |
| Flucytosine | 8 | 4.9 | 4.2 |
| Digoxin | 7 | 420 | 40.0 |
| Ethosuximide | 0.7 | 49 | 48.0 |

When a drug follows linear kinetics its elimination half-life is found to remain constant, does not depend on the dose of the drug or its concentration. When a drug follows non-linear kinetics, its elimination half-life and clearance change with a change in dose or concentration.

**(c) Biological half-life**

In the case of an ideal CRDD system, the rate of drug absorption should be equal to the rate of drug elimination. If the biological half-life($t_{1/2}$) of a drug is small (less than 2 hours), then more amount of drug would be present in a single dose of the controlled release dosage form. Drugs having $t_{1/2}$ in the range of 2-4 hours are ideal candidates for controlled release system. Drugs with long half-life should not be formulated into controlled release dosage form.

**(d) Metabolism**

Drug-selected for controlled release system should be completely metabolized, but the rate of metabolism should not be too rapid. A drug which encourages or inhibits metabolism is a poor candidate; because steady states are challenging to achieve.

**(e) Drug-Protein Binding**

The drugs can bind to the components like blood cells and plasma proteins and also to tissue proteins and macromolecules. Drug-protein binding is a reversible process. As the free drug concentration in the blood declines, the drug-protein complex dissociates and liberates the free drug to maintain equilibrium. Due to high molecular size, a protein bound drug is unable to enter into hepatocytes; as a result, the metabolism of the drug is reduced. The bound drug is not presented as a substrate for liver enzymes there by the rate of metabolism is further reduced. The glomerular capillaries do not permit the way of plasma-protein anddrug-protein complexes. Hence, the only unbound drug is eliminated. The elimination half-life of drugs usually increases when the percent of the bound drug to plasma increases. Such drugs should not be formulated as sustained/controlled release formulations.

**(f) Dosage form index**

Dosage form index is defined as the ratio of $C_{ss.max}$ to $C_{ss.min}$. Its value must be nearer to unity.

## Pharmacodynamic Properties of the Drug

(a) **Therapeutic range:** For controlled release drug delivery system, a drug should have its therapeutic range wide enough so that any variation in the release rate do not produce its concentration beyond this level.

(b) **Therapeutic index:** It is the most widely used parameter to measure the margin of safety of a drug. Therapeutic index = $TD_{50}$ /$ED_{50}$. The longer the value of the therapeutic index, the safer is the drug. A drug is considered to be safe, if its therapeutic index value is greater than 10. Drugs with a very small value of therapeutic index are not suitable candidates for the formulation of sustained release products.

(c) **Plasma concentration-response relationship:** Drugs such as reserpine whose pharmacological activity is independent of its concentration are poor candidates for the controlled-release system.

## Bibliography


1. Allen, L.V., Popvich, G.N., & Ansel, H.C. (2004). Ansel's Pharmaceutical dosage forms and drug delivery system.
2. Banker S G, Rhodes TC. Modern Pharmaceutics. Marcel Dekker Inc., New York, 2002: 575.
3. Bhargava A, Rathore RPS, Tanwar YS, Gupta S and Bhaduka G. Oral sustained release dosage form: an opportunity to prolong the release of drug. Int J Adv Res Pharm Bio Sci, 3(1), 2013, 7- 14.
4. Chauhan MJ and Patel SA. A concise review on sustained drug delivery system and its opportunities. Am J Pharm Tech Res, 2012;2(2): 227-238.
5. Chugh I, Seth N, Rana AC and Gupta S. Oral sustained release drug delivery system: an overview. Int Res J Pharm, 2012;3(5): 57-62.
6. Cristina M, Aranzaz;u Z and Jose ML. Critical factors in the release of drugs from sustained release hydrophilic matrices. J Control Rel,2011; 154: 2011, 2-19.
7. Dusane AR, Gaikwad PD, Bankar VH and Pawar SP. A review on: sustained released technology. Int J Res Ayu Pharm, 2011;2(6): 1701-1708.
8. John, C., & Morten, C. (2002). The Science of Dosage Form Design Aulton: Modified release peroral dosage forms. Churchill Livingstone.
9. Kamboj S and Gupta GD. Matrix Tablets: An important tool for oral controlled release dosage forms. Pharmainfonet, 2009;7, 1-9.
10. Kar RK, Mohapatra S and Barik BB. Design andcharacterizationof controlled release matrix tablets of Zidovudine. Asian J Pharm Cli Res, 2009;2: 54.
11. Kube RS, Kadam VS, Shendarkar GR, Jadhav SB and Bharkad VB. Sustained release drug delivery system: review. Int J Res Pharm Biotech,2015; 3(3): 246 -251.
12. Kumar S, Shashikant and Bharat P. Sustained release drug delivery system: a review. Int J Inst Pharm Life Sci, 20122(3): 356-376.
13. Lapidus H and Lordi NG. Studies on controlled release formulations. J Pharm Sci, 1968;57, 1292.

14. Leon Lachman, Herbert A. Liberman, Joseph L. Kang, The Theory and Practice of Industrial Pharmacy, Third Edition, Varghese Publishing House, Bombay, Sustained Release Dosage Forms, 419-428.

15. Mali AD and Bathe AS. A review on sustained release drug delivery system. GCC J Sci Tech,2015; 1(4): 107-123.

16. Mamidala R, Ramana V, Lingam M, Gannu R and Rao MY. Review article factors influencing the design and performance of oral sustained/controlled release dosage form. Int J Pharm Sci Nanotechnology,2009; 2, 583.

17. Mohd Abdul Hadi, Raghavendra Rao NG. Novel Technologies in Formulations: An Overview. World Journal of Pharmaceutical Research. 2012, 1(3): 452.

18. Nalla C, Gopinath H, Debjit B, Williamkeri I and Reddy TA. Modified release dosage forms. J Chem Pharm Sci,2013; 6(1): 13-21.

19. Patel Khyati, Dr. Patel Upendra, Bhimani Bhavin, Patel Ghanshyam. Extended Oral Drug Delivery System. International Journal of Pharmaceutical Research and Bioscience. 2012, 1(3): 2.

20. Patel PN, Patel MM, Rathod DM, Patel JN,Modasiya MMK. Sustain Release Drug Delivery: A Theoretical Prospective. J Pharm Res, 2012; (8): 4165-4168.

21. Patnaik AN, Nagarjuna T and Thulasiramaraju TV. Sustained release drug delivery system: a modern formulation approach. Int J Res Pharm Nano Sci,2013; 2(5): 586- 601

22. Ratilal Dusane Abhijit, Gaikwad Priti D, Bankar Vidyadhar H, Pawar Sunil P. A Review on: Sustained Released Technology. International Journal of Research in Ayurveda and Pharmacy. 2011, 2(6): 1.

23. Robinson, J.R., & Lee, V.H. (1987). Controlled drug delivery. Marcel Dekker.

24. Salsa T, Veiga F and Pina ME. Oral controlled release dosage form. I. Cellulose ether polymers in hydrophilic matrices. Drug Develop Ind Pharm,1997; 23: 929-938.

25. Sara J Risch, Science by Design, P. O. Box 39390, Edina, MN-55439. Encapsulation; Overview of Uses and Techniques. Chapter 1. 1995, 590: 1-6.

26. Shamma SP, Haranath C, Reddy CPS andSowmya C. An overview on SR tablet and itstechnology. Int J Pharm Drug Ana,2014; 2(9):740-747.

27. Shargel, L., & Yu, A.B.C. (1999). Modified release drug products. In: Applied Biopharmaceutics and Pharmacokinetics. McGraw Hill.

28. Swabrick, J., & Boylan, J.C. (1996). Encyclopedia of pharmaceutical technology. Newyork: Marcel Dekker.

29. Theeuwes, F. Elementary Osmotic Pump. J Pharm Sci, 1975;64, 1987–1991.

30. Thombre NA, Aher AS, Wadkar AV and Kshirsagar SJ. A review on sustained release oral drug delivery system. Int J Pharm Res Sch, 2015;4(2): 361-371.

31. Ummadi S, Shravani B, Rao NGR, Reddy MS and Nayak BS. Overview on controlled release dosage form. Int J Pharm Sci, 2013;3(4): 258-269.

# Exercise

## A. Multiple Choice Questions

1.  Which of the following statements is incorrect?
    - (a)   Controlled release formulation can provide a location specific action
    - (b)   Controlled release formulation can provide a local action
    - (c)   Controlled release formulation cannot provide a location specific action
    - (d)   Controlled release formulation increases duration of action

2.  Which of the following statements is correct?
    - (a)   Therapeutic window of a drug is the ratio of $LD_{50}$ to $ED_{50}$
    - (b)   Therapeutic window of a drug is the ratio of $ED_{50}$ to $LD_{50}$
    - (c)   Therapeutic window of a drug is its duration of action
    - (d)   Therapeutic window of a drug is its dosing frequency

3.  Which of the following statements is correct?
    - (a)   Controlled release formulation can reduce the tolerability
    - (b)   Controlled release formulation can improve the tolerability
    - (c)   Controlled release formulation can increase the potential first-pass clearance
    - (d)   Controlled release formulation can extend the product's life cycle

4.  Which of the following statements is incorrect?
    - (a)   CR dosage form cannot provide the scope of dose adjustment
    - (b)   CR dosage form can cause dose dumping
    - (c)   CR dosage form can delay the onset of action of the drug
    - (d)   CR dosage form fails to delay the onset of action of the drug

5.  Which of the following statements is correct?
    - (a)   Drug having short biological half-life is suitable for CR dosage form.
    - (b)   Drug having long biological half-life is suitable for CR dosage form.
    - (c)   Drug having narrow therapeutic window is suitable for CR dosage form.
    - (d)   Drug having large dose size is suitable for CR dosage form.

6.  Which of the following statements is correct?
    - (a)   Drugs absorbed mainly in lower intestine are suitable for designing CR dosage form
    - (b)   Drugs with large elimination rate are suitable for designing CR dosage form
    - (c)   Drugs which is immediately absorbed are suitable for designing CR dosage form
    - (d)   Drugs with undesirable side effects are suitable for designing CR dosage form

7.  Which of the following statements is correct?
    - (a)   Stimuli-induced systems are dissolution-controlled CR system
    - (b)   Stimuli-induced systems are erosion-controlled CR system
    - (c)   Hybrid system contains drug in a release controlled-matrix
    - (d)   Hybrid system contains drug in a matrix which is again coated with a polymer

8. Which of the following is a biopharmaceutical factor?
   (a) Therapeutic range
   (b) Elimination half-life
   (c) Drug pKa and ionization at physiological pH
   (d) Rate of metabolism

7. Which of the following is pharmacodynamic factor?
   (a) Mechanism and site of drug absorption
   (b) Route of drug administration
   (c) Rate of metabolism
   (d) Plasma concentration-response relationship

9. Which of the following is pharmacokinetic factor?
   (a) Dosage form index
   (b) Therapeutic index
   (c) Mechanism and site of absorption
   (d) Therapeutic range

10. Which of the following statements is correct?
    (a) In case of dissolution-controlled matrix penetration of the medium is controlled by porosity of the tablet matrix.
    (b) In case of dissolution-controlled matrix penetration of the medium is controlled by presence of hydrophilic material in the tablet matrix.
    (c) In case of dissolution-controlled matrix penetration of the medium is controlled by particle surface.
    (d) All of the above.

11. Which of the following statements is correct?
    (a) In nonporous reservoir system, drug molecules are released through micropores by diffusion.
    (b) In nonporous reservoir system, drug molecules diffuse through polymer membrane.
    (c) In nonporous reservoir system, drug molecules diffuse from lower concentration to higher concentration.
    (d) None of the above.

12. Which of the following statements is correct?
    (a) The release of the drug from ion-exchange resin is independent on the pH and electrolyte concentration in its surroundings.
    (b) The release of the drug from ion-exchange resin is dependent on the pH and electrolyte concentration in its surroundings.
    (c) The release of the drug from ion-exchange resin is independent on the properties of resin itself.
    (d) The release of the drug from ion-exchange resin is independent on the rigidity of resin itself.

13. Which of the following statements is not correct?
    (a)  To prepare osmotic tablet drug layer and/or sweller layer is to be formed,
    (b)  To prepare osmotic tablet membrane(s) need to be formed
    (c)  To prepare osmotic tablet microscopic holes are to be formed
    (d)  None of the above

14. Diffusibility of drug from a matrix tablet depends on?
    (a)  Molecular weight of the polymer used
    (b)  Method of preparation of the polymer
    (c)  Molecular weight of the drug
    (d)  Average weight of the tablet

15. Which of the following statements is correct?
    (a)  Solubility of a drug is its thermodynamic property.
    (b)  Solubility of a drug is not its thermodynamic property.
    (c)  Absorption of a drug into system circulation from GIT is independent of the solubility of the drug in gastric fluid.
    (d)  None of the above.

16. Which of the following statements is correct?
    (a)  For better absorption of drug in GIT, the drug must be smaller in size.
    (b)  For better absorption of drug in GIT, the drug must have adequate aqueous solubility.
    (c)  For better absorption of drug in GIT, the drug must be available in ionized form.
    (d)  For better absorption of drug in GIT, the drug must not be smaller in size.

17. Which of the following statements is correct?
    (a)  Highest value of partition coefficient would be 10.
    (b)  Highest value of partition coefficient would be 100.
    (c)  Highest value of partition coefficient would be 1.
    (d)  None of the above.

18. Which of the following statements is correct?
    (a)  Erythromycin estolate tablet is a conventional dosage form.
    (b)  Erythromycin estolate tablet is a sustained release dosage form.
    (c)  Erythromycin estolate tablet is a controlled release dosage form.
    (d)  Erythromycin estolate tablet is a modified release dosage form.

19. Which of the following statements is correct?
    (a)  The rate of drug release from a reservoir system is directly proportional to the diffusion coefficient of the drug.
    (b)  The rate of drug release from a reservoir system is not proportional to the area.

(c)  The rate of drug release from a reservoir system is directly proportional to the diffusion path length.

(d)  The rate of drug release from a reservoir system is independent on partition coefficient of the drug.

## B. Short Questions

1. Define controlled-release dosage form.  What are modified-release and delayed-release dosage form?
2. Briefly justify the reason for development of controlled release dosage form.
3. Define minimum therapeutic index, maximum safe concentration and therapeutic window.
4. What is site specific targeting, receptor targeting and extended release dosage form?
5. Briefly mention the advantages and disadvantages of controlled release dosage form.
6. What are the characteristics of the drug to be considered for selection of a drug for CR dosage form?
7. Explain dissolution-controlled release systems.
8. Explain diffusion-controlled release systems.
9. Write a note about CR dosage form using the principle of ion-exchange.
10. What do you understand by osmosis-based formulation for controlled drug delivery?

## C. Long Questions

1. Discuss why CR dosage form is more beneficial.
2. Explain the rationale of controlled-release dosage form.
3. Explain with relevant example the approaches used for designing CR dosage form.
4. Explain the concepts or approaches used to design controlled drug delivery system. Classify the CR drug delivery systems.
5. Write down the principle of dissolution-controlled release. Write notes on diffusion-controlled matrix and reservoir systems.
6. Write down briefly the effect of molecular weight, diffusion coefficient, apparent partition coefficient of drugs, and its route of administration on the design of CR dosage form.
7. Explain the effect of following characteristics on CR dosage form design: (1) aqueous solubility of drug, (2) pKa-value and ionization of drug at physiological pH, (3) stability of drug.
8. Explain the pharmacokinetic properties with respect to dose, release rate, and absorption rate of drug suitable for CR dosage form.

9. Explain the pharmacokinetic properties with respect to absorption window, distribution, and metabolism of drug suitable for CR dosage form.
10. Explain the biological half-life, drug-protein binding, therapeutic range, therapeutic index, and plasma concentration-response relationship of a drug selected for CR dosage form.

# CHAPTER 2

# Polymers

*Introduction, classification, properties, advantages and application of polymers in formulation of controlled release drug delivery systems.*

## Introduction

The word polymer has been derived from Greek words, *poly* means 'many' and *mers* mean 'parts or units of high molecular mass'. Since the beginning of life, polymers have existed in natural forms such as DNA, RNA, proteins, and polysaccharides. These play crucial roles in plant and animal life. From the earliest times, man has used naturally-occurring polymers for making clothes, decoration, shelter, tools, weapons, writing materials and other requirements. The origin of today's polymer industry has been commonly accepted as being the nineteenth century, and the important discoveries concerning the modification of certain natural polymers have taken place. In the eighteenth century, Thomas Hancock gave an idea of a modification of natural rubber through blending with certain additives. Later on, Charles Goodyear improved the properties of natural rubber through vulcanization process with sulphur. Bakelite was the first synthetic polymer produced in 1909 and after that, the synthetic fibre and rayon were developed in 1911. The systematic study of polymer science started only about a century back with the pioneering work of Herman Staudinger. Staudinger has given a new definition of the polymer. In 1919, he first published the concept that *high molecular mass compounds were composed of long covalently bonded molecules.*

Polymers are high molecular weight substances composed of large number of low molecular weight species called *monomers*. Thus, the term polymer can be defined as a *macromolecule with high molecular mass composed of considerable number of smaller molecules (monomers) joined together.* The polymers are characterized by:

- Variable molecular weight (depending on the source or mode of synthesis or extraction),
- Low specific gravity,
- Greater resistance to erosion and corrosion.

The advantages of polymeric materials over other materials is that they can be tailor-made; that is, polymers can be synthesized as per the requirement such as soft or rigid or tough, transparent or opaque, light or heavy, crystalline or amorphous, etc. For example, there are different varieties of polyethylene  [$(CH_2-CH_2)n$]- low density, medium density and high density (abbreviated as LDPE, MDPE, and HDPE). In our lives, polymers now find applications as major class of materials such as plastics, fibers, rubbers, rexin (artificial leather) and explosives. Polymerization is *the combination of two or more monomer sunder the definite condition of temperature, pressure, and in the presence of a suitable catalyst, etc.* The formation of the new macromolecule with the characteristic – C–C– linkages is called polymer. The condition for a monomer to be polymerized is the functionality. The functionality of a monomer is defined as *the number of reactive or bonding sites available in the molecule* such as carbon-carbon multiple bonds, condensable functional groups such as hydroxyl, carboxyl, amine, halogen group, etc. Carbon-carbon double bond is called bi-functional because when the double bond is broken, two single bonds are available for the combination; for example, ethylene can be polymerized but not ethane (**Fig. 2.1**).

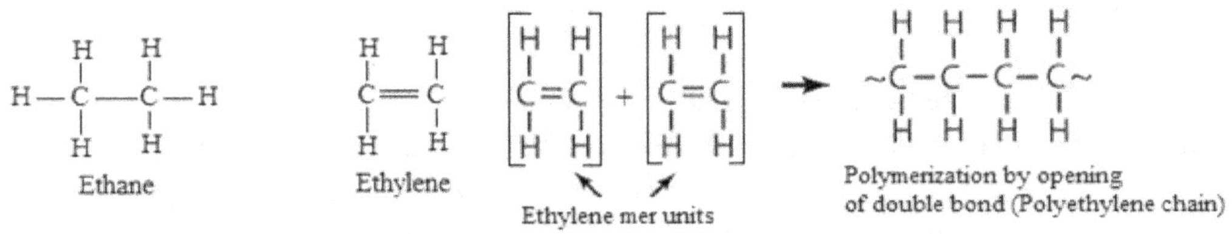

**Fig. 2.1:** Polymerization of ethylene monomer units by -c-c- bond into polyethylene due to presence of double bond, while the ethane is completely saturated compound hence, can't be polymerized.

## Classification of Polymers

The polymer is a common name of a vast number of materials of high molecular weight. These materials exist in many form and numbers. The polymer can have different chemical structure, physical properties, mechanical behavior, thermal characteristics, etc. By these properties, polymers can be classified in different ways, which is shown in **Fig. 2.2.**

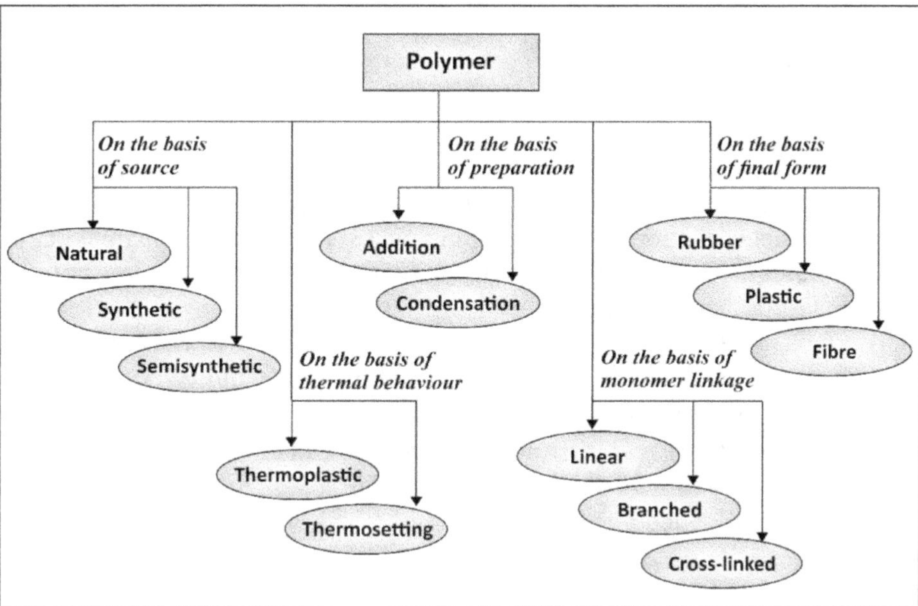

**Fig. 2.2:** Classification of polymers.

1. **Based on Origin:** By their existence in nature, polymers have been classified into three types.
    (i) *Natural polymer*: The polymers occurring in nature are called natural polymer.These are also known as biopolymers. For example, natural rubber, natural silk, cellulose, starch, proteins, etc.
    (ii) *Semi-synthetic polymer*: These are the chemically modified natural polymers such as hydrogenated natural rubber, cellulose acetate, cellulose nitrate, methyl cellulose, etc.
    (iii) *Synthetic polymer*: The polymers which have been synthesized in the laboratory are known as synthetic polymers. These are also known as human made polymers. For example, polyvinyl alcohol, polyethylene, polystyrene, polysulfone, etc.
2. **Based on Thermal Response:** By thermal response, polymers can be classified into two groups;
    (i) *Thermoplastic polymers*: These can be softened or plasticized repeatedly on the application of heat (thermal energy), without much change in properties if certain precautions are taken. Examples are polyolefins, nylons, linear polyesters and polyethers, PVC, sealing wax, etc.
    (ii) *Thermosetting polymers*: Some polymers experience certain chemical changes on heating and convert themselves into an infusible mass. The curing or setting process is due to a chemical reaction which leads to further growth and cross-linking of the polymer chain molecules and ultimately

produces giant molecules, for example, Phenolic resins, urea, epoxy resins, diene rubbers, etc.

3. **Based on Mode of Formation:** By mode of formation, polymers can be classified into two types.

   (i) *Addition polymers*: These polymers are formed from olefinic, diolefins, vinyl and related monomers. These are formed as a result of the simple addition of monomer molecules in quick succession by a chain reaction. This process is called *addition polymerization*. Examples are polyethylene, polypropylene, and polystyrene.

   (ii) *Condensation polymers*: These are formed from intermolecular reactions between bifunctional or polyfunctional monomer molecules having reactive functional groups such as $-NH_2$, $-NCO$, $-OH$, $-COOH$, etc.

4. **Based on Line structure:** Bystructure, polymers can be classified into three types.

   (i) *Linear polymer*: If the monomer units are combined in a linear pattern, the polymer is called linear polymer.

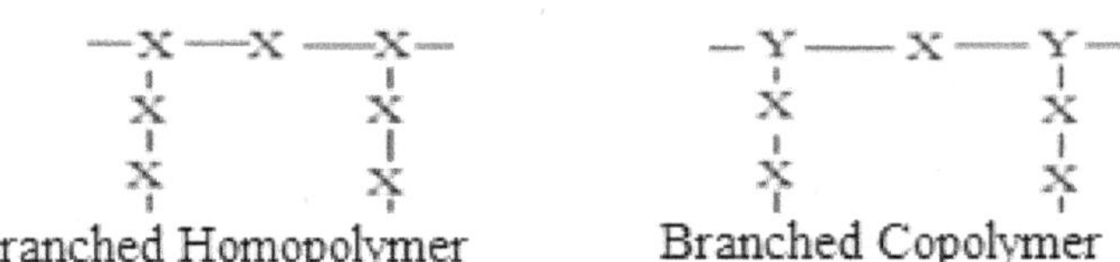

Linear Homopolymer                    Linear Copolymer

   (ii) *Branched polymer*: The branched polymer is formed when the monomers are joined together in a branched manner.

Branched Homopolymer          Branched Copolymer

   (iii) *Cross-linked polymer*: When the monomers are joined together in a branched chain with cross-linking fashion, the polymer formed is called cross-linked polymer.

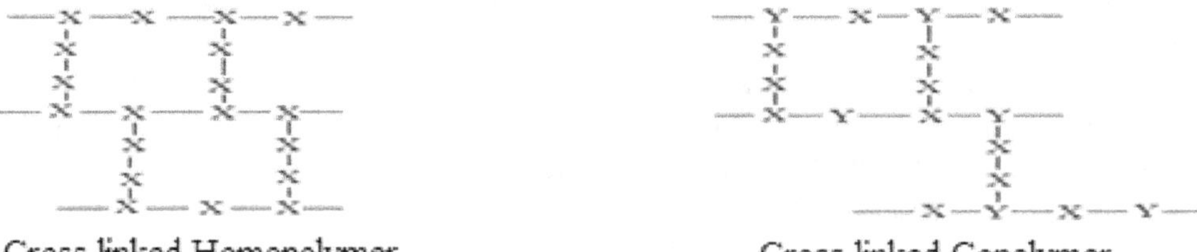

Cross linked Homopolymer                    Cross linked Copolymer

When the monomers are joined together in a branched chain with cross-linking fashion, the polymer formed is called cross-linked polymer.

5. **Based on the ultimate form and use:** Based on the ultimate form and use the polymers can be classified into three groups.

   (i) ***Rubber or Elastomer*:** These are high molecular weight polymers with long flexible chain but joined with weak intermolecular forces. For this reason, these polymers exhibit tensile strength ranging from 300 – 3000 psi and can elongate at break ranging from 300 to 1000%. Examples of these kind of polymers are natural rubber and synthetic rubber.

   (ii) ***Plastics*:** These are relatively tough and are of high molecular weight. Plastics can be moulded with or without application of heat. These are much stronger than rubber. Plastics exhibit tensile strength ranging from 4000 to 15000 psi and elongation at break ranging from 20 to 200% or more. Polyethylene, polypropylene, PVC, polystyrene, etc. are common examples of plastic.

   (iii) ***Fibers*:** Fibers are long chain polymers. These are characterized by highly crystalline regions which result mainly from secondary forces. These are much less elastic than plastics and elastomers. These have a high tensile strength ranging from 20000 to 150000 psi. These are light in weight and can absorb moisture.

## Classification of Polymers by their Physical Properties

Polymers can be classified into various categories by different parameters. For example, source, thermal response, chemical structure, etc. which have mentioned earlier. Below the polymers have been classified by their physical properties, such as the type of chain, tactility, crystallinity, polarity, etc. (**Fig. 2.3**)

   (i) **Isotactic polymer:** In this type of polymer, the specific groups are arranged on the same side of the main chain.

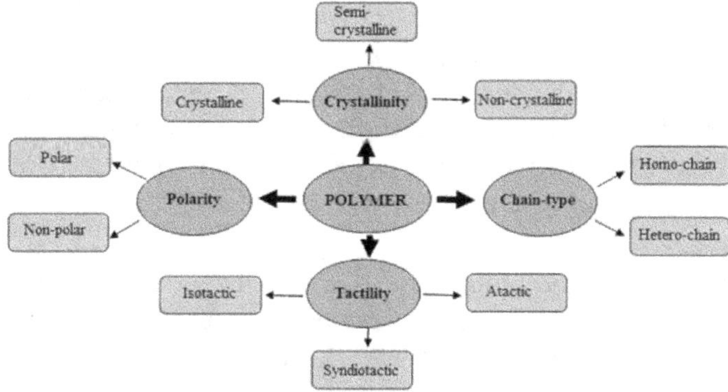


**Fig. 2.3:** Classification of polymers on the basis of physical properties.

(ii)   **Syndiotactic polymer:** If the side groups (specific groups) are arranged alternately, it is called syndiotactic polymer.

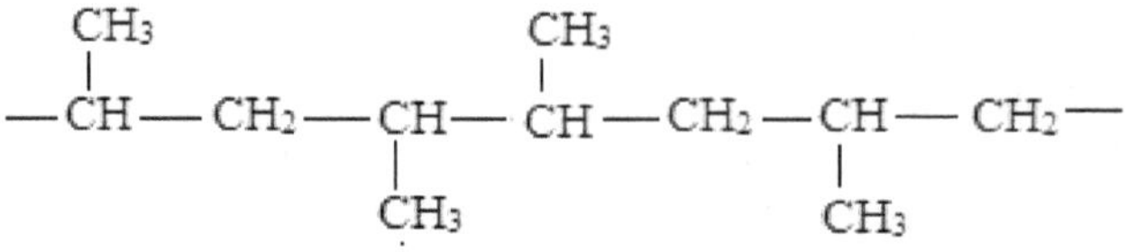

$$\overset{\overset{\displaystyle CH_3}{|}}{-CH}-CH_2-CH-\overset{\overset{\displaystyle CH_3}{|}}{CH}-CH_2-CH-CH_2-$$

Syndiotic Polypropene

(iii)  **Atactic polymer:** If the specific groups (side groups) are arranged in an irregular fashion (randomly) around the main chain, it is called atactic polymer. This type of polymers is adequately strong and are more elastic.

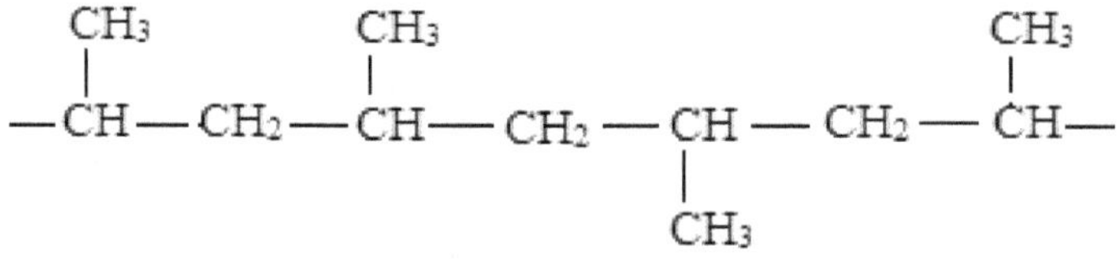

$$\overset{\overset{\displaystyle CH_3}{|}}{-CH}-CH_2-\overset{\overset{\displaystyle CH_3}{|}}{CH}-CH_2-CH-CH_2-\overset{\overset{\displaystyle CH_3}{|}}{CH}-$$

Atactic Polypropene

## Properties of Polymers

Thermal, physical and mechanical properties of polymers depend on their molecular structure, molecular weight, linearity, intra- and inter-molecular interactions. Hence, different polymers exhibit different properties.

## Physical Properties

### Crystallinity & Melting point

A polymer with linear chain can pack together in regular arrays, for example, polypropylene chain pack in such a way that a regular lattice or crystalline form is produced. When polypropylene is exposed to higher temperature, the polymer starts melting and at a particular temperature whole polymer substance melt. This range of temperature is relatively narrow. For example, polybutylene terephthalate and polyethylene terephthalate are a crystalline polymer. These melt at 220°C and 250°C to 260°C respectively.

There are some polymers whose structures are so irregular that the formation of the crystalline structure is thermodynamically impossible. These form glass-like structure. Glass is not crystalline, amorphous substance. In case of amorphous polymer structure is formed due to either its own structural irregularity or rapid cooling of the polymer melt in which crystallization could not take place because of quenching. During rapid cooling rotation around a single bond of the polymer is very difficult at low temperature. As a result, the polymer molecules could not arrange themselves in a regular or orderly manner, an amorphous structure is formed. These polymers do not have a sharp melting point; they remain soft over a wide range of temperature. For example, polystyrene and polyvinyl acetate are an amorphous polymer and their melting range are $35^\circ - 85^\circ$C and $70^\circ - 115^\circ$C respectively.

Stiffness and polymer strength of polymer increase with their crystallinity due to their increase intermolecular interaction.

### Optical properties

The optical properties of polymers change from transparent to opaque with an increase of crystallinity. Amorphous polymers are transparent. Such a change in optical properties is due to the differences in their refractive indices. Refractive index indicates the level of light scattering.

### Diffusivity

Crystallinity increases the barrier property of the polymer. Any substance whether drug or solvent of small molecular size usually cannot penetrate or diffuse through crystals of the polymer. Thus, crystalline polymers exhibit more durability and protect the internal component from attacking molecules (barrier properties). Diffusion and solubility of a polymer depend on its degree or level of crystallinity.

On the other hand, less crystalline or an amorphous polymer is suitable when release of drug is necessary. Crystallinity in a given polymer depends on;

- Its topology and isomerism. Isomerism refers to linear versus branched, isotactic versus atactic.
- Molecular weight
- Intermolecular forces
- Pendant groups (bulky versus small group)
- Rate of cooling
- Stretching mode (uniaxial versus biaxial)

Good barrier property of polymers is useful pharmaceutically for coating the pharmaceutical products (tablets, granules) and for making packaging products.

### Anisotropy

Anisotropy refers to the difference in properties along longitudinal and transverse directions. This happens due to the crystalline character of a molecule. Some polymers are having complete or partial crystallinity behave like an anisotropic material.

## Thermal Properties

### Thermal Transitions

Order of thermal transitions in the polymer may be different. That is, the change in volume with change of temperature may follow first or second order transition. When a crystalline polymer melts its volume increases significantly as the solid is entirely transformed into liquid. The melting temperature $(T_m)$ represents a first-order thermal transition in the polymer.

While an amorphous polymer melts, its volume changes gradually over a wide range of temperature and the melting temperature $(T_m)$ represents a second-order thermal transition in the polymer. This change of melting temperature is alternatively *called glass transition temperature* $(T_g)$. The type of the polymer (crystalline or amorphous) can be identified by examining the peaks (an endothermic and a baseline shift) obtained in differential scanning calorimetry (DSC) analysis of the polymer.

**Glass transition temperature**

Glass transition temperature $(T_g)$ represents the molecular motion of the polymer chain. Many factors influence, $T_g$. Thus, it is not an absolute property. Amorphous polymers are hard, stiff, and glassy at a temperature well below the transition temperature. However, these polymers may not be brittle. At temperature well above the transition temperature, the amorphous polymers become rubbery, and these may flow. The glass transition temperature of linear organic polymers may vary from $-100°C$ to above $300°C$. Some organic polymers having $T_g$ more than $300°C$ may decompose at a temperature below their $T_g$.

The glass transition temperature of polymers is important for pharmaceutical formulations, solid dosage form for making a chewable dosage form pharmaceutically acceptable polymers which can be soft and flexible at $37°C$ (temperature of mouth) can be used as chewable matrix.

This has been mentioned earlier that the glass transition temperature depends on many factors, some are mentioned below;

- **Length of the polymer chain:** Space in between the polymer chain ends is called free volume. As the free volume increases, the portion of polymer acquires more freedom to move. This affects the temperature at which the movement of the polymer occurs. For example, polyethylene may be of two types –high density and low density. Hence, the size of free volume inside their structure is also different. At a given weight, low-density polymer occupies more volume compared to high-density counter-part. Polymers of long-chain have smaller free volume than their shorter counter parts. If the free volume is more, the $T_g$ value is less. A polymer having short chains or lower molecular weight exhibits lower $T_g$ values.

- **Side groups of polymer side chain:** The groups attached to the side chain of a polymer may be polar or bulky. These may produce steric hindrance. Thus, to make a segmental motion in a polymer containing large groups, higher temperature is required. For example, polypropylene contains methyl groups, and polystyrene contains phenyl groups. Due to the larger size of the phenyl group, the Tg value of polystyrene is much higher, about $100°C$; while $T_g$ value of polypropylene is $-20°C$.

  Strong intermolecular interaction is found within the polymers having polar side groups. This strong interaction disturbs the segmental movement of the polymer chain. For example, the structural difference between polyethylene and polyvinylchloride (PVC) is that in polyvinyl chloride, chlorine is attached in place of hydrogen, and in polyethylene there is hydrogen. Chlorine is more polar than hydrogen. Hence, the glass transition temperature ($T_g$ value) of polyvinyl chloride is much higher (100°C) than that of polyethylene (–120°C).

- **The flexibility of polymer chain:** Flexible chain possesses higher entropy than rigid chain; that is, the tendency of motion is more inflexible chain than the rigid one. In other words, the polymer having a flexible chain can behave as a liquid while polymer with rigid chain behaves as solid. The flexibility of polymer can be affected by the groups such as phenyl, amide, sulphone and carbonyl present either in the backbone or as a side group hanging on the backbone of the polymer. For example, the structure of polyethylene adipate and polyethylene terephthalate are very similar. However, phenylene is present in polyethylene terephthalate; while butylene is present in polyethylene adipate. As a result, the $T_g$ value of polyethylene adipate is 69°C while that of polyethylene terephthalate is –70°C, making a difference in $T_g$ values of 100°C.

- **Polymer chain branching:** When a polymer has a linear chain, its free volume is less. However, the free volume becomes more if the polymer has a branched chain. Thus, the $T_g$ values of linear chain polymer are expected to be higher. Moreover, branching in a polymer restricts the polymer to segmental motion; hence its $T_g$ value is expected to be higher. Therefore, the effect of branching on the $T_g$ value of a polymer can be assessed only when the complete structure of the polymer is known.

- **Polymer chain cross-linking:** The entropy of a linear chain polymer is higher than that of a cross-linked chain polymer. Thus, the linear chain polymer is expected to move, and their $T_g$ values would be less. Now by adding cross-links to a linear chain, the extent of movement of the chain can be reduced, and this results in the reduction of entropy at a particular temperature. As a result, the $T_g$ value goes high. Hence, $T_g$ values would be very high with an increase in the extent of cross-linking in a polymer. This increase of $T_g$ value can go to the extent that before showing any segmental motion the polymer starts decomposing.

- **Processing rate:** Before preparing any polymer product, it is necessary to process the polymer at various temperatures or pressures that can significantly affect the molecular motion in the polymer. The Tg value of a given polymer can be evaluated with the help of the rate of processes such as heating, cooling, loading, etc. As per kinetics, if the rate of these processes is high (fast heating or fast cooling or fast loading), the polymer chain would not move to the expected extent. These polymers practically behave as rigid chains which have a lower tendency to move and higher $T_g$ values. Thus, if a polymer is heated at a different heating rate and measured by using differential scanning calorimeter, the observed $T_g$ value may be different from the expected $T_g$ value. This indicates that heating rate should be consistent and adjusted in such a way that it does not change the expected motion and its $T_g$ value.

- **Plasticizer:** The entropy and mobility of a polymer molecule can be increased by plasticizer molecule. Thus, the plasticized polymer can result to lower Tg value with greater mobility, and non-plasticized polymer does not have this ability. Plasticizer generally mixed with the polymer are sodium lauryl sulfate, glyceryl monostearate, triethyl citrate, etc.

## Mechanical Properties

Mechanical properties of a polymer depending on their molecular structure, molecular weight, and inter-molecular forces. When these are kept under stress, they resist differently. The mechanical properties of polymers include;

- ➢ Tensile strength: ability to resist against stretching or the resistance of a polymer to breaking under tension.
- ➢ Compressive strength: the strength of the compacted polymer; in other words, a polymer can withstand loads tending to reduce size.
- ➢ Flexural strength: it is also known as bend strength or modulus of rupture it is the ability of the material to bend.
- ➢ Impact strength: it is the resistance of a polymer to fracture under a sudden impact or shock; it is the ability to withstand sudden stress.
- ➢ Fatigue: it refers to the weakening of a material caused by repeatedly applied loads or dynamic loading.

Under applied stress the mechanical properties of a polymer increase with increasing molecular weight of the polymer. With the increasing molecular weight their intermolecular interaction increases. A flexible polymer can be stretched better; while compression strength of a rigid polymer is more. If the polymers are exposed to loads, they will deform. Their strengths can be measured by measuring their deformation. Fibrous or highly cross-linked polymers show the elastic property. The slope of the stress-strain curve becomes steeper when the intermolecular forces within a fibrous polymer increase or when the density of cross-linking within a cross-linked polymer increases. The slope of the curve becomes sharper when the modulus becomes higher. To express the strength of a polymer either the modulus or stiffness can be used. Some polymers do not show sharp breaking point. For example, tough plastics continue to deform under lower stresses before finally breaking. On the other hand, rubbers or elastomers show different behavior; this depends on the extent of cross-linking or curing.

For example, stretching of a rubber band. However, highly cross-linked rubber shows very low deformation at their breaking point. Cross-linking changes the properties of rubber and can make a hardened plastic or even fiber. Whatever may be the type of polymer whether rubber, plastic, or fiber, some amount of energy is required to break the polymer. The area under the stress/strain curve depends on the toughness of the polymer. Tough plastic yields a larger area under the curve (**Fig. 2.4**).

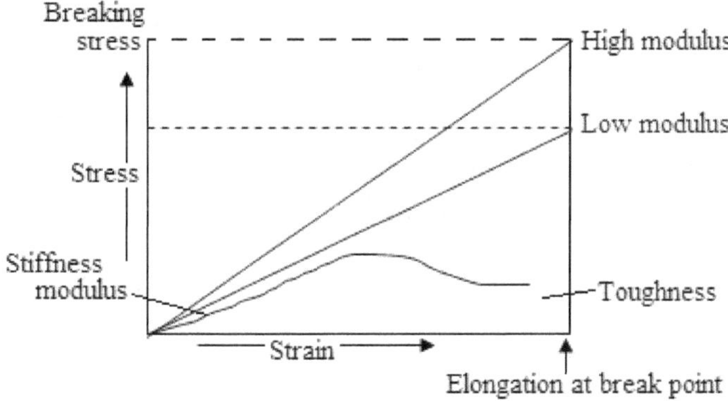


**Fig. 2.4:** Stress-strain curve of polymer

## Viscoelastic properties

Mechanical properties of a polymer are measured at a fixed rate of loading, at a particular temperature, or relative humidity, etc. The polymer is neither an elastic nor a pure fluid material. Their elastic behavior proves that they can store energy. On the other hand, their elastic behavior shows that the polymers can disperse the stored energy. Hence, it can be said that most of the polymers are a viscoelastic material. For example, polyvinyl chloride (PVC) has a glass transition temperature $(T_g)$, 100°C. This indicates that PVC behaves like a solid or glass at a temperature below 100°C and behaves like a fluid at a temperature above 100°C. Thus, a product made of PVC can be satisfactorily used at room temperature, well below its $T_g$ (100°C); but its solid or elastic behavior may change if it is kept under the loaded condition for a long time. During this long period of time, the intermolecular forces within the polymer become weaker and hence, the polymer becomes softer.

There are two methods to measure viscoelastic properties of a polymer

1. **Creep test:** In this test the polymer is loaded with a certain weight and its deformation is measured with time.
2. **Stress relaxation test:** In this test the polymer is deformed to a certain extent, then its stress (internal stress) relaxation is measured with time.

## Molecular weight

It has been discussed earlier that mechanical properties of polymers increase with the increase of their molecular weights. With increased molecular weight the polymer behaves as solid, and it becomes difficult to handle the polymer melts or their solutions. The polymers have a property called *entanglement* which controls the flow property of polymer melt or solution. The polymer chains entangle more into each other with the increase in molecular weight. As a result, the polymer lose its flow property in the solid state (as a melt) or in a liquid state (as a solution). Hence, for satisfactory performance either in the form of melt or solution, the polymer should have a particular range of molecular weight.

## Advantages

- Cheap to make
- Because of their different properties, these have various applications.
- Provide scopes tomake the polymer and the product.
- Some polymers can be recycled, melted down and made into something else which saves valuable natural resources.
- If polymers are used instead of wood, a lesser number of trees will have to be cut down.

## Disadvantages

- Near polymer-producing industrial area, habitation may be preferred.
- Plastic products are appeared to be cheaper than the natural materials.
- Made from oil, a non-renewable resource.
- Most plastics are not biodegradable; so, there is a problem of how to get rid of them.
- Landfill sites are unpleasant.
- Give off toxic fumes when they burn.
- Sorting types of polymers for recycling can be expensive.

## Application of Polymers in Formulation of Controlled Release Drug Delivery Systems

A drug delivery system is a device that delivers the therapeutic agent (drug) at the desired site at a desired rate. In other words, it releases the drug timely at a right location of the body so that the drug can show its therapeutic effect. The use of polymers has been increasing day by day in pharmaceutical applications particularly in making drug delivery systems. Millions of patients have been getting benefit from advanced drug delivery systems. These delivery systems contain polymer for different purposes. For example, the polymers have been used as binders in tablets, viscosity, and flow control agents in liquids, suspensions and emulsions; it is also usedin film coatings, etc. After administration, the drug is absorbed into the systemic circulation following steps mentioned below:

- ➢ Diffusion of the drug through the matrix of the dosage form.
- ➢ Dissolution of the drug in the fluid of the gastrointestinal tract.
- ➢ Diffusion of the drug through the aqueous fluid of GIT to the surrounding tissue, such as the villi of the small intestine.
- ➢ Absorption of the drug across the wall of the GIT.
- ➢ Entry into the systemic circulation and deposition at the required site of action.

To modify the release characteristics of a formulation such as controlled release dosage forms there are several strategies by which controlled release dosage forms may be formulated. All of which involve the use of polymers and a range of geometries to control the rate at which the drug diffuses from the dosage form and hence dissolves in the biological fluids. Some systems involve the modification of the solubility of the therapeutic agent (by chemical modification or insoluble salt formation) or involve the use of slowly dissolving polymers. There are the methods involved in diffusion-controlled release systems:

(A) Reservoir systems,

(B) Matrix systems and

(C) Miscellaneous diffusion-controlled drug release systems.

(A) **Reservoir systems:** In these systems the drug-containing core is detached from the biological fluids by a water-insoluble polymeric coat or layer, liable on the geometry of the drug delivery system. Examples of polymers that are commonly used as the polymeric coated layers include, ethylcellulose, poly (ethylenevinyl acetate), silicone and various acrylate copolymers.

A diagrammatic representation of the design and operation of a reservoir system is shown in **Fig. 2.5**.

Drug release from these systems occurs by some steps, initially involving the partitioning of the drug into the polymeric coat layer. The drug then diffuses from the inner to the outer side of the coat-layer due to the difference in concentration gradient and at this stage partitions into the surrounding biological media. Mathematically, the rate of drug diffusion (termed the flux, J) across the polymeric coat/layer may be defined as the product of the diffusion coefficient (D) and the concentration gradient $\left(\dfrac{dC}{dx}\right)$ as follows:

$$J = -D\left(\frac{dC}{dx}\right) \qquad .....(2.1)$$

Assuming steady state condition, the above equation may be integrated to produce Equation 2:

$$J = -D\,\frac{\Delta C}{h} \qquad .....(2.2)$$

Where h is the polymer coating/layer thickness. Based on equation 1 and 2, the rate of drug release $\dfrac{dM}{dt}$ can be expressed as;

$$\frac{dM}{dt} = \frac{D_m A\, K}{h} \qquad .....(2.3)$$

Where, D, is the diffusion coefficient of the drug withinthe polymer membrane,

A is the surface area of the dosage form, and

K is the partition coefficient of the drug (between the polymeric coat/layer and the biological solution).

The partition coefficient is frequently expressed as the ratio of the solubility of the drug in the polymeric phase to that in aqueous solution.

Equation 3 specifically relates to the diffusion of the therapeutic agent through the polymeric matrix however in the biological environment one other factor must be considered, namely the diffusion of the drug through the hydrodynamic (unstirred) diffusion layer.

This is a stagnant layer of fluid that is present on the surface of the drug delivery system through which the drug must diffuse before entry into the main bulk of the biological fluids. To facilitate these considerations, Equation 3must be expanded.

The rate of drug release per unit area of the dosage form $\left(\dfrac{M}{t}\right)$ may be described as;

$$\frac{M}{t} = \frac{C_p K D_d D_m}{K D_d h_m + D_m h_d} \qquad\qquad .....(2.4)$$

Where, $C_p$ = saturation solubility of the drug in polymer coat/layer,

K = partition coefficient,

$D_d$ = Diffusion coefficient of the drug in the hydrodynamic layer,

$D_m$ = diffusion coefficient of the drug in the polymer coat/layer,

$h_d$ = thickness of the polymer coat/layer, and

$h_m$ = thickness of the hydrodynamic layer

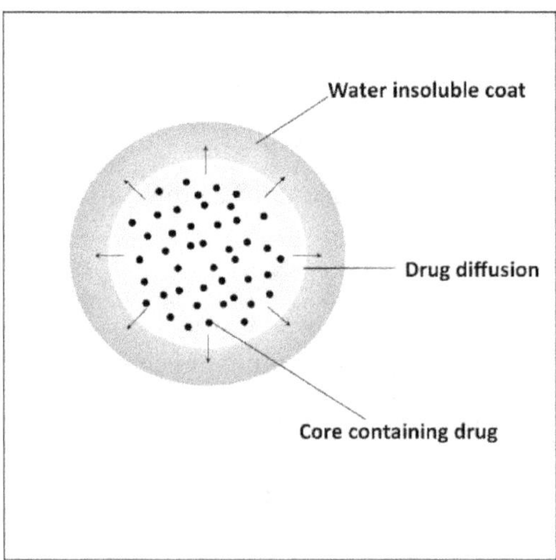


**Fig. 2.5:** Schematic diagram of reservoir system.

The equation 4 defines the parameters that can influence the subsequent delivery of therapeutic agents and is consequently used to design the drug release. Several drug delivery systems have been designed to provide reservoir-controlled drug release. Some commonly used and essential are discussed below.

Similarly, there are some methods by which the systems such as, pellets, spheres and tablets may be produced, and these are coated with an insoluble polymeric coating using conventional spray/film coating techniques, such as pan coating, air suspension coating. Alternatively, planar (laminated) drug delivery systems, such as transdermal patches, are prepared using extrusion or film coating techniques.

All reservoir systems follow a common design. For example, the drug core is enclosed within a polymeric barrier. The selection of the composition of the polymeric membrane is doneby the physicochemical properties of the drug; such as, the ability of the drug to diffuse through the polymer coating at an appropriate rate, the method of manufacture and the route of administration to the patient.

***Occusert system:*** The drug can be delivered to the eye for the treatment of disorders of the eye; such as glaucoma, using conventional drug delivery systems, such as drops, ointments. The rapid clearance of drugs from the surface of the eye due to blinking and tear flow is the primary disadvantage of such conventional dosage form.

The efficiency of ocular drug delivery system may be improved through the use of polymeric implants. These are implanted under the lower cul-de-sac of the eye. The Occusert represents one such example that has been designed to release either 20 µg/h or 40 µg/h of a drug such as a pilocarpine for a seven days' period. The Occusert is an ellipsoidal shaped implant that is composed of several layers, diagrammatic representations of which are shown in **Fig. 2.6**.

In this system drug (pilocarpine) is dispersed within a polymer (alginic acid) matrix which is sandwiched between two layers each composed of poly (ethylene-co-vinyl acetate) — the layers of the alginic acid act as the rate controlling membranes. The fourth layer is composed of an opaque, annular ring that is placed below the rate controlling layer. Both the rate controlling membranes and the drug-containing matrix is transparent. The function of this ring is to provide visibility of the device after installation. Drug releases from this delivery system occur by diffusion.

Initially tear (lachrymal) fluid diffuses through the rate controlling membranes and enters into the inner alginate matrix where dissolution of pilocarpine occurs. Now in the molecular state, pilocarpine diffuses from the region of high concentration (the drug-polymer matrix) to the lachrymal fluid through the rate controlling membrane. If the release of drug from this system is zero order; it can be expressed mathematically using equation 5 (modification of equation 4).

$$\frac{dM}{dt} = \frac{DKC_s}{h} \qquad\qquad .....(2.5)$$

Where, $\frac{dM}{dt}$ is the rate of release of the drug,

D is the diffusion coefficient of the drug through the polymeric rate controlling membrane,

K is the membrane: solution partition coefficient,

Cs is the saturated concentration of drug in the lachrymal fluid within the alginic acid matrix, and h is the thickness of the rate controlling layer.

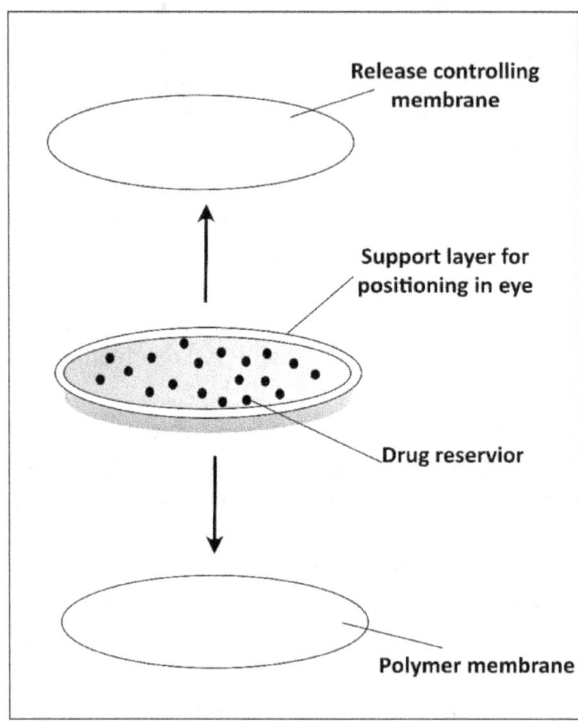


**Fig. 2.6:** Diagrammatic representation of occusert for ocular drug delivery.

There are two features of the Occusert system that are important for determining the subsequent performance,

➢  the thickness/composition of the rate controlling membrane, and

➢  the selection of the salt form of the drug.

However, there are some reservoir-controlled drug delivery systems (water impermeable), the rate controlling membrane is designed to help and control the rate of diffusion of tear fluid into the inner drug-polymer layer of the device. This is the most critical design component for some reasons.

➢  Drug release may only occur whenever a saturated solution of the drug is present within the alginic acid layer,and therefore the rate of ingress of fluid will influence the subsequent rate of dissolution of pilocarpine.

> Secondly, the choice of the drug salt will directly affect the saturated drug solubility.

It is worth noting that the zero-order release of the drug only occurs whenever a saturated solution of the drug is maintained within the inner polymer matrix and therefore, the use of a solubledrug or its salt.The increase of the rate of release of the drug, would ensure that the duration of zero-order release is reduced. Whenever insufficient drug remains within the alginic acid layer to maintain a saturated drug solution, the drugis released according to first order kinetics. According to Equation 5 the rate of release of the drug may be altered by modification of the thickness of the rate controlling membranes.

***Transdermal Patches***: The reservoir systems for controlled drug delivery may be provided through the transdermal delivery system. In transdermal drug delivery system, the drug diffuses through the skin and is ultimately absorbed into the systemic circulation. It is known that the skin protects the body from the entrance of possibly dangerous chemicals and therefore, only a limited number of therapeutic agents possess the appropriate physicochemical properties to cross this anatomical barrier. Three main anatomical barriers restrict the diffusion of drug through the skin;

- the *stratum corneum* (a keratinized layer at the outermost region of the skin),
- the viable epidermis and
- the dermis into which the microcirculation may be found.

Since long, topical formulations have been used for the treatment of localized disorders, such as infection, itching, inflammation, etc. However, the skin can be used as a portal for the controlled delivery of drugs into the systemic circulation. Penetration of drug occurs in a series of stages;

> drug penetration from the dosage form into the *stratum corneum,*

> diffusion through the *stratum corneum,*

> partitioning into and diffusion through the lower layers of the epidermis,

> partitioning into the dermis and diffusion to the walls of the microcirculation.

> partitioning into the microcirculation and distribution of the drug through the systemic circulation to the target organ.

Although three layers resist the drug diffusion, the major barrier to drug absorption is the stratum corneum.

There are several transdermal therapeutic systems (TDDS) including reservoir membrane designs. A typical reservoir transdermal therapeuticsystem is shown in **Fig. 2.7.**

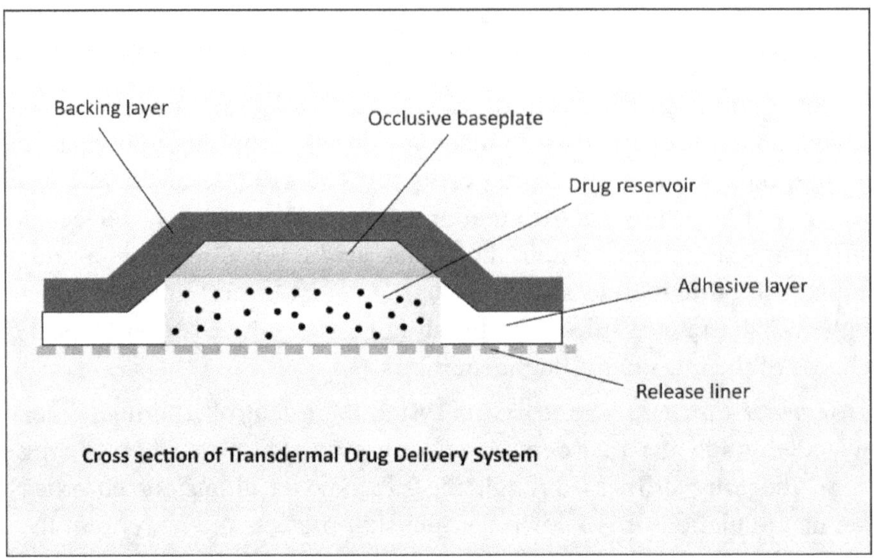


**Fig. 2.7:** Cross section of transdermal patch.

The drug delivery system is composed of several layers, such as a metallic backing layer, which is impermeable to drug. It prevents drug loss. Besides, the system contains the drug reservoir, arate controlling membrane and an adhesive layer. This facilitates the location and retention of the drug on the skin. The system also contains a release liner, which is present on the surface of the adhesive layer and is removed before use. The mechanism of drug release is similar to other reservoir-controlled drug delivery systems and involves the following steps:

- Dissolution of the drug within the reservoir matrix.
- Diffusion of the drug to and partitioning into the membrane.
- Drug diffusion within the membrane and partitioning into the adhesive layer.
- Drug diffusion within the adhesive and partitioning into the *stratum corneum.*

The control of drug release from these systems depends on the physicochemical properties of the other layers. For example, the drug is dissolved or dispersed in a matrix may be a solid polymer or a viscous paste containing silicone oil or other compatible liquids. The fundamental importance to the design of these systems is the composition of the rate controlling membrane. Drug diffusion into the adjacent adhesive layer is the rate-limiting step. Also, the selection of adhesive is important which facilitates the diffusion of the drug.

Commonly used adhesives are silicones and acrylate copolymers. The rate of release of drug from transdermal reservoir systems may be conveniently described by the following equation:

$$\frac{dM}{dt} = \frac{K_m/_r \, K_a/_m \, D_a D_m}{K_m/_r \, D_m h_a + K_a/_m \, D_a h_m}$$

Where, $C_R$ is the drug concentration present in the matrix,

$K_m/_r$ and $K_a/_m$ are the reservoir/membrane and membrane/adhesive partition coefficients,

$D_m$ and $D_a$ are the diffusion coefficients of the drug in the rate controlling membrane and the adhesive layer, $h_a$ and $h_m$ are the thicknesses of the rate controlling membrane and the adhesive layer.

**(B) Matrix Systems:** In matrix designed drug delivery systems, the drug is homogeneously dispersed or dissolved in a polymeric medium. The manufactureof matrix designed drug delivery systems is more candid and may be done using a number of different approaches; for examples:

1. **Mixing of a polymer with the drug particles and directly compressed into tablets:** The direct compression method has been used in several studies for the production of matrix-controlled release systems. For example, the tablets of dihydrocodeine bitartrate can be produced by direct compression of the drug with poly (ethylene oxide). Cellulose derivatives, such as HPMC or sodium carboxycellulose have been used for the preparation of controlled release dosage forms. These two polymers have been used to design the required drug release rate. Other approaches used include the compression of cellulose derivatives with acrylate derivatives such as Eudragit E100, and a multilayered tablet has been prepared by using the combination of poly (ethylene oxide) with HPMC.

2. **Dissolving the drug and polymer in an suitable solvent followed by removal of the solvent.** For the production of matrix drug delivery systems, this method has been examined by several authors. In some cases, the drug is dissolved/dispersed within a polymer solution, then cast into an appropriate mold, and the solvent is removed. In addition to the physicochemical parameters of the drug, the solvent used for the solubilization of the polymer and the rate of removal of solvent have been reported to affect drug release. Matrix drug-containing systems have also been used as drug release coatings for medical devices. Schierholtz, J. M. and co-workers described the release of antimicrobial substances such as ciprofloxacin, fosfomycin, gentamicin and flucloxacillin from polyurethane that had been prepared by a solvent evaporation method. Similarly, the physicochemical and antimicrobial properties of PVP-I containing poly($\varepsilon$-caprolactone) films, prepared by solvent evaporation for use as coatings for medical devices, were described by Jones, D. S., and coworkers. Two methods have received considerable attention for the production of microparticles by spray drying and by evaporation of the (emulsion) solvent.

3. **Mixing of a drug into a polymer by polymerization of a drug-monomer mixture or by hydrogel swelling within a drug solution:** Chemically crosslinked hydrogels have been used as a matrix for controlled drug delivery has received considerable attention in the pharmaceutical and related sciences. The drugs can be incorporated into these systems by either polymerization and crosslinking of the monomer in the presence of dissolved or dispersed drug or by immersion of the crosslinked hydrogel in a drug solution — this result drug absorption into the polymer matrix. There are several examples of the production of drug-loaded hydrogels by immersion swelling in a drug solution; for example, the incorporation of model drugs within crosslinked poly (vinyl alcohol), the incorporation of gentamicin within radiation-crosslinked poly (2-methoxyethyl acrylate-co-dimethyl acrylamide) and poly(2-methoxyethyl acrylate-co-acrylamide) hydrogels, the formulation of insulin-loaded poly (acryloyl-hydroxyethylstarch)-PLGA microspheres, the incorporation of gentamicin sulfate within interpenetrating polymer networks composed of poly(acrylic acid) and gelatin and the loading of hydrogel contact lenses with a range of therapeutic agents commonly administered to the eye. It has been reported that the uptake of the drug is dependent on the chemical properties and the degree of crosslinking of the hydrogel and the selection of solvent in which the hydrogel is immersed. The physicochemical properties of the drug and the subsequent release of the drug depend on the amount of drug incorporated and the type of and degree of crosslinking within the hydrogel.

4. **Curing a polymer in the presence of dissolved/dispersed drug:** Certain polymers, such as silicone may be formulated to prepare implantable dosage forms; for example, intravaginal rings or medicated medical devices. These systems are prepared by crosslinking of polydimethylsiloxane at an elevated temperature in the presence of acatalyst. For several decades medicated intravaginal silicone drug delivery systems have been used clinically for contraceptive purposes and the synchronization of estrus in farm animals. Recently these systems have been reformulated for the treatment of symptoms of the menopause, for the controlled delivery of oxybutynin (for the treatment of urinary incontinence) and for the delivery of nonoxynol-9 to prevent transmission of sexually transmitted diseases.

Thus, the matrix drug delivery systems contain drug either in dissolved or in the dispersed state within a polymeric matrix. Diffusion of the drug over the polymeric matrix is the rate-controlling step and is, therefore, responsible for the resultant therapeutic actions. To understand the mathematical aspects of drug release from matrix systems, it is essential to consider the nature of drug release. The **Fig. 2.8** shows that the drug is initially dispersed throughout the dosage form. After ingestion/insertion the drug which is present at the surface of the drug delivery system starts diffusing from the matrix into the adjacent biological fluids. This initial release is poorly controlled and is referred to as the burst effect. Then, drug release takes place by diffusion through the matrix and dissolution in the surrounding fluids. As a result, two major consequences are observed: (1) it can be assumed that the drug delivery system is composed of an infinite number of layers containing the drug. Therefore, as drug diffusion proceeds from the outside of the device, each sequential release of drug results in the production of a drug-free zone, often termed the zone of depletion, as shown in **Fig. 2.8.**

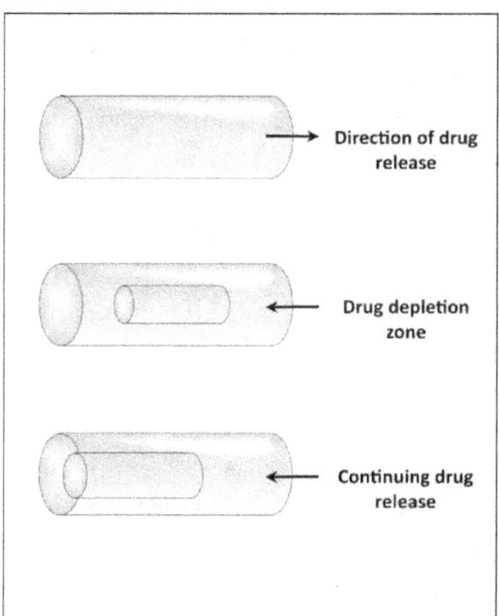


**Fig. 2.8:** Drug release from insoluble polymer.

Roseman, T. J., and Higuchi, W. I. illustrated the release of a steroid, medroxy progesterone acetate, from silicone cylinders. (2)The amount of drug released from matrix systems decreases with time (due to the increasing diffusional path length), unlike reservoir type systems in which zeroorder release of drug occurs. Higuchi, T. derived an expression to a model drug release from these systems based on the following assumptions:

➢ Sink conditions are operative and therefore drug release is controlled by the delivery system.
➢ A pseudo-steady state is sustained during drug release.
➢ The diffusion coefficient of the drug through the delivery system remains constant.
➢ The diameter of drug particles (if present) is less than the average distance of drug diffusion through the matrix.
➢ There is no interaction among the drug and the matrix.

**(C) Miscellaneous diffusion controlled drug release system**
- ***Ophthalmic Drug Delivery:*** Polymer exhibits favorable biological behavior such as bioadhesive, permeability-enhancing properties, and

physicochemical characteristics, which make it a unique material for the design of suitable ocular drug delivery. Due to the elastic properties, polymer hydrogels provide better acceptability, concerning the solid or semisolid formulation. Ophthalmic delivery systems, such as suspensions or ointments, ophthalmic chitosan gels improve adhesion to the mucin, which coats the conjunctiva and the corneal surface of the eye, and increase precorneal drug residence times, showing down drug elimination by the lachrymal flow. Also, its penetration enhancement has a more targeted effect and allows lower doses of the drugs. On the hand, polymer-based colloidal system has been found to work as a transmucosal drug carrier. These either facilitate the transport of drugs to the inner eye (a chitosan-coated colloidal system containing indomethacin) or accumulates into the corneal/conjunctival epithelia (chitosan nanoparticulate containing cyclosporine). The microparticulate drug carrier (microspheres) is thought of a promising delivery system for topical administration of acyclovir to the eye. High molecular weight (1930 kd) chitosan has been used to increase the efficacy and duration of action of the ofloxacin.

- *Gene delivery*: Gene delivery systems comprise viral vectors, cationic liposomes, polycation complexes, and microencapsulated systems. For gene delivery, viral vectors are found advantageous because these are highly efficient and have a wide range of cellular targets. When used *in vivo*, these provide immune responses and oncogenic effects. To overcome the limitations of viral vectors, non-viral delivery systems are considered for gene therapy. The non-viral delivery system has advantages such as ease of preparation, cell/tissue targeting, low immune response, unrestricted plasmid size, and large-scale reproducible production.

  The polymer has been used as a carrier of DNA for gene delivery system. The polymer can also be used as oral gene carrier because of its adhesive and transport properties in the GI tract. Mac Laughlin et al. showed that plasmid DNA containing cytomegalovirus promoter sequence and a luciferase reporter gene can be delivered *in vivo* by chitosan and depolymerized chitosan oligomers to express a luciferase gene in the intestinal tract.

- *Intratumoral and local drug delivery*: In recent times intratumoral and local drug delivery strategies have gained momentum as a promising drug delivery system in cancer therapy. Polymer films can be fabricated to deliver paclitaxel at the tumor site in therapeutically effective concentration. Paclitaxel can be loaded at 31% (w/w) in films, which may be translucent and flexible. Polymer films containing paclitaxel are obtained by casting method with high loading efficiencies, and the chemical integrity of the molecule would be unaltered during the preparation.

- ***Oral drug delivery:*** Oral delivery of diazepam coated with polymer films has been investigated in rabbits. The results specified that a film composed of a 1:0.5 drug-polymer mixture might be an effective dosage form that is equivalent to the commercial and traditional tablet dosage forms. The capacity of the polymer to form films may permit its use in the formulation of film dosage forms, as an alternative to pharmaceutical tablets. The pH sensitivity, coupled with the reactivity of the primary amine groups, make polymer a unique polymer for oral drug delivery applications.

- ***Nasal drug delivery:*** The nasal mucosa presents an ideal site for bioadhesive drug delivery systems. Polymer-based drug delivery systems, such as microspheres, liposomes and gels have been found to have good bioadhesive characteristics and swell easily when in contact with the nasal mucosa increasing the bioavailability and residence time of the drugs to the nasal route. Various polymer salts such as chitosan lactate, chitosan aspartate, chitosan glutamate, and chitosan hydrochloride are good candidates for the nasal sustained release of vancomycin hydrochloride. Nasal administration of Diphtheria Toxoid incorporated into chitosan microparticles results in a protective systemic and local immune response against Diphtheria Toxoid with enhanced IgG production. Nasal formulations have induced significant serum IgG responses similar to secretory IgA levels. This is superior to parenteral administration of the vaccine. Nasal absorption of insulin after administration into polymer powder has been found to be the most effective formulation for nasal drug delivery of insulin in sheep compared to chitosan nanoparticles and chitosan solution.

- ***Buccal drug delivery:*** The polymer is excellent to be used for buccal delivery because it has muco/bioadhesive properties and can act as an absorption enhancer. Buccal tablets of chlorhexidine diacetate give prolonged release of the drug in the buccal cavity with the improved antimicrobial activity of the drug. Polymer microparticles with no drug combined have antimicrobial activity due to the polymer. The buccal bilayered devices (bilaminated films, palavered tablets) using a mixture of drugs (nifedipine and propranolol hydrochloride) and chitosan, with or without anionic crosslinking polymers (polycarbophil, sodium alginate, gellan gum) has promising potential for use in controlled delivery in the oral cavity.

- ***Gastrointestinal drug delivery:*** Polymer granules having internal cavities prepared by de-acidification when added to acidic and neutral media are found buoyant and provide a controlled release of the drug prednisolone. Floating hollow microcapsules of melatonin showed gastro-retentive controlled-release delivery system. The release of the drug from these microcapsules is greatly retarded up to 1.75 to 6.7 hours in the simulated gastric fluid. Mucoadhesive microcapsules of metoclopramide and glipizide loaded with chitosan have been found to remain in the stomach for more than 10 hours.

- *Vaginal drug delivery*: By introducing thioglycolic acid into the primary amino groups of chitosan, the polymer is modified. The microspheres containing the polymer and embedded with clotrimazole, an imidazole derivative, is widely used for the treatment of mycotic infections of the genitourinary tract. By introducing thiol groups, the mucoadhesive properties of the polymer are strongly improved and the residence time on the vaginal mucosa tissue (26 times longer than the corresponding unmodified polymer) in increased. This guarantees a controlled drug release in the treatment of mycotic infections. Vaginal tablets of a polymer containing metronidazole and acriflavine have shown adequate release and good adhesion properties.

- *Colonic drug delivery*: For specific delivery of insulin to the colon, the polymer has been used. The chitosan capsules are coated with an enteric coating (hydroxy propyl methyl cellulose phthalate). Apart from insulin, these contain various additional absorption enhancer and an enzyme inhibitor. It has been found that capsules specifically disintegrate in the colonic region.

  It has been suggested that this disintegration is due to either the lower pH in the ascending colon as compared to the terminal ileum or to the presence of a bacterial enzyme, which can degrade the polymer.

- *Multiparticulate drug delivery system*: H. Steckel and F. Mindermann-Nogly prepared chitosan pellets using the extrusion/spheronization technology. Microcrystalline cellulose was used as an additive in concentrations ranging from 0- 70 %. The powder mixture was extruded using water and diluted acetic acid in different powder to liquid ratios. The study showed that chitosan pellets with a maximum of 50 % (m/m) could be produced with demineralized water as the granulating fluid. The mass fraction of chitosan within in the pellets could be increased to 100% by using dilute acetic acid for the granulation step.

  ➢ Other potential applications include
  ➢ Conversion of oil and other liquids to solids for ease of handling
  ➢ Taste and odor masking
  ➢ To delay the volatilization
  ➢ Safe handling of toxic substances

- **Novel Drug Delivery systems:** To deliver drugs efficiently to specific organs novel drug delivery systems have been developed. For this purpose, a range of organic systems such as micelles (fig 2.9) (liposomes, and polymeric nanoparticles) have been designed. In recent times, significant advances in drug-delivery systems have facilitated more effective drug administration for the following purposes:

> ➤ To reduce drug degradation and loss,
> ➤ To prevent harmful side-effects,
> ➤ To increase the bioavailability various drugs, and
> ➤ To formulate drug targeting systems.

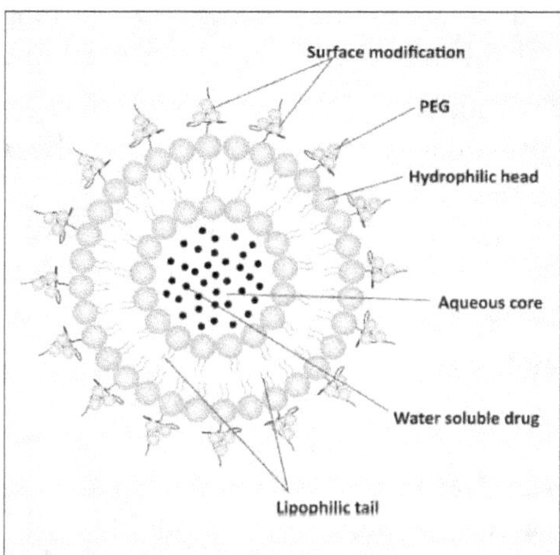


**Fig. 2.9:** Schematic representation of drug carrier- micelle.

Among the several drug carriers, microparticles (**Fig. 2.10**) made of insoluble or biodegradable natural and synthetic polymers are being used.

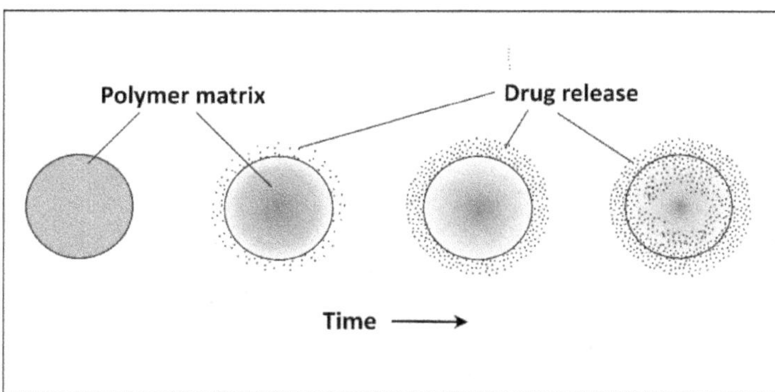


**Fig. 2.10:** Drug release from typical matrix release system.

- **Drug Delivery carriers:** Colloidal drug carrier systems show greater potential as a drug delivery system. These contain polymers, micellar solutions, vesicle, and liquid crystal dispersions, as well as nanoparticles dispersions (10–400 nm). During the development of these formulations, the major problem is to produce the systems with optimized drug loading and release properties, long shelf-life and low toxicity. The drug incorporated into the microstructure of the system, may participate and influence the system due to molecular interactions; if the drug possesses amphiphilic and mesogenic properties. In aqueous solutions, micelles are formed by self-assembly of amphiphilic block copolymers (5 – 50 nm), and these are very important for drug delivery applications. In the core of block copolymer micelles, the drugs can be physically entrapped and transported at concentrations that can exceed their intrinsic solubility in water.

- Moreover, the hydrophilic blocks can form hydrogen bonds with the aqueous medium and produces a tight shell around the micellar core. Thus, the contents of the hydrophobic core are effectively protected against hydrolysis and enzymatic degradation. Substitution of block copolymer micelles with specific ligand is a promising strategy to a broader range of sites of activity with a much higher selectivity.

- **Controlled drug delivery:** Controlled drug delivery formulation is a device, which is designed, prepared and used to release a drug at a predictable rate inside the body when administered by a parenteral or non-parenteral route. Controlled Drug Delivery (CDD) takes place when a polymer, whether natural or synthetic, is judiciously combined with a drug or other active agent; so that the active agent is released from the formulation in a predesigned manner. There may be three types of release pattern – (1) the active agent may be released constantly over a long period, (2) it may be cyclic over a long period, or (3) it may be triggered by the environment or other external events.

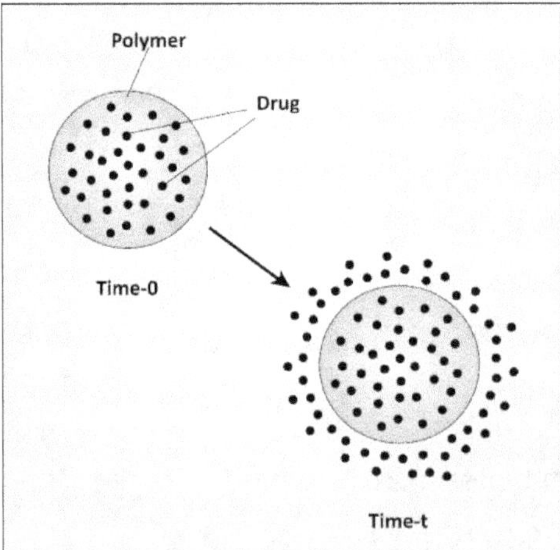


**Fig. 2.11:** Schematic representation of controlled release system.

Schematic representation of controlled drug delivery is shown in **Fig. 2.11**. The method used to prepare controlled-release formulation depends on the mechanism that controls the release of the drug from the delivery device – 1. Diffusion, 2. Osmosis, or 3. Polymer erosion.

- **Biomaterials for Delivery Systems:** In the earlier times, the polymers were mainly used for non-biological purposes, because of their physical properties, for example:

    1. Poly (urethanes) for **elasticity**.
    2. Poly (siloxanes) or silicones for **insulating ability**.
    3. Poly (methyl methacrylate) for **physical strength and transparency**.
    4. Poly (vinyl alcohol) for **hydrophilicity and strength**.
    5. Poly (ethylene) for **toughness and lack of swelling**.
    6. Poly (vinyl pyrrolidone) for **suspension capabilities**.

The polymers must be chemically inert and free from leachable impurities with appropriate physical structure, minimal undesired aging, and be readily processable. Polylactides and polyglycolides had been initially used as absorbable suture material, and these polymers were subsequently used in controlled drug delivery systems. The most important advantage of these polymers is that these degrade and produce biologically acceptable molecules. These degradation products are metabolized and removed from the body through normal metabolic pathways. However, biodegradable materials do produce degradation by-products that may have or may not have adverse reactions within the biological system. These degradation products must be tested thoroughly; because there are some factors that may affect the biodegradation of the original materials.

The biodegradation of polymer is shown schematically below;

Polymers have the applications other than in controlled drug delivery systems. There are traditional pharmaceutical formulations in which polymers have been used. Most common and critical applications are;

- **As binder in making granules for tablet:** Compression of granules prepare tablets. For conversion of powders to granules, a suitable binder is required. Most commonly used polymers are starch, gelatine, acacia, PVP, guar gum, etc. Each of these polymers has specific adhesive property and solubility characteristics. Depending on the requirement a suitable polymer is used as a binder.

- **To coat the tablets:** Conventionally tablets may be used for the immediate release of the drug in the stomach. Such tablets may be uncoated and coated depending on the taste of the drug. If the taste of the drug is bland and free from obnoxious odor, it is prepared and used as uncoated. Some drugs such as erythromycin are absorbed in the intestine (enteric coated); hence their tablets should be coated with such polymer which is soluble in alkaline medium. For coating of tablets, suitable polymer is used.

- **As binder in making granules:** For increasing tapped density of powders to prepare capsules.

  For encapsulation one of the important factors is bulk density or tapped density. Some drugs have low bulk density; hence difficult to fill in capsule shell. For this reason, the drug powders should be granulated to increase the bulk density; so that it can be easily filled in the capsule of the desired size.

- **To increase the viscosity/consistency of liquid formulations:** The viscosity of suspension formulation can be increased by adding Newtonian or non-Newtonian fluid in the preparation; so that the dispersed particles can be suspended for more extended period. The desired suspension formulation should be thixotropic; that is shear thinning. An ideal suspension could disperse the suspended particles on storage, while on shaking it can pour the suspension at the desired rate. Thus, pseudoplastic or a mixture of plastic and pseudoplastic polymers can be used as the suspending agent.

- **To adjust the pourability of the suspension:** Pourability of a suspension depends on consistency and viscosity of the suspending medium. As mentioned above a suitable concentration of pseudoplastic polymer is used to prepare the suspension.

- **To adjust the consistency of emulsion, ointment, cream, and paste:** The consistency of ointment, the cream should be such that the consistency of the preparation is high enough to hold the dispersed particles or globules firmly. The cream or ointment should not pour easily, but it could be spread smoothly. The consistency of an emulsion is relatively less than that cream or ointment. The consistency of a paste is more than that of cream or ointment. Polymers having suitable characteristics are used for the preparation of these preparations.

- **To prepare different types of gels:** The term "Gel" was introduced in the late 1800 to name some semisolid material according to pharmacological, rather than molecular criteria. The U.S.P. defines gels as a semisolid system consisting of dispersion made up of either small inorganic particle or large organic molecule enclosing and interpenetrated by a liquid. The inorganic particles form a three-dimensional "house of cards" structure. Gels are semisolid systems in which a liquid phase is constrained within a three-dimensional polymeric matrix (consisting of natural or synthetic gums) in which a high degree of physical (or sometimes chemical) crosslinking has been introduced. Some of these systems are as clear as water in appearance, visually aesthetically pleasing as in gelatine deserts and other are turbid. The clarity range is from clear to a whitish translucent. The polymers are used between 0.5-15% and in most of the cases they are usually at the concentration between 0.5-2%. Gels are usually clear, transparent, semisolids, containing the solubilized active substances.

- **To mask the unpleasant taste of a drug:** A large number of natural and synthetic polymers are available. Polymers commonly used in taste masking applications can be divided into two groups: soluble and insoluble in water. Taste-masking layer can be prepared by combining the water-insoluble and water-soluble polymers with a different ratio (for example ethyl cellulose and hypromellose). Water-soluble polymers are substances that dissolve, disperse or swell in water and thus modify the physical properties of aqueous systems in the form of gelation or thickening. Traditionally, water-soluble polymers used for taste masking are cellulose ethers (hydroxypropylmethyl cellulose and methyl cellulose) and synthetic vinyl polymers. The most effective taste masking results are obtained by using polymers or their mixtures which are insoluble at neutral pH. For taste masking applications, methacrylic copolymers and ethyl cellulose are widely used.

- **To improve the stability of the drug:** Membrane systems provide stability of a drug. For example, erythromycin, mesalazine, naproxen, omeprazole, amino salicylic acid, etc. degrade in acid medium. To protect it from acid, the tablet of erythromycin is coated with an acid resistant anionic polymer and release the drug in the intestine at higher pH. Table 2.1 below summarizes pharmaceutical applications of some common polymers.

**Table 2.1:** Pharmaceutical application of some common polymers.

| Polymer | Applications |
| --- | --- |
| **Water-soluble synthetic polymers** <br> Poly(acrylic acid) <br> Poly (ethylene oxide) <br> Poly (vinyl pyrrolidone) <br> Polyacrylamide <br><br> Poly (ethylene glycol) | Cosmetic, pharmaceuticals, immobilization of cationic drugs <br> Coagulant, flocculant, the swelling agent <br> Tablet binder, tablet coating <br> Coagulant, absorbent, gel electrophoresis to separate proteins <br> by molecular weight <br> plasticizer, suppositories base |
| **Cellulose-based polymer** <br> Ethyl cellulose <br><br> Carboxymethyl cellulose <br> Hydroxyethyl and hydroxypropyl cellulose <br> Hydroxypropyl methyl cellulose <br> Cellulose acetate phthalate | Water-insoluble but dispersible in water, aqueous coating for sustained-release formulations <br> Super-disintegrating agent, emulsion stabilizer <br> Water-soluble, tablet coating <br> Tablet binder, tablet coating, preparation of capsule shell <br> Enteric coating |
| **Hydrocolloids** <br> Alginic acid <br><br> Carrageenan <br> Chitosan | Thickening and suspending agent in suspension, paste, cream, gel; binder and disintegrant; stabilizer in o/w emulsion <br> Viscosity modifier; modified release formulation <br> Cosmetics; controlled-release dosage form; rapid-release dosage form; mucoadhesive dosage form |

| Polymer | Applications |
|---|---|
| **Water-insoluble biodegradablepolymers** (Lactide-co-glycolide) polymers | Microparticle, nanoparticle preparation for protein delivery |
| **Starch-based polymer** Starch Sodium starch glycolate | Glidant, diluent, disintegrant, binder in tablet and capsule; Super-disintegrant in tablet and capsule |
| **Plastic and rubber** Polyurethane Silicones Polycarbonate Polychloroprene Poly (vinyl acetate) Polyethylene Polystyrene Polypropylene Poly (methyl methacrylate) | The backing membrane of the transdermal patch; biomedical engineering Adhesive in TDDS; implants; Biomedical and pharmaceutical products Biomedical and pharmaceutical products Binder for chewing gum The backing membrane of TDDS, wrapping, packaging, containers Petri dishes containers for cell culture Containers, heat shrinkable film, packaging Hard contact lenses |

# Bibliography


1. Priyanka Shinde. Methods, types and applications of pharmaceutical polymers. World Journal of Pharmacy and Pharmaceutical Sciences. 2017;6(8):784-97.
2. Pawar Dipali Sanjay PPV, Dhanawade Pooja Pandit, Dongare Sujata Dattaprasad and Mali Savita Shivaji. Polymers Used in Pharmaceuticals: A Brief Review. International Journal of Pharma And Chemical Research. 2016;2(4):233-8.
3. P. JJaR. Role of biodegradable polymers in drug delivery. International journal of current pharmaceutical research. 2012;4(4).
4. Ankita R ABaBK. Polymers in a Drug Delivery System-A review. International Journal of Pharmaceutical Research and Development. 2002;2(8).
5. Denis L GPaCV. Biomedical and Pharmaceutical Polymer. published by Pharmaceutical press. 2011:1-148.
6. Sharma R, Singla N, Mehta S, Gaba T, Rawal RK, Rao HS, et al. Recent advances in polymer drug conjugates. Mini reviews in medicinal chemistry. 2015;15(9):751-61.
7. Souery WN, Bishop CJ. Clinically advancing and promising polymer-based therapeutics. Acta biomaterialia. 2018;67:1-20.
8. Haag R, Kratz F. Polymer therapeutics: concepts and applications. Angewandte Chemie (International ed in English). 2006;45(8):1198-215.
9. Duncan R. Polymer therapeutics at a crossroads? Finding the path for improved translation in the twenty-first century. Journal of drug targeting. 2017;25(9-10):759-80.

10. Kamaly N, Yameen B, Wu J, Farokhzad OC. Degradable Controlled-Release Polymers and Polymeric Nanoparticles: Mechanisms of Controlling Drug Release. Chem Rev. 2016;116(4):2602-63.

11. Hunter AC, Elsom J, Wibroe PP, Moghimi SM. Polymeric particulate technologies for oral drug delivery and targeting: a pathophysiological perspective. Nanomedicine : nanotechnology, biology, and medicine. 2012;8 Suppl 1:S5-20.

12. Narang AS, Chang RK, IIussain MA. Pharmaceutical development and regulatory considerations for nanoparticles and nanoparticulate drug delivery systems. Journal of pharmaceutical sciences. 2013;102(11):3867-82.

13. De Robertis S, Bonferoni MC, Elviri L, Sandri G, Caramella C, Bettini R. Advances in oral controlled drug delivery: the role of drug-polymer and interpolymer non-covalent interactions. Expert opinion on drug delivery. 2015;12(3):441-53.

14. Balaure PC, Grumezescu AM. Smart synthetic polymer nanocarriers for controlled and site-specific drug delivery. Current topics in medicinal chemistry. 2015;15(15):1424-90.

15. Fleige E, Quadir MA, Haag R. Stimuli-responsive polymeric nanocarriers for the controlled transport of active compounds: concepts and applications. Advanced drug delivery reviews. 2012;64(9):866-84.

16. Meirelles LMA, Raffin FN. Clay and Polymer-Based Composites Applied to Drug Release: A Scientific and Technological Prospection. Journal of pharmacy & pharmaceutical sciences : a publication of the Canadian Society for Pharmaceutical Sciences, Societe canadienne des sciences pharmaceutiques. 2017;20(0):115-34.

17. Mauri E, Papa S, Masi M, Veglianese P, Rossi F. Novel functionalization strategies to improve drug delivery from polymers. Expert opinion on drug delivery. 2017;14(11):1305-13.

18. Stankovic M, Frijlink HW, Hinrichs WL. Polymeric formulations for drug release prepared by hot melt extrusion: application and characterization. Drug discovery today. 2015;20(7):812-23.

19. Movassaghian S, Merkel OM, Torchilin VP. Applications of polymer micelles for imaging and drug delivery. Wiley interdisciplinary reviews Nanomedicine and nanobiotechnology. 2015;7(5):691-707.

20. Torchilin VP. Targeted polymeric micelles for delivery of poorly soluble drugs. Cellular and molecular life sciences : CMLS. 2004;61(19-20):2549-59.

21. Bae Y, Nishiyama N, Fukushima S, Koyama H, Yasuhiro M, Kataoka K. Preparation and biological characterization of polymeric micelle drug carriers with intracellular pH-triggered drug release property: tumor permeability, controlled subcellular drug distribution, and enhanced in vivo antitumor efficacy. Bioconjug Chem. 2005;16(1):122-30.


# Exercise

## A. Multiple Choice Questions

1. A polymer may be characterized by
   (a) Molecular weight
   (b) Low specific gravity
   (c) Greater resistance to erosion and corrosion
   (d) All of the above

2. Polymerization is the union of two or more monomers under the definite condition of
   - (a) Temperature
   - (b) Pressure
   - (c) Presence of a suitable catalyst
   - (d) All of the above

3. Which of the following statements is not correct?
   - (a) Based on the source, the polymer may be natural
   - (b) Based on the source, the polymer may be thermoplastic
   - (c) Based on the source, the polymer may be semi-synthetic
   - (d) Based on the source, the polymer may be synthetic

4. Which of the following statements is not correct?
   - (a) Based on the line structure, the polymer may be natural
   - (b) Based on the source, the polymer may be linear
   - (c) Based on the source, the polymer may be branched
   - (d) Based on the source, the polymer may be cross-linked

5. Which of the following statements is not correct?
   - (a) The crystallinity of a polymer depends on its topology and isomerism
   - (b) The crystallinity of a polymer depends on its molecular weight
   - (c) The crystallinity of a polymer depends on its tensile strength
   - (d) The crystallinity of a polymer depends on its glass transition temperature

6. Which of the following statements is correct?
   - (a) Glass transition temperature of the polymer depends on the flexibility of its chain
   - (b) Glass transition temperature of the polymer depends on the source
   - (c) Glass transition temperature of the polymer depends on thermal transitions
   - (d) Glass transition temperature of the polymer depends on its diffusivity

7. Which of the following statements is correct?
   - (a) Stiffness and strength of polymers decreases with their crystallinity
   - (b) Stiffness and strength of polymers increases with their crystallinity
   - (c) Stiffness and strength of polymers increases with the plasticizer present
   - (d) None of the above

8. Which of the following statements is correct?
   - (a) The tensile strength of a polymer is the ability to resist against stretching
   - (b) The tensile strength of a polymer is the strength of a compacted polymer
   - (c) The tensile strength of a polymer is the ability of the polymer to bend
   - (d) The tensile strength of a polymer is the ability to withstand load tending to reduce the size

9. Which of the following statements is correct?
   - (a) Optical property is a mechanical property of the polymer
   - (b) Anisotropy is a mechanical property of the polymer
   - (c) Tensile strength is a mechanical property of the polymer
   - (d) The thermal transition is a mechanical property of the polymer

10. Which of the following statements is correct?
    (a) Plasticizer decreases entropy and mobility of a polymer
    (b) Plasticizer increases entropy and mobility of a polymer
    (c) Plasticizer increases the glass transition temperature of a polymer
    (d) Plasticizer increases branching of the polymer chain

11. Which of the following statements is correct?
    (a) Compressive strength is not a mechanical property of the polymer
    (b) Flexural strength is a mechanical property of the polymer
    (c) Impact strength is not a mechanical property of the polymer
    (d) None of the above

12. Which of the following statements is correct?
    (a) Compressive strength is the ability of a polymer to withstand loads tending to reduce the size
    (b) Compressive strength is the ability of a polymer to bend
    (c) Compressive strength is the ability of a polymer to withstand sudden shock
    (d) None of the above

13. Which of the following statements is correct?
    (a) Highly cross-linked rubbers show very high deformation at their breaking point
    (b) Highly cross-linked rubbers show moderate deformation at their breaking point
    (c) Highly cross-linked rubbers show very low deformation at their breaking point
    (d) Highly cross-linked rubbers show no deformation at their breaking point

14. Creep test is related to
    (a) The viscosity of a polymer
    (b) The elasticity of a polymer
    (c) The consistency of a polymer
    (d) Viscoelasticity of a polymer

15. Which of the following statements is correct?
    (a) The rate of release of drug from a transdermal system depends on saturation solubility of the drug
    (b) The rate of release of drug from a transdermal system depends on the diffusion coefficient of the drug
    (c) The rate of release of drug from a transdermal system depends on partition coefficient of the drug
    (d) All of the above

16. Which of the following statements is correct?
    (a) Novel drug delivery system is developed to prevent harmful side-effects
    (b) Novel drug delivery system is developed to increase the bioavailability of the drug
    (c) Novel drug delivery system is developed for drug targeting
    (d) All of the above

17. The mechanism of release of drug from the controlled-drug delivery is
    - (a) Diffusion
    - (b) Osmosis
    - (c) Polymer erosion
    - (d) All of the above
18. Which of the following statements is correct?
    - (a) Poly (urethane) provides elastic property
    - (b) Silicones provide insulating property
    - (c) Poly vinyl pyrrolidone is used for suspension capability
    - (d) All of the above
19. The polymeris used to
    - (a) Increase the viscosity of the suspension
    - (b) Adjust the pH of the suspension
    - (c) Control the moisture content in the granules
    - (d) Increase the pourability of a liquid formulation
20. Which of the following statements is correct?
    - (a) The molecular weight of a polymer is low
    - (b) The specific gravity of a polymer is high
    - (c) The polymer is liable to erosion and corrosion
    - (d) None of the above

## B. Short Questions

1. Classify the polymers by thermal response, mode of formation, and the basis of their origin.
2. Classify the polymers by their physical properties.
3. Explain briefly thermal properties of the polymer.
4. Write down the advantages and disadvantages of the polymer.
5. Why Occusert is used? Write a note on Occusert.
6. Discuss the transdermal patches.
7. Write notes on multi-particulate drug delivery system and buccal drug delivery system.
8. Write a short note on drug delivery carrier and vaginal drug delivery.
9. Explain how various types of gel are prepared and how the unpleasant taste can be masked by using polymer.

## C. Long Questions

1. Discuss in detail the thermal properties of the polymer.
2. Discuss in detail the mechanical properties of the polymer.
3. Classify the polymer.
4. Discuss briefly the different approaches of the matrix system.
5. Write down the pharmaceutical applications of the polymer.
6. Discuss how the polymers are used in ophthalmic drug delivery, nasal drug delivery, and in controlled drug delivery.

Chapter 3

# Microencapsulation

---

*Definition, advantages and disadvantages, microspheres /microcapsules, microparticles, methods of microencapsulation, applications*

---

## Introduction

The term 'microencapsulation' is used to describe some techniques used for the production of particulate carriers, in the size range from nanometre (nm) to millimeter (mm), in which a solid or liquid is entrapped within a polymer coat or matrix. Apart from pharmaceuticals, this technology has been used by some other industries including food, household products, and agrochemicals; perhaps, most notably for the manufacture of carbonless carbon paper. To develop this product, the National Cash Register Co. in the 1950s developed the first microencapsulation technique (coacervation/phase separation), for the production of pressure-sensitive dye-containing microcapsules (Green and Schleicher, 1956).

Microencapsulation techniques are widely used in the development and production of improved drug- and food-delivery systems; and to enhance the stability of the material, reduce adverse or toxic effects, or to extend the release of material for different applications in different fields of manufacturing. Till this time, the use of some exciting and promising therapeutic materials has been limited clinically because of their restrictive physicochemical properties, which are necessary to be administered frequently. Appropriate microencapsulation techniques should be designed to overcome their intrinsic inconveniences. During the past two decades, pharmaceutical technologists have successfully developed the controlled release formulations to sustain/maintain adequate and effective plasma drug levels over a prolonged period by designing oral or parenteral microparticulate delivery systems. The ultimate objective is to control and extend the release of drug from the microparticles without affecting or modifying the normal biological characteristics of the drug in the body after administration and absorption. In the past decade, ongoing efforts have been made to develop drug carriers particularly to the intended target organ; so that the total amount of drug administered can be reduced and the therapeutic efficacy is increased. The site-specific microparticulate delivery systems can maintain an effective concentration of drug for a more extended period in the target tissue and result in decreased side effects associated with lower plasma concentrations in the peripheral blood circulation. The application of microparticles for drug delivery is not limited to any specific illness; rather they can be widely used in many situations where continuous/controlled/targeted drug administration is essential. The shell can be matrix, single layer or multilayer, and can consist of one kind or several kinds of materials. The capsule can be permeable, semipermeable, or impermeable. Many materials such as gums, carbohydrates, cellulose, lipids, inorganic materials, and proteins can be used for making the wall. The selection of wall/coat materials depends on the physicochemical properties of the core materials, the process of making the microcapsules, and the desired properties of the product. Biodegradable polymers have been widely used in microcapsules for drug delivery to provide controlled release of encapsulated drugs. The size of microcapsules is typically several hundred nanometers to a few thousand micrometers. Their surface may be smooth or rough; the shape may be spherical or irregular. The microcapsules can be solid as free-flowing powders or suspended in water, depending on the applications and stability of the capsules and the encapsulated ingredients. Microparticles are usually formed by the controlled precipitation of polymers and can be divided into the following groups:

- Microcapsule (spherical geometry with a continuous core region surrounded by a continuous shell; reservoir systems);
- Microsphere (spherical matrix with dispersed or dissolved entrapped drug; matrix systems); and
- Irregular geometry with a number of small droplets or particles of the core material.

## Definition

In the development of a new pharmaceutical product, optimization of the drug release of per-oral dosage forms in the absorption window of the active ingredient is the primary responsibility of the development scientist. Microencapsulation is a simple and economic technique to enclose bioactive materials, such as drugs and cells, within a semipermeable polymeric material.

Microencapsulation may be defined as *a process of packing small droplets of liquids, gas or fine solid particles into a thin film of polymer(s)*. It can be simply said that microcapsule is a small spherical particle or globule surrounded by a uniform wall. The material present within the microcapsule is called the core or internal phase or fill. The wall is sometimes called a shell or coating or membrane. The size range of most microcapsules ranges from 1 μm to 1 mm. The microcapsule may have multiple walls.

The method of microencapsulation depends on the physical and chemical properties of the material to be encapsulated. The core may be a crystal, an irregularly shaped adsorbent particle, an emulsion, a suspension of solids, or a suspension of smaller microcapsules.

## Advantages

The primary advantages of microencapsulation are;
- Can delay or sustain the release of the drug from the formulation,
- Can be used as controlled and targeted drug delivery.
- Reduces the frequency of administration and avoids peak and valley effects in blood level,
- The total dose of the drug can be lowered.
- Biocompatible,
- Relatively stable in special cases.
- Can prevent side effects related to the presence of the drug in the stomach; hence, the risk of side effects can also be reduced.
- The unpleasant odor and taste of drug can be masked.
- Provides prolong action of the dosage form.
- Can modify the physical characteristics of a material which is frequently required in formulations.
- Can protect the drug from degradation in the acidic environment of the stomach; thus does not allow the drug to degrade (oxidation).
- Liquids can be handled as solids.
- Method of preparation is not difficult.
- Allows safe and convenient handling of toxic substances.

## Disadvantages

- Cross-reaction between the core material and wall of the shell may take place.
- Difficult to achieve continuous and uniform film.
- Shelf-life of hygroscopic material may be reduced.
- May increase the cost of production.
- More skill and knowledge are required for this advanced and complex technology.

## Microspheres

The oral route is the most common and convenient route of drug administration. Drugs with short half-lives and easily absorbed from the GIT are quickly eliminated from the body. To overcome these problems oral controlled drug delivery systems have been developed. Such a delivery system releases the drug slowly in the GI tract and can maintain a steady drug level in the serum for more extended period. However, lower bioavailability may also result due to incomplete release of the drug and a shorter residence time of dosage forms in the upper gastrointestinal tract. Thus, efforts to improve the bioavailability of drug from oral dosage form have been growing day by day in pharmaceutical industries.

There are various approaches to deliver a drug substance at the target site in a sustained or controlled release way. One of these approaches is microspheres as carriers for drugs. The behavior of the drug in the body can be controlled by coupling the drug to a carrier particle. The clearance kinetics, tissue distribution, metabolism and cellular interaction of the drug is influenced effectively by the behavior of the carrier. This pharmacodynamic behavior may be used to enhance the therapeutic effect of the drug. The main purpose of any drug delivery system is to administer a therapeutic amount of drug to the proper site in the body to achieve the required plasma drug concentration promptly, and then to maintain the drug concentration in circulating blood.

This has been mentioned earlier that microspheres are small spherical particles. These are sometimes called microparticles. Microspheres can be manufactured using various natural, and synthetic materials, called polymer. Glass microspheres, polymer microspheres, and ceramic microspheres are commercially available. The density of solid and hollow microspheres vary widely. Accordingly, their applications are different. Hollow microspheres are typically used as additives to lower the density of a material. Depending on the type of material used to prepare (material of construction) and their size range solid microspheres have several applications.

Two most common types of polymer microspheres are prepared with polyethylene and polystyrene. Polystyrene microspheres are usually prepared for biomedical applications. These can help the processes such as cell sorting and immunoprecipitation. Polystyrene can adsorb proteins and ligands readily and permanently. Thus, polystyrene microspheres are suitable for medical research and biological laboratory experiments.

Usually, polyethylene microspheres are used as permanent or temporary filler. Polyethylene melts at a lower temperature; hence these microspheres can create porous structures in ceramics and other materials. Polyethylene microspheres are widely used in flow visualization and fluid flow analysis, microscopy techniques, health sciences, process troubleshooting, and numerous research applications; because these are highly spherical, available in colored and fluorescent forms. Charged polyethylene microspheres are also used in the electronic paper for digital displays.

Glass microspheres have limited applications in medical technology; these are mainly used as filler for weight reduction, retro-reflector for highway safety, an additive for cosmetics and adhesives.

Ceramic microspheres are commonly used as grinding media. Microspheres vary widely in quality, sphericity, uniformity of particle and particle size distribution. For each application, the appropriate microsphere is to be selected. There are different methods for the preparation of microspheres. This provides the scopes to control different aspects of drug administration. As a result, the following benefits are achieved –

1. Accurate delivery of small quantity of the potent drugs is possible,
2. Reduced drug concentration at the site other than the target site, and

3. The protection of the labile compound before and after the administration and before their appearance at the site of action.

Microspheres are free-flowing powders made of proteins or synthetic polymers which are biodegradable and ideally their particle size is less than 200μm.

## Characteristics of Microspheres

**Table 3.1:** Basic Characteristics of microsphere

| S. No. | Parameter | Measurable Quantity |
|--------|-----------|---------------------|
| 1. | Size | Diameter, Uniformity, Distribution characteristics |
| 2. | Composition | Density, Refractive index, Hydrophobicity, Hydrophilicity, Non-specific binding, Autofluorescence |
| 3. | Surface chemistry | Reactive groups, Level of functionalization, Charge |
| 4. | Special properties | Visible dye/fluorophore, Super-paramagnetic |

## Advantages

1. Constant and prolonged therapeutic effect can be achieved.
2. Dosing frequency can be reduced and thereby, the patient compliance is improved.
3. Could be injected into the body due to the spherical shape and smaller size.
4. Better drug utilization can improve the bioavailability and reduce the incidence or intensity of adverse effects.
5. Morphology of microsphere allows a controllable variation in degradation and drug release.

## Disadvantages

Some of the disadvantages are
1. The drug release from the formulations may be modified.
2. The release rate of the controlled release dosage form may vary due to factors like food and the rate of transit through gut.
3. Due to the dose difference, the release rate can differ.
4. Controlled release formulations generally contain a higher drug load, and thus, any loss of integrity of the release characteristics of the dosage form may lead to potential toxicity.
5. Dosage forms of this kind should not be crushed or chewed.

## Methods of Preparation

### Spray Drying

In Spray Drying method, the polymer is first dissolved in a suitable volatile organic solvent such as dichloromethane, acetone, etc. The drug in the solid form is dispersed in the polymer solution using a high-speed homogenizer.

This dispersion is then atomized in a stream of hot air. The atomization leads to the formation of the small droplets or the fine mist from which the solvent evaporates instantaneously leading to the formation of the microspheres in size range 1-100µm. Microparticles are separated from the hot air using the cyclone separator, while the trace of solvent is removed by vacuum drying. One of the significant advantages of this process is the feasibility of operation under aseptic conditions. This process is rapid and leads to the formation of porous microparticles.

### Solvent Evaporation

These processes are carried out in a liquid manufacturing vehicle. The microcapsule coating material is dispersed in a volatile solvent which is immiscible with the liquid manufacturing vehicle phase. Before microencapsulation, the core material is dissolved or dispersed in the coating polymer solution. With agitation, the core material or the mixture of materials is thoroughly dissolved/dispersed in the liquid manufacturing vehicle phase to obtain the appropriate size microcapsule. The solution/dispersion is then heated; if necessary, to evaporate the solvent for the polymer of the core material is dispersed in the polymer solution, polymer shrinks around the core. If the core material is dissolved in the coating polymer solution, matrix-type microcapsules are formed. The core may be either water soluble or water insoluble materials. Solvent evaporation involves the formation of an emulsion between polymer solution and an immiscible continuous phase whether aqueous (o/w) or non-aqueous(w/o) (fig 3.1).

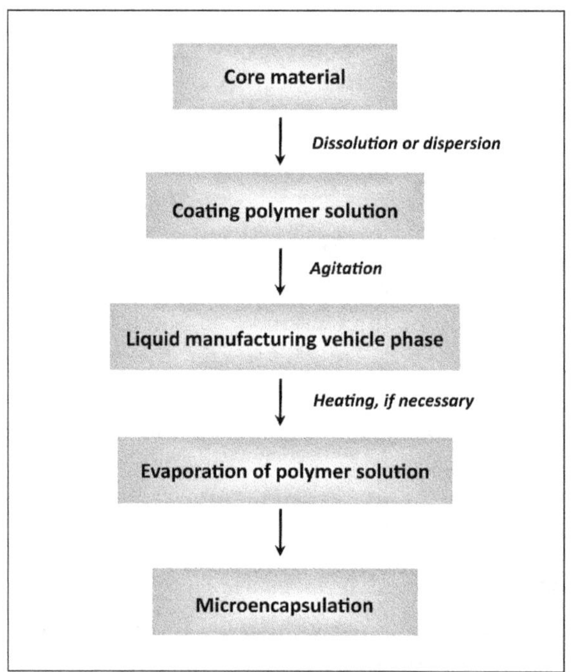



**Fig. 3.1:** Schematic representation of micro-encapsulation via solvent evaporation method.

## Microcapsules

The biological cell is a common and real example of the natural microcapsule. The cellular components are protected from the outer environment by its wall or cell membrane. The cell membrane does not allow all the materials to freely enter into the cell or all the inner components of the cell to exit; because the cell membrane is selectively permeable. Thus, it can control the influx and release of metabolites. The encapsulated material in a microcapsule is called core, or fill, or internal phase. The encapsulating matrix is called shell, coating, wall material or membrane.

The core can be any form – crystalline, amorphous fine solids, emulsion or suspension, or even smaller microcapsules. The shell may be matrix, single layer, multilayer, and can consist of one or several types of materials (fig 3.2). It may be permeable, semi-permeable and impermeable. Various materials such as gums, carbohydrates, celluloses, lipids, proteins, and inorganic salts are used to prepare shell. The selection of coating material depends on

- The physicochemical properties of the core materials,
- The process of making the microcapsules, and
- Desired release characteristics of the core material.

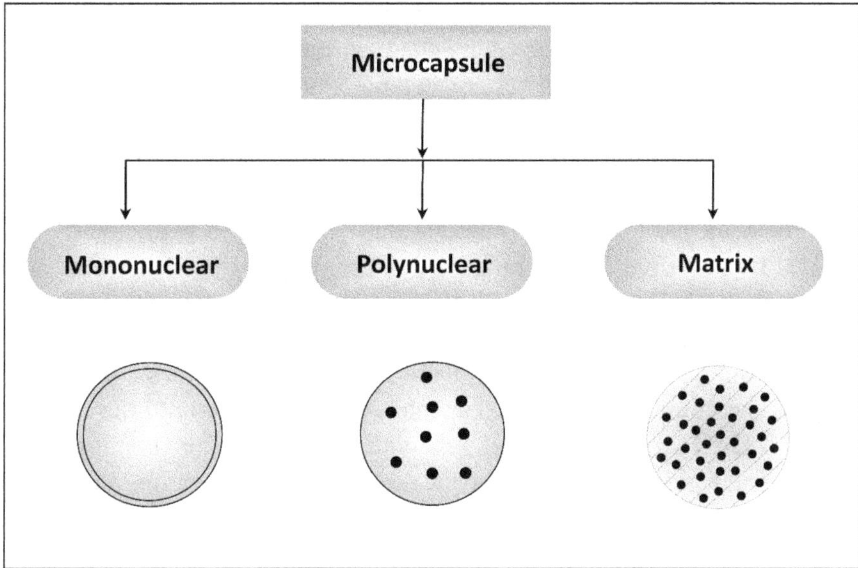


**Fig. 3.2:** Morphology of microsphere.

Biodegradable polymers have been widely used in microcapsules for delivery of drugs to providecontrolled release of encapsulated drugs. The size of microcapsules may range several hundred nanometres to a few thousand micrometers. The surface of microcapsules may be rough or smooth. The shape of these may be spherical or irregular. Depending on the applications and stability of the capsules and the encapsulated ingredients the microcapsules may be free-flowing solid powders or suspended in water. The properties of the microcapsules such as average size, size distribution, surface morphology, inner structure, and ingredient distribution will affect the following release profile.

Microcapsules are prepared to

> ➢ protect active ingredients,
> ➢ reduce nutritional loss,
> ➢ mask or preserve flavors,
> ➢ control the release of encapsulated materials,
> ➢ reduce drug dosage,
> ➢ deliver drugs to specific locations, and to
> ➢ make easy handling encapsulated material.

In the cosmetic industry, microcapsules are used to gain the sustained release of deodorants and perfumes.

Complete impermeability to the encapsulated gases or liquids is difficult to achieve, due to the small size and thin wall thickness of typical microcapsules. However, the durability of core materials can be improved by using suitable coating materials and capsule size. For the release of the core material, the capsule wall is required to be opened. It can be done from outside by mechanical means, such as by shearing, chewing or crushing, or from inside, such as by heating above the boiling point of the core material. The coat can also be destroyed by dissolving, melting or burning. To prevent leaking of the encapsulated materials, the solubility parameter of the polymer should be opposite to that of the core material. Alternatively, controlled release of the encapsulated materials can be achieved through permeation through the shell wall, and the permeability of the wall can be modified by cross-linking of the polymer used. Generally, the release profile is influenced by the physicochemical properties of the core material, such as diffusivity, partition coefficient, and vapor pressure. The release of the content of the capsule depends on the material used to make the coating, thickness, porosity and on the reactivity of the coating material. If the capsule wall is permeable to the core material, the release is regulated by the wall thickness and porosity. This is most important for providing sustained release of the inside content, which is commonly desired in therapeutic treatment.

In contrast, opening the microcapsule wall provides immediate burst release. The capsule wall can also be semipermeable, allowing small molecules entering inside but preventing contents inside from leaving, which can be used for encapsulating cells. For drug delivery applications, the capsule wall should be biocompatible, and biodegradability can be used to tune the release.

Many factors, such as can control the release of drugs from biodegradable polymers

> ➢ Biodegradation kinetics of the polymer,

> Properties of polymers and drugs,
> Compatibility between polymers and drugs, and
> The shape of the microcapsules.

Liposomes are hollow microcapsules of phospholipids that are formed spontaneously when phospholipids are dispersed in water. To encapsulate material in the core of liposomes, phospholipids are usually dissolved in organic solvents, such as chloroform, and mixed with a solution containing the material to be encapsulated. The solvent is evaporated to form dry lipid film, which is then hydrated in a buffer solution to form liposomes. The size range is from 25 nm to several micrometers in diameter.

Aqueous or lipid-soluble materials can be entrapped in liposomes, which have been used to deliver vaccines, hormones, enzymes, and vitamins. The encapsulated ingredients can be released from liposomes by heating above the transition temperature of the phospholipids, typically around 50°C. Above the transition temperature, the liposome bilayer is broken, and the content is released immediately. The electrostatic charge, pH, permeability, and stability of liposomes can be controlled better than for other types of microcapsules — however, poor encapsulation efficiency and the lack of a continuous production process limit large-scale use. The use of organic solvents is also a concern for some applications — both the lipid and ingredients to be encapsulated can be lost during the solvent evaporation process. Recently microfluidic techniques have been developed that allow high-efficiency encapsulation into liposomes in a solvent-free continuous process. However, another challenge is that the liposomes must be kept in dilute aqueous suspension, which is not favorable for large-scale production, storage, and shipping.

## Microparticles

Microparticulate drug delivery system is one of the processes to provide the sustained and controlled delivery of drug to long periods of time. These are small particles of solids or small droplets of liquids surrounded by walls of natural and synthetic polymer films of varying thickness and degree of permeability. The wall or coat acts as a release rate controlling substance and has a diameter within the range of 0.1μm-200μm. In earlier times, albumin microspheres are used in drug delivery system as suggested by Kramer in 1974. In 1997, Java Krishna and Catha proposed the use of microspheres as sustained release vehicles. There are also reports about using hemoglobin as natural, biodegradable carriers for drugs for microparticulate administration. Microparticles have been proved to be an ideal way of preparing sustained and controlled release dosage forms. These are also used to deliver drugs which are difficult to deliver due to limited solubility in water. In such drugs the attainment of high Cmax, Tmax, and Area under the curve is problematic. Thus, a need exists for immediate release products containing these agents. Microsphere-based formulations can be formulated to provide a constant drug concentration in the blood or to target drugs to specific cells or organs.   Depending   on the size of the core material a particular method is selected. Table 3.2 shows the suitability of the method based on the approximate size range of core material. The maximum size for micro coating is 5000μm; however, for micro coating the particle size would be more than 5000μm.

**Table 3.2:** Application of microencapsulation method based on the particle size of the core

| Method of Microencapsulation | Type of Core material | Approx. particle size |
|---|---|---|
| Spray drying and congealing | Solids and liquids | 600 μm |
| Solvent evaporation | Solids and liquids | 5 - 5000μm |
| Multi-orifice centrifugal | Solids and liquids | 1 – 5000μm |
| Coacervation-phase separation | Solids and liquids | 2 - 5000μm |
| Air suspension | Solids | 35 - 5000μm |
| Pan coating | Solids | 600 - 5000μm |

**Advantages of Microparticles**

Recently, controlled release delivery system has become a very useful tool in the pharmaceutical field. A wide range of advantages to chronic diseases such as rheumatoid arthritis, osteoarthritis, and musculoskeletal disorders including degenerative joint conditions demand long-term therapy. Following advantages have been noted with this type of dosage forms;

1. Provides effective delivery of drugs which are insoluble or sparingly soluble in water.
2. They give the products which exhibit immediate release properties and can give 80% or more of the active agent in about 10 minutes or less. Ex. Nimesulide.
3. The technique provides the way for improving the taste of an active agent.
4. They increased the relative bioavailability of drugs.
5. The formulation of microparticles also provides the method of targeting drug delivery to specific sites.
6. The microparticles hold great potential in reducing the dosage frequency and toxicity of various drugs.
7. Microparticles in the form of microcapsules can also be used as a carrier for drugs and vaccines as diagnostic agents & in surgical procedures.
8. They can also be used to produce amorphous drugs with desirable physical properties.
9. They also caused the reduction of the local side effects ex. GI irritation etc. of drugs on oral ingestion.
10. They provide the sustained release formulation with a lower dose of the drug to maintain plasma concentration & improved patient compliance.

11. The PH triggered microparticles are used in immunization, transfection & gene therapy.
12. Parenteral microparticles have the advantage of administering a high concentration of water-soluble drugs without severe osmotic effects at the site of administration.
13. They also have an advantage of being stored in dry particle or suspension form with little or no loss of activity over an extended storage period.
14. They are useful in the administration of effervescent dosage form of medicaments to an individual unable to chew. Ex. Debilitated patients are having difficulty in swallowing solids and the elderly.
15. In contrast, smaller microparticles need to be prepared for application to other sites such as the eye, lung, and joints.

## Methods of Microencapsulation

This has been mentioned earlier that microencapsulation is a technology or method for enveloping small droplets of liquids, gases or fine solid particles with natural or synthetic polymers. Biological

There are many methods of microcncapsulation, such as

1. Dipping or centrifuging,
2. Air suspension coating or fluidized bed coating,
3. Spray drying,
4. Spray chilling or cooling,
5. Co-crystallization,
6. Liposome entrapment,
7. Coacervation,
8. Emulsification/solvent evaporation or extraction,
9. Interfacial polymerization.

Most of these methods are physical techniques. No chemical reaction takes place. One typical method involving chemical reaction is interfacial polymerization. The selection of a method depends on the following factors;

➤ Econo
➤ mics,
➤ Properties of the core
➤ Wall material,
➤ Microcapsule size,
➤ Application and
➤ Release mechanism.

**1. Dipping or Centrifugation method:** In this method, the droplets of core material are exposed to high-speed rotation with the film forming liquid material. The droplets are then hardened. By this method, uniformly coated and relatively large capsules are produced. The diameter of the capsules may be up to 8 mm. For example, kerosene can be encapsulated by using a solution of polyvinyl alcohol and sodium alginate in water or glycerine. The capsules can be hardened in calcium chloride solution.

2. **Fluidized bed coating:** In this method, the fine core materials are suspended in a vertical current of air, and the solution of coat material is sprayed over the suspended particles. Once the solvent is evaporated out, the coat is deposited onto the core material.

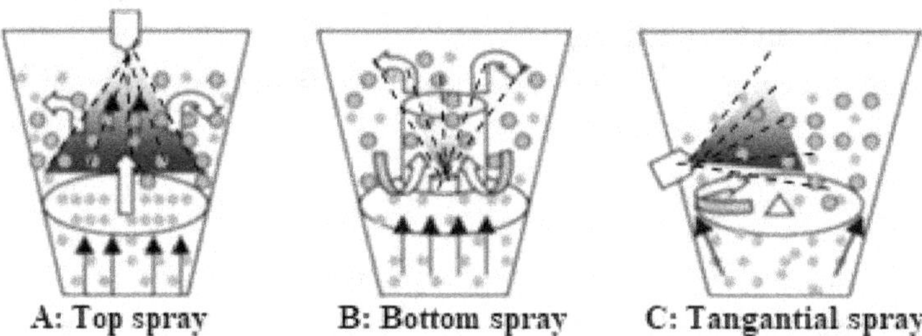



**Fig. 3.3:** Schematic diagram of three types fluidized bed coating techniques.

To achieve the desired thickness, the process can be repeated. By using this method, the minimum size of the coated particle obtained can be up to 100μm. However, the smaller particles may aggregate or may be carried away by the exhaust air (**fig 3.3**). This method is generally used to encapsulate pharmaceutical materials, seeds, and food stuffs.

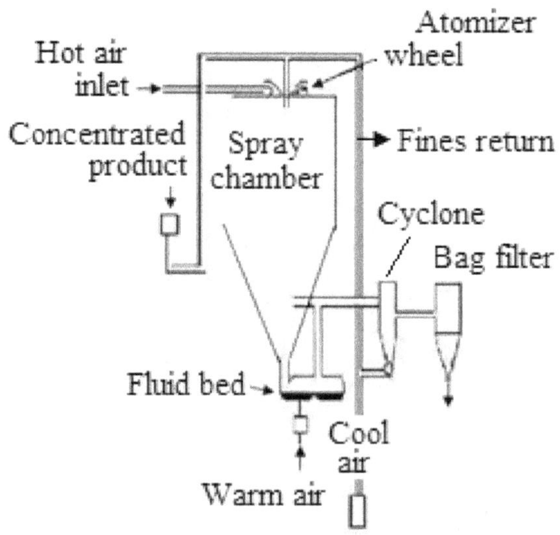



**Fig 3.4:** Schematic diagram of spray dryer.

3. **Spray drying:** In this method, an emulsion or suspension is sprayed in a stream of hot gas, generally air and in some cases inert gas such as nitrogen within a chamber. Polymers are dissolved in a suitable solvent containing the additives to be encapsulated. During spraying, the atomized droplets shrink as the solvent evaporates, leaving the core surrounded by polymer. The microcapsules obtained are solid and free-flowing. The core material

may be sprayed from an inner nozzle and the encapsulating material from a concentric ring nozzle.

This method is mainly used for encapsulating flavors in the food industry due to its low cost, about 30-50 times cheaper than freeze-drying. However, the high temperature in spray drying creates stability problems for some thermo-labile materials. An alternative to spray drying is spray chilling or cooling.

Spray drying is a physico mechanical method commonly used for microencapsulation. In this method, an active material is dissolved or suspended in a melt or polymer solution, sprayed over hot or normal air-stream. The particles are dried and collected. Particles produced in this process usually are in size range of 1-150 μm. In this process, an emulsion is prepared from the liquid product mixed with a carrier substance and a filmogen solution. This emulsion is then sprayed into small droplets in hot air. In high temperature, the solvent evaporates leading to a solid matrix around the particles the second phase remains as a coat. The small droplets of the product are stored in the carrier substance and embedded in the film open. The main parameters of the process are;

- The core material,
- The coating material,
- The temperatures of drying air/gas of inlet and outlet,
- The air/gas flow rate,
- The distribution of temperature and humidity inside the dryer,
- The time of contact with hot air/gas, and
- The geometry of the drying chamber.

It is desired that the wall material with low viscosity should have good emulsifying and film-forming properties at high solid concentrations, can be easily dried and chemically inert. An advantage of this process is the short processing time. The short contact-time with hot air allows using this method to encapsulate sensitive materials. It includes heat sensitivity, water sensitivity; in the case of oxygen sensitive materials, it is better to use nitrogen gas in place of air. However, some of the low-boiling point aromatic substances can be destroyed in the spray drying process. The fig. 3.4 represents the schematic diagram of a spray drier.

The high temperature in spray drying is problematic for some the materials which are not stable at a higher temperature. However, it is the main method used for encapsulating flavours in the food industry due to its low cost; about 30-50 times cheaper than freeze-drying.

4. **Spray chilling or cooling:** The spray chilling or cooling is an alternate method to spray drying. A hot emulsion or suspension containing molten coating material and the aqueous or solid core material is sprayed into a chamber containing cool air or liquid. The cooling solidifies the coating material, resulting in microcapsules. Spray chilling or cooling can be used to encapsulate water-soluble ingredients, such as water-soluble vitamins and enzymes.

A variation of the method includes solvent extraction during cooling. For example, droplets of polymer/drug solution can be sprayed into liquid nitrogen containing frozen ethanol, and hardened at about −80°C wherein solvent extraction occurs. By this method, proteins can be encapsulated in polymer micro-particles without significant loss of biological activity. There is another approach to the drying process, freeze-drying or lyophilization. The atomized droplets can be frozen, in liquid nitrogen, and the solvent can be removed by sublimation in a vacuum.

A heated emulsion or suspension containing molten coating material and the aqueous or solid core material is sprayed into a chamber containing cool air or liquid. Due to cooling the coating material solidifies and the microcapsules are produced. Spray chilling or cooling method can be used to encapsulate water-soluble ingredients, such as water-soluble vitamins and enzymes. An alternative to this method includes solvent extraction while cooling. For example, the droplets of polymer/drug solution can be sprayed into liquid nitrogen containing frozen ethanol, and hardened at −80°C wherein solvent extraction occurs. Proteins can be encapsulated in polymer micro-particles without significant loss of biological activity. There is another approach to the drying process, freeze-drying or lyophilization.

5. **Co-crystallization:** This is a process to encapsulate ingredients between sucrose crystals. The sucrose crystals are solid, monoclinic, and spherical; as such are not suitable for encapsulation. Aggregates of the crystals form when they are spontaneously crystallized from a supersaturated solution. The crystals aggregate in size range of 3 to 30 μm and can entrap materials. First, the sucrose syrup is concentrated to the point of supersaturation, then the material to be encapsulated is added, and the syrup is mixed to induce nucleation and agglomeration. It is essential to control the rates of nucleation and crystallization during the process. Various types of flavors can be encapsulated by this method.

Liposomes are hollow microcapsules of phospholipids that form spontaneously when phospholipids are dispersed in water. To encapsulate material in the core of liposomes, phospholipids are usually dissolved in organic solvents, such as chloroform; then mixed with a solution containing the material to be encapsulated. The solvent is evaporated to form dry lipid film, which is then hydrated in a buffer solution to form liposomes. The size range of the liposomes formed varies from 25 nm to several micrometers in diameter.

Aqueous or lipid-soluble materials can be entrapped in liposomes. Liposomes have been used to deliver vaccines, hormones, enzymes, and vitamins. The content of the liposome can be released by heating above the transition temperature of the phospholipids, around 50°C. Above the transition temperature, the liposome bilayer is broken, and the content is released immediately. The electrostatic charge, pH, permeability, and stability of liposomes can be more easily controlled compared to other types of microcapsules. The poor encapsulation efficiency and the lack of a continuous production process limit large-scale use. For some applications, the use of organic solvents is also a problem. Both the lipid and ingredients to be encapsulated can be lost during the solvent evaporation process. Recently microfluidic techniques have been developed that provides high-efficiency encapsulation into liposomes in a solvent-free continuous process. However, another problem is the storage of liposomes. The liposomes must be kept in dilute aqueous suspension, which is not suitable for large-scale production, storage, and shipping.

6. **Liposome entrapment:** Liposomes are hollow microcapsules of phospholipids. Liposomes are formed spontaneously when phospholipids are dispersed in water. To encapsulate material in the core of liposomes, phospholipids are usually dissolved in organic solvents, such as chloroform, and mixed with a solution containing the material to be encapsulated. The solvent is then evaporated to form a dry lipid film. The film is then hydrated in a buffer solution to form liposomes. The size range of liposomes varies from 25 nm to several micrometers in diameter. Aqueous or lipid-soluble materials such as vaccines, hormones, enzymes, and vitamins can be entrapped in liposomes and can be delivered. The encapsulated ingredients are released from liposomes by heating above the transition temperature of the phospholipids, around 50°C. Above the transition temperature, the liposome bilayer ruptures and the content are released immediately. Compared to other types of microcapsules, the following properties of liposomes can be more easily controlled;

   ➢ electrostatic charge,
   ➢ pH,
   ➢ permeability, and
   ➢ stability

However, the major limitation of large-scale manufacture of liposomes is (1) poor encapsulation efficiency and (2) lack of a continuous production process. The use of organic solvents is also a concern for some applications. During the solvent evaporation process, both the lipid and ingredients to be encapsulated can be lost. The recently developed microfluidic technique allows high-efficiency encapsulation into liposomes in a solvent-free continuous process. However, another problem is that the liposomes must be kept in dilute aqueous suspension, which is not feasible for large-scale production, storage, and shipping.

7. **Coacervation-Phase separation:** Coacervate refers to a small spherical droplet of separate organic molecules, specifically, lipid molecules. It is held together by hydrophobic forces from the surrounding liquid. Coacervates measure 1 – 100 μm, possess osmotic properties and can be formed spontaneously from certain dilute organic solutions.

Their name has been derived from the Latin word coacervare, which means to assemble together or cluster. These were considered to play a significant role in the evolution of cells and, therefore, of life itself. Once formed in water, organic chemicals do not necessarily remain uniformly dispersed but may separate into layers or droplets. The droplets formed to contain a colloid, rich in organic compounds and are surrounded by a tight layer of water molecules. These are known as Coacervates. Their structures have been first investigated by the Dutch chemist H.G. Bungenberg de Jong, in 1932. A wide variety of solutions can produce the coacervates; for example, coacervates are formed spontaneously when a protein, such as gelatine, interacts with gum arabic. These are important and interesting. They provide a locally segregated environment, also in that their boundaries allow the selective absorption of simple organic molecules from the surrounding medium. Schematic diagram of the processes involved in the coacervation technique is presented in fig. 3.5.

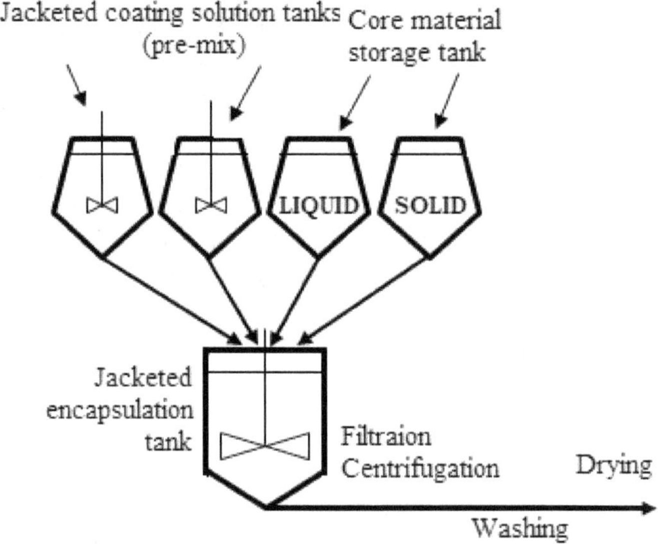


**Fig. 3.5:** Flow diagram of coacervation technique

The general method of coacervation-phase separation technique involves three steps which are to be performed with continuous stirring:

1. Formation of three immiscible chemical phases,
2. Deposition of coating over the core material, and
3. Rigidization of the coating.

For coacervation, two methods are available, namely simple and complex processes.

- In simple coacervation, a de-solvation agent is added for phase separation.
- Whereas, complex coacervation involves complexation between two oppositely charged polymers.

1. **Phase separation:** The core material is dispersed in a continuous phase in which the polymer is dissolved. The polymer is then gradually deposited onto the core material by inducing precipitation by adding non-solvent for the polymer, adjusting pH, ionic strength or temperature. Precipitants or nonsolvent commonly used include silicone oil, vegetable oil, light liquid paraffin, and low molecular weight polybutadiene. When phase separation takes place, very fine coacervate droplets appear at first, and they tend to coat solid dispersed particles. The droplets coalesce until a coherent coacervate phase appears surrounding the solid particles. Finally, the coating is solidified by heating, crosslinking or removing solvents by exposing to an excess amount of another nonsolvent, such as hexane, heptane, and diethyl ether. The microcapsules are collected by filtration or centrifugation, washed with solvents, and then dried. Since the method is complicated and expensive, so it is not broadly used in industry. In this step three immiscible chemical phases – manufacturing solvent/vehicle (a liquid phase), core material phase, and a coating material phase. The core material is dispersed in the solution of polymer (coating material) phase. The solvent or mixture of solvents used to dissolve polymer is the liquid manufacturing vehicle phase. The coating polymer is made immiscible in the liquid phase by using any of the phase separation techniques;

    1. By changing the temperature of the polymer solution,
    2. By adding a suitable salt or nonsolvent or an incompatible
    3. By initiating polymer-polymer interaction. Phase separation is a physicochemical process of preparing microcapsules.

It allows producing particles of 2 – 5000µm size. There may be a liquid core. The polymers form two distinct liquid phases. One phase is rich in polymer and designed to act as the capsule shell, while the other is rich in the incompatible polymer. The incompatible polymer is used in the system to cause the formation of two phases. It is not designed to be part of the final capsule shell, although a small amount may remain entrapped in the final capsule as an impurity. The process is normally carried out in organic solvents and used to encapsulate solids with a finite degree of water solubility.

Coacervation is efficient and can produce microcapsules with a broad range of sizes. Another disadvantage of coacervation is that formation of large aggregates is difficult to be avoided; since extremely sticky coacervate droplets frequently adhere to each other beforecomplete phase separation.

2. **Deposition of coating over the core material/ Interfacial Polymerisation:** In this step, the coating polymer present in the solution starts depositing over the core material.This is done by utilizing any one of the three methods mentioned above. The coating material and core material are mixed in manufacturing vehicle by controlled stirring. The coating polymer in solution state deposits rapidly around the core particle if the polymer is adsorbed at the interface of the core and manufacturing liquid. In fact, for effective coating, the adsorption of coating polymer is essential. However, to achieve continuous deposition of the polymer,

total interfacial free energy of the system must be reduced. This is possible, by decreasing the surface area of the coating material during coalescence of the liquid polymer droplets. Although this method allows encapsulating both the liquid and solid, the chemistry of the polymerization is different. This method is widespread in industrial use, but it cannot be used to encapsulate sensitive drugs/actives.

3. **Rigidization of coating:** The coating of core particles needs to be solidified or rigidized. This is accomplished by using any of the three methods:

 (a)  changing the temperature,

 (b)  cross-linking,

 (c)  desolvation.

Once the coating is rigidized, the microcapsules are collected, washed to remove the solvent till the residual solvent is within the limit, and dried. Rigidization of the microcapsules takes place under any one or more of the following conditions.

 **(a) Change of temperature:** Microcapsules of N-acetyl þ-aminophenol are prepared with ethyl cellulose, a water-insoluble polymer by using the temperature-solubility characteristics of the polymer (ethyl cellulose) in cyclohexane. At room temperature, ethyl cellulose is insoluble in cyclohexane but soluble at a higher temperature. A 2% dispersion of ethylcellulose in hot cyclohexane is heated to almost boiling to prepare a clear solution. To this solution, finely powdered N-acetyl þ-aminophenol is dispersed with constant stirring. The core-to-coat ratio (as on a dried basis) is maintained at 2:1. The mixture is allowed to cool with continuous stirring. With the decrease in temperature, the phase separation/coacervation of ethylcellulose would take place along with the formation of microcapsules containing N-acetyl þ-aminophenol. When the temperature of the mixture is further reduced to room temperature, the microcapsules formed will solidify. The stirring would be continued until the microcapsules formed are completely solidified. After solidification, the microcapsules are separated from cyclohexane and collected through decantation, filtration, and centrifugation.

 The microcapsules collected should be washed with cold water until the residual solvent is found within the permissible limits.

 **(b) Cross-linking/addition of incompatible polymer:** When microcapsules are prepared by adding an incompatible polymer to the mixture of immiscible core and solution of the polymer. The solidification of coating polymer takes place by chemical cross-linking. For example, methylene blue HCl can be coated with ethylcellulose, and the microcapsules are solidified by cross-linking with liquid polybutadiene. A 2% solution of ethylcellulose is prepared with toluene. Crystalline powder of methylene blue HCl is dispersed in the solution by stirring. Methylene blue HCl is insoluble in toluene. Usually, the ratio of methylene blue HCl to ethylcellulose is maintained at 4:1(that is, for 4g methylene blue HCl per g of ethylcellulose should be taken). Phase separation/coacervation is done by slow addition of liquid polybutadiene with continuous stirring. Usually, 25g of polybutadiene is required per g of ethylcellulose. Polybutadiene is soluble in toluene but is incompatible with ethylcellulose.

**(c)** **Addition of a nonsolvent:** In this method, a liquid in which the polymer is not soluble is added to the polymer solution. As a result, phase separation occurs, and the polymer present in soluble form becomes insoluble. At this point, if there is any insoluble material is present in the system, the polymer gets deposited onto the insoluble particles. This phenomenon is utilized in microencapsulation. For example, methyl scopolamine hydrobromide (core material) can be coated with cellulose acetate butyrate (coating material) as follows. The core to coating material ratio would be 2:1. Cellulose acetate butyrate is dissolved in methyl ethyl ketone; in this solution, methyl scopolamine hydrobromide powders are dispersed with continuous stirring. The temperature of the system is maintained at $55 \pm 1°C$. To this mixture, if isopropyl ether, in which the coating material is not soluble, is added slowly with continuous stirring the phase separation will start, and the polymer will deposit over the dispersed core particles to make microcapsule. Once the microencapsulation process is completed, the mixture is slowly cooled to room temperature. The microcapsules formed are separated by centrifugation; these are washed with isopropyl ether and then dried under vacuum.

**(d)** **Addition of salt:** If a water-soluble inorganic salt is added to an aqueous solution of a polymer, phase separation would take place. This phenomenon can be utilized in microencapsulation. For example, an oil-soluble vitamin can be encapsulated by a water-soluble polymer, gelatin using sodium sulfate, an inorganic salt. A solution of the vitamin in corn oil is emulsified in a 10% solution of gelatin in water. The gelatin must be of highest quality with an isoelectric point at about pH 8.9 and prepared from pig-skin. The emulsion should be prepared by using 20g of oil phase with 100g of the aqueous phase. During emulsification, the temperature of the system is maintained at $50 \pm 1°C$, and the droplet size of the oil phase is maintained at a desired size range with continuous and controlled (rpm) stirring. Then a 20% solution of salt ($Na_2SO_4$) is slowly added to the system under stirring to effect phase separation. Gelatin will be deposited over the oil droplets and microcapsules would be formed. The volume of salt solution to be added depends on the volume of the emulsion; usually at a ratio of 1:2.5. The mixture is then transferred to 7% solution of the salt maintained at $19 \pm 0.5°C$ with continuous stirring. The volume of this salt solution would be about 10 times of that of the mixture being transferred. Thus, the microcapsules formed are rigidized. The microcapsules are filtered, washed with chilled water repeated until the salt is removed completely; then, the product is dried using spray drying method.

(e) **In-situ polymerization:** Similar to interfacial polymerization, the *in-situ* polymerization involves preparing the wall of a capsule through polymerization of monomers which are added to the encapsulation reactor. However, reactive agents are not added to the core material. Polymerization occurs exclusively in the continuous phase side of the interface formed by the dispersed core material and continuous phases. A low weight pre polymer is produced in a polymerization process and during growing in size, it deposits onto the surface of the dispersed core material being encapsulated, and polymerization with cross-linking continues to take place. Thus, a solid capsule shell is produced.

8. **Emulsification/solvent evaporation or extraction:** This method is mainly used to encapsulate hydrophobic materials through oil-in-water (o/w) emulsification process. The polymer solution is prepared by dissolving it in a water-immiscible and volatile organic solvent, and the material to be encapsulated is dissolved or suspended in the polymer solution. The mixture is then emulsified into water containing emulsifier as shown in **fig. 3.6.** The volatile organic solvent present in the emulsion is removed by evaporation at high temperature or under reduced pressure or by extraction in a large amount of water. Thus, the solid particles are separated. The rate of solvent removal can affect the morphology of the final particles, and such rate is determined by:

> temperature,
> polymer solubility,
> solvent, and
> pressure.

The microparticles are then collected and dried to remove the residual solvent. However, this method is only effective for hydrophobic materials; since hydrophilic materials may not be dissolved in the organic solvent and diffuse out or partition from the dispersed oil phase into the aqueous phase. To encapsulate hydrophilic materials, oil-in-oil (o/o) emulsification is used. In this method, the water-miscible organic solvent is used to dissolve the polymer and hydrophilic materials to be encapsulated, and hydrophobic oils are used as the continuous phase. A cosolvent can be added to the dispersed phase to facilitate solubilization the hydrophilic material. Alternatively, the hydrophilic material can be dispersed as fine particles in the dispersed phase. Multiple emulsion such as water-in-oil-in-water (w/o/w) methods is used for most of the water-soluble materials. An aqueous solution of hydrophilic materials is emulsified into an organic solvent in which the polymer is dissolved to form the primary water-in-oil (w/o) emulsion. The primary emulsion is then added to water containing a suitable emulsifier under vigorous mixing. This produces the w/o/w emulsion. To obtain micro-particles, the solvent is removed by evaporation or extraction.

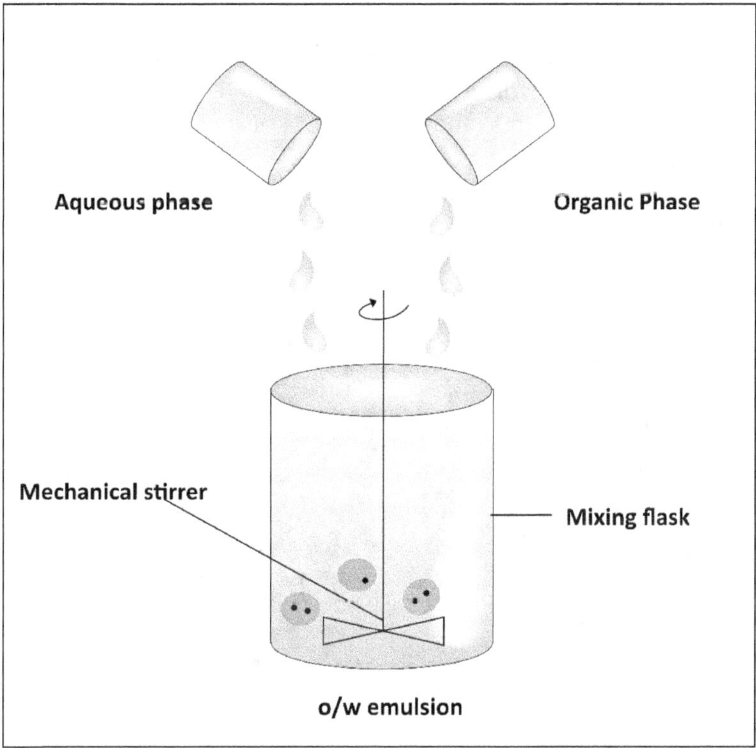


**Fig. 3.6:** Schematic representation of emulsification/solvent evaporation technique.

### Freeze-drying or lyophilization

The atomized droplets can be frozen, such as in liquid nitrogen, and the solvent can be removed by sublimation in a vacuum. Co-crystallization is a process to encapsulate ingredients between sucrose crystals. Sucrose crystals are solid, monoclinic and spherical and not suitable for encapsulation. Aggregates of the crystals are formed when they are spontaneously crystallized from a supersaturated solution. The crystal aggregates are in size range of 3 to 30 µm and can entrap materials. A supersaturated solution of sucrose is prepared first, then the material to be encapsulated is added, and the syrup is mixed to induce nucleation and agglomeration. During the process, it is necessary to control the rates of nucleation and crystallization. Various types of flavors can be encapsulated by this method.

### Spray congealing

In spray congealing method the fluid is atomized and sprayed into an environment maintained at a temperature below the melting point of the carrier material. The atomization results to the formation of molten droplets. The temperature in the chamber is then reduced. As a result, the molten droplets solidify upon cooling, and the final microparticles are produced.

## Pan coating

Pan coating is widely used in the pharmaceutical industry. With this method tablets, capsules, multi-particulates, and drug crystals are coated. The coating is a process in which a coating solution is applied to the surfaces of solid core material such as tablets in a coating pan. The tablet surfaces become covered with a polymeric film. Before the tablet surface dries, the applied coating changes from a sticky liquid to tacky semisolid, and finally to a non-sticky film.

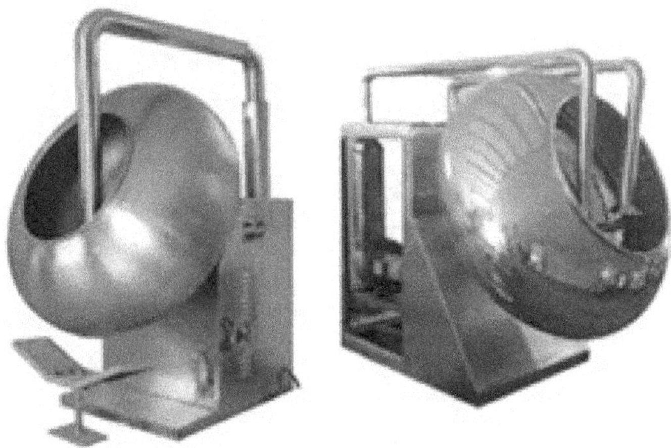

**Fig. 3.7:** Diagram of typical coating pans.

The entire coating process is conducted in a series of mechanically operated coating pans. The smaller pans of about 12 inch diameter are used for experimental, developmental, and pilot plant operations, and the larger once are used for industrial production. Some pans contain baffles rectangularly to the circumference. Microcapsules can be applied by padding, coating, spraying, immersion or exhaustion.

A suitable binder is required for all these methods. The binder may be acrylic, polyurethane, silicone, starch, sucrose, etc. Its role is to fix the core materials onto the coating film and to hold them in place during use. The fig. 3.7 represents the diagrams of typical and conventional coating pans.

## Air suspension coating

In the air suspension coating or fluidized bed coating, fine solid core materials are suspended by a vertical current of air, and the solution of coating material is sprayed. The solvent is evaporated, and a layer of the coating material is deposited onto the core material. The process can be repeated to achieve the desired film thickness. The size of the particle coated by this technique usually large varies with a minimum of 100 µm. Smaller particles tend to aggregate or are carried away by the exhaust air. The technique has been used to encapsulate pharmaceuticals, seeds, and foodstuffs. The morphology of various types of microcapsules is shown in fig 3.8.

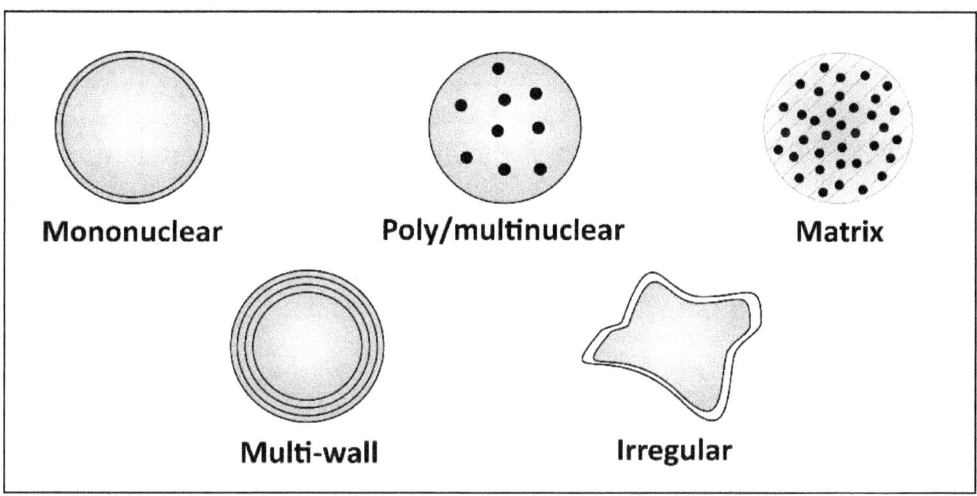


**Fig. 3.8:** Morphology of microsphere.

For efficient and effective coating of particles (microencapsulation) by this method following processing variables must be considered;

> ➢ Solubility, volatility, crystallinity, density, surface area, melting point, friability and flowability of the core material.
> ➢ Concentration of the coating material.
> ➢ The rate of application of coating material.
> ➢ Volume of air necessary for support and fluidization of the core material.
> ➢ The total amount of coating material required for coating.
> ➢ Inlet and outlet temperature during operation.

Various coating materials can be used in this method for microencapsulation. The coating material can be used in the form of solution, dispersion, emulsion or in the form of hot melt through suitable equipment. The amount of coating material may vary from 455g to 4.45kg. This process is generally used to encapsulate solid core material. However, this method can be used to encapsulate liquid material, if a lower amount of coating material is required and by coating the solid sorbents are pre-treated with liquid sorbates. Air suspension method can be used both for microencapsulation and microencapsulation. The **table 3.3** provides the list of some coating materials commonly used for various processes.

**Table 3.3:** Coating materials commonly used for different methods

| Coating material | A | B | C | D | E | F |
|---|---|---|---|---|---|---|
| Water-soluble resins | | | | | | |
| Gelatin | √ | √ | √ | √ | √ | √ |
| Gum arabic | | √ | √ | √ | √ | √ |
| Starch | | √ | √ | √ | √ | |

**Table 3.3** *Contd...*

| Coating material | A | B | C | D | E | F |
|---|---|---|---|---|---|---|
| Polyvinylpyrrolidone | ∫ | ∫ | ∫ | ∫ | ∫ | |
| Carboxymethyl cellulose | | ∫ | ∫ | ∫ | ∫ | |
| Hydroxyethyl cellulose | | ∫ | ∫ | ∫ | ∫ | ∫ |
| Methylcellulose | | ∫ | ∫ | ∫ | ∫ | |
| Polyvinyl alcohol | ∫ | ∫ | ∫ | ∫ | ∫ | ∫ |
| Polyacrylic acid | | ∫ | ∫ | ∫ | ∫ | ∫ |
| Water-insoluble resins | | | | | | |
| Polyethylene | ∫ | | | | ∫ | ∫ |
| Ethylcellulose | | ∫ | ∫ | ∫ | ∫ | ∫ |
| Polymethacrylate | | ∫ | ∫ | ∫ | ∫ | ∫ |
| Polyamide (Nylon) | | | | | ∫ | ∫ |
| Poly(ethylene-vinyl acetate) | ∫ | ∫ | ∫ | ∫ | | ∫ |
| Cellulose nitrate | ∫ | ∫ | ∫ | ∫ | | ∫ |
| Silicones | | | ∫ | ∫ | | |
| Poly(lactide-co-glycolide) | | ∫ | ∫ | | | ∫ |
| Enteric resins | | | | | | |
| Shellac | | ∫ | ∫ | ∫ | ∫ | |
| Cellulose acetate phthalate | ∫ | ∫ | ∫ | ∫ | ∫ | ∫ |
| Zein | ∫ | | | | ∫ | |
| Lipids and waxes | | | | | | |
| Paraffin | ∫ | ∫ | ∫ | ∫ | ∫ | |
| Carnauba wax | | | ∫ | ∫ | ∫ | |
| Spermaceti | | ∫ | ∫ | ∫ | ∫ | |
| Beeswax | | | ∫ | ∫ | ∫ | |
| Stearic acid | | | ∫ | ∫ | | |
| Stearyl alcohol | | | ∫ | ∫ | ∫ | |
| Glyceryl stearate | | | ∫ | ∫ | ∫ | |

A – Multi-orifice Centrifugal, B – Phase Separation Coacervation, C – Pan coating, D – Spray Drying & congealing, E – Air suspension, F – Solvent evaporation

## Using liquid and supercritical carbon dioxide

Compressed carbon dioxide in the liquid or supercritical state can be used as an efficient solvent in microencapsulation processes. Carbon dioxide is non-toxic, non-flammable, and not expensive also. The high volatility of carbon dioxide allows it to be easily separated from polymeric materials by lowering pressure. The supercritical fluid state is attained when the temperature and pressure of a substance are above its critical temperature and pressure. For carbon dioxide, the critical temperature is 31°C, and the critical pressure is 74 bar, as shown in fig 3.9. Above the critical temperature, the density can be continuously varied from gas-like to liquid-like substance without undergoing a phase transition. Supercritical fluids display a hybrid of the properties that are typical for a liquid and a gas. This includes the ability to dissolve solids, miscibility with permanent gases, high diffusivity, and low viscosity. Since, the solubility parameter, dependent on density, the solvating power of a supercritical fluid, can be fine-tuned by adjusting pressure or temperature. It is a good solvent for many non-polar volatile materials. Carbon dioxide is a poor solvent for most highly polar or high molecular weight materials under moderate pressure and temperature. Generally, the solubility of a substance in supercritical fluid increases with vapor pressure, with gases being completely miscible. Organic solvents, such as methanol, can be added to increase the solvent power of supercritical carbon dioxide.

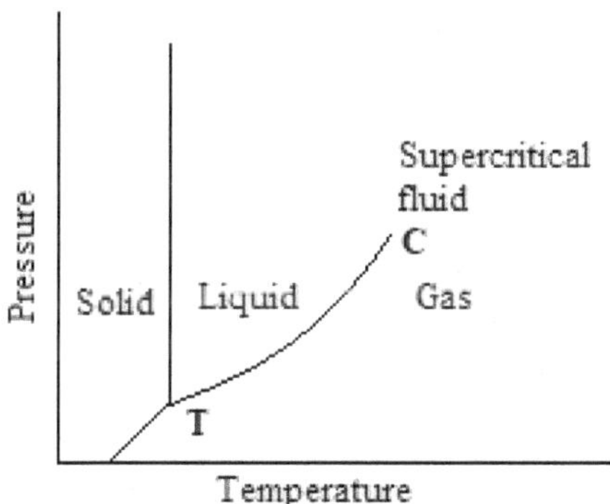


**Fig. 3.9:** Phase diagram of carbon dioxide.

Supercritical carbon dioxide can be used as a medium for polymer synthesis and processing. It has poor solvent power for most polar and high molecular weight substances; but can be used for polymer fractionation, extraction, purification, and polymer particle formation by anti-solvent precipitation. Low cohesive energy density polymers, such as fluorocarbons and silicones, have appreciable solubility in $CO_2$ at moderate temperature and pressure. Due to the high solubility of fluorinated polymers in $CO_2$, it has used in coatings, lithography, and in formation of water-in-$CO_2$ emulsions. Supercritical $CO_2$ is an excellent nonsolvating, porogenic (porosity loving) diluent for synthesizing porous polymers. Although elevated pressure and specialized equipment are required, supercritical carbon dioxide is used, because it evaporates easily and it is not harmful. Most of the polymers partially dissolve in carbon dioxide; but it has substantial solubility in many polymers, as a result of the glass transition temperature (Tg) of polymers or plasticization decrease, even at moderate pressure. The Tg, a thermodynamic effect, reduces due to intermolecular interaction between $CO_2$ and polymer. If the interaction is stronger, it can enhance the depression. The glass transition temperature of polystyrene was reduced by up to 50°C when exposed to $CO_2$ under the pressure of the only 25 bar. When the polymer is exposed to supercritical carbon dioxide, the polymer swells, and the free volume present in the polymer is increased; as a result, the additives diffuse into the polymer significantly. For example, dimethyl phthalate can diffuse into poly (vinyl chloride) 6 times more under supercritical $CO_2$ than without $CO_2$.

Generally, three steps are followed for the impregnation –

1. The polymer materials are exposed to supercritical CO2 for a while;

2. The solution of additives in $CO_2$ is introduced, and the solute is transferred from $CO_2$ to the polymer, and

3. $CO_2$ is released, and the solute is trapped in the polymer material. However, the diffusion of additives in the polymer may be promoted under supercritical CO2, if a cosolvent is used. The application of polymer products can be adversely affected by its impurities, such as unreacted monomers, residual solvents, catalysts, and by-products since these impurities can change the taste, color, toxicity or thermophysical properties of polymers through plasticization or depolymerization. Hence, strict regulations should be implemented to fix the permissible levels of various impurities. Usually, polymers are purified by vacuum, steam stripping, or solvent extraction; in certain cases, these methods cannot remove the residual impurities sufficiently within the permissible levels. Supercritical extraction from polymers can produce high-purity, high-quality products with lower energy cost. When the polymer is exposed to supercritical carbon dioxide, the impurities can diffuse out of polymer significantly.

## Materials required for Microencapsulation

There are various substances which are used to entrap, or coat or encapsulate solids, liquids, or gases of different types, origin, and properties. However, not all, some of these materials have been considered as 'generally recognized as safe' (GRAS). Here, categories of materials based on their source are given below in **table 3.4**.

**Table 3.4:** Origin, type of polymers used in microencapsulation

| Origin | Polymers | | |
|---|---|---|---|
| | Carbohydrate | Protein | Lipids |
| Plant | Starch Derivatives Cellulose Derivatives Plant exudates Gum arabic Gum karaya Mesquite gum Plant extract Galactomannans Soluble soybeans Polysaccharides | Gluten (Corn) Isolates (pea, soy) | Fatty acids/alcohol Glycerides Waxes Phospholipids |

**Table 3.4** *Contd...*

| Origin | Polymers | | |
|--------|----------|--|--|
| | **Carbohydrate** | **Protein** | **Lipids** |
| Marine | Carrageenan<br>Alginate | | |
| Microbial/<br>animal | Xanthan<br>Gellan<br>Dextran<br>Chitosan | Caseins<br>Whey proteins<br>Gelatin | Fatty acids/alcohols<br>Glycerides<br>Waxes<br>Phospholipids<br>(Shellac) |

Based on the active ingredients and the polymer used the actual method of microencapsulation is selected. The table 5 provides the names of the materials used for microencapsulation.

**Table 3.5:** Application of polymeric materials, active constituents and method of microencapsulation used.

| Active | Polymer | Method |
|--------|---------|--------|
| Vitamins<br>Vitamin C,<br>Synthetic ascorbic acid | Maltodextrin<br>Maltodextrin | Spray drying |
| Vitamin C | Tripolyphosphate/chitosan | Spray drying |
| Vitamin E | Starch | High-pressure homogenization |
| Vitamin A acetate<br>dissolved in coconut oil | hi-CAP 100 (starch<br>octenyl succinate, OSA-starch) | High-pressure homogenization<br>O/w emulsion, spray drying |
| Folic acid | Alginate-pectin | Coacervation |
| Aroma/flavor<br>European pear aroma | cyclodextrin (CD),<br>soybean soluble<br>polysaccharide (SSPS),<br>highly branched cyclic<br>dextrin (HBCD) | Spray-drying, freeze drying |
| Oregano, citronella,<br>and<br>marjoram flavors | Milk-protein based matrices:<br>Milk-protein based matrices:<br>WPC, skimmed milk<br>powder (SMP) | Milk-protein based matrices:<br>Spray-drying |
| Limonene | Gum arabic-sucrose-gelatin | Freeze-drying |
| Cardamom oil | Mesquite gum | Spray-drying |
| Probiotics<br>Bifidobacterium lactis | Hydrated gellan, xanthan<br>gums | Extrusion |
| Bifidobacterium PL1 | Starch | Spray coating, spray-drying |
| Lactobacillus<br>Acidophilus<br>Bifidobacterium.<br>lactis | Alginate/Hi-MaizeTM starch | Emulsion |

**Table 3.5** *Contd...*

| Active | Polymer | Method |
|---|---|---|
| Lactobacillus. acidophilus 547B. bifidum ATCC 1994, Lactobacillus casei | Alginate/CaCl2/chitosan | |
| Bifidobacterium. breve R070Bifidobacterium. Longum R023 | Milk fat, denatured whey protein | Emulsion, spray-drying |
| Lactobacillus sp. | Gum arabic (GA), gellan gum (GG), mesquite gum (MG), moreover, binary mixtures | Interfacial polymerization Highest |
| Lipids Conjugated linoleic acid (CLA) | Whey protein concentrate (WPC), gum arabic (GA), blend WPC/maltodextrin 10DE (1:1, w/w) | Spray-drying |
| Linoleic acid | Gum arabic | spray-drying |
| Lipids: oleic acid, linoleic acid, stearic acid | Potato starch, waxy maize starch, tapioca starch | Microwave heating |
| Oil Vegetable oil | Maltodextrin/GA, 3/2, w/w | Spray drying and Agglomeration in an air-fluidized bed |
| Fish oil | (a) Modified cellulose, skim milk powder, a mixture of fish gelatin/corn starch (b) Methylcellulose (MC), hydroxypropyl methylcellulose (HPMC), maltodextrin (c) High oil retention; especially MC improved the stability and concentration in the powder (d) Modified starch | Spray-drying<br><br>Layer-by-layer deposition and spray drying |
| Mixtures Ferrous sulfate+ascorbic acid | Liposomes | Pro-liposome and micro fluidization |
| Iron (ferric pyrophosphate), iodine (potassium iodate), Vitamin A (retinyl palmitate) | Hydrogenated palm fat | Spray cooling |

**Table 3.5** *Contd...*

| Active | Polymer | Method |
|---|---|---|
| Chito-oligo saccharide | Polyglycerol monostearate (PGMS) | |
| Anthocyanin pigments of black carrot | Maltodextrins: | Spray-drying |
| Isoflavone, b galactosidase | Medium-chain triacylglycerol (MCT), polyglycerol monostearate (PGMS) | |
| Allyl isothiocyanate – AIT (pathogens inhibitor) | Gum arabic | |
| IgY | Whey protein concentrates (WPC-34, 50 and 80); whey protein isolate (WPI) | Emulsification, heat gelation |

The polymers may be classified into two categories based on their source – natural and synthetic. Synthetic polymers may be biodegradable and non-biodegradable.

Names of some polymers of each category are mentioned below;

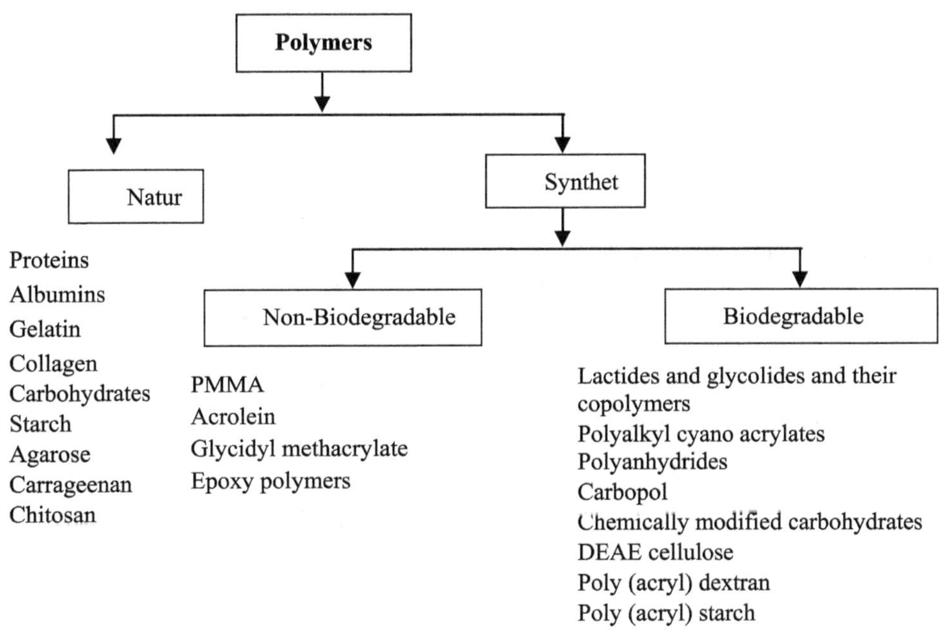

# Bibliography


1. Abraham, G. A.; Gallardo, A.; San Roman, J.; Fernandez-Mayoralas, A.; Zurita, M.; Vaquero, J. J. Biomed. Mater. Res. 2003, 64A(4), 638–647.

2. Alagusundaram M, Chetty MS, Umashankari C. Microspheres as a Novel drug delivery system; A review.; Int J Chem. Tech. 2009 12: 526-534.

3. Allen LV, Popovich NG, Ansel HC. Pharmaceutical Dosage Forms and Drug Delivery Systems. Delhi, India: BI Publication, 2005, 8: 265.

4. Carrasquillo, K. G.; Stanley, A. M.; Aponte-Carro, J. C.; De Jesus, P.; Costantino, H. R.; Bosques, C. J.; Griebenow, K. J. Controlled Release 2001, 76(3), 199–208.

5. Champagne, C. P.; Fustier, P. Curr. Opin. Biotechnol. 2007, 18, 184–190.

6. Collins AE and Deasy PB. Bioadhesive lozenge for the improved delivery of cetylpyridinium chloride J. Pharm. sci, 1990, 79:116-120.

7. Desai, K. G. H.; Park, H. J. Drying Technol. 2005, 23, 1361–1394.

8. Gharsallaoui, A.; Roudaut, G.; Chambin, O.; Voilley, A.; Saurel, R. Food Res. Int. 2007, 40, 1107–1121.

9. Ghulam Murtaza, Mahmood Ahamed, Naveed Akhtar and Fatima Rasool. A comparative study of various microencapsulation techniques: effect of polymer viscosity on microcapsule characteristics. Pak. J. Pharm. Sci. 2009, 3:291-300.

10. Khawla A, Abu izza, Lucila Garcia-Contreras, Robert Lu D. (Selection of better method for the preparation of microspheres by applying hierarchy process). J. Pharm Sci., 1996; 85: 144-149.

11. Kreitz M, Brannon-peppas L, Mathiowitz E. (Microencapsulation Encyclopedia of controlled drug delivery). John Wiley Sons publishers, 1999; 493-553.

12. Leon, L, Herbert AL, Joseph LK. The Theory and Practice of Industrial Pharmacy. Varghese Publishing House. 1990, 3: 412-428.

13. Li, M.; Rouaud, O.; Poncelet, D. Int. J. Pharm. 2008, 363, 26–39.

14. Liang, M. T.; Davies, N. M.; Toth, I. Int. J. Pharm. 2005, 301, 247–254.

15. Lopez, CR, Portero A, Vila-Jato, JC, Alonso MJ. Design and Evaluation of chitosan/ Ethylcellulose mucoadhesive bilayered devices for buccal drug delivery. J. Control. Re, 1998, 55: 143-152.

16. Lu W and Park TG, Protein release from poly (lactic-co-glycolic acid) microspheres: protein stability problems. PDA J Pharm Sci Technol, 1995, 49:13-19.

17. Murua, A.; Portero, A.; Orive, G.; Hern´andez, R. M.; Castro, M. d.; Pedraz, J. L.; J. Controlled Release 2008, 132, 76–83.

18. Ngo, A. T.; Karam, P.; Fuller, E.; Burger, M.; Cosa, G. J. Am. Chem. Soc. 2008, 130, 457–459.

19. Park, J. H.; Ye, M.; Park, K. Molecules 2005, 10, 146–161.

20. Passerini, N.; Craig, D. Q. M. J. Pharm. Pharmacol. 2002, 54(7), 913–919.

## Exercise

### A. Multiple Choice Questions

1. Which of the following statements is correct?
   - (a) Microcapsules are not biocompatible.
   - (b) Total dose of a drug remains same in microparticle
   - (c) Microparticles can modify the physical characteristics of a drug
   - (d) Shelf-life of hygroscopic drug can be increased.

2. Which of the following statements is correct?
   - (a) Microcapsules are intended only for oral administration
   - (b) Microcapsules can be administered through injection
   - (c) Microcapsules are not spherical bodies
   - (d) Microcapsule does not change the bioavailability of drug

3. Which of the following statements is correct?
   - (a) The drug release from microcapsules cannot be modified.
   - (b) Microcapsules should be crushed.
   - (c) The release rate from microcapsules does not differ due to dose difference.
   - (d) Constant and prolonged therapeutic effect can be achieved.

4. Selection of coat material for microencapsulation depends on
   - (a) Physicochemical properties of core material
   - (b) Size of the microcapsules
   - (c) Physicochemical properties of excipient
   - (d) None of the above

5. Microencapsulation technique is widely used to
   - (a) Enlarge the particle size of the drug
   - (b) Improve or enhance the stability of the drug
   - (c) Provide traditional dosage form
   - (d) Eliminate the adverse effect of the drug

6. Microencapsulation technique is
   - (a) Suitable for safe handling of toxic substances
   - (b) Unsuitable for safe handling of toxic substances
   - (c) Difficult to practice
   - (d) Capable to increase shelf-life of hygroscopic drug

7. Which of the following statements is correct?
   - (a) Microencapsulation technique does not allow any reaction between core and coat material to take place
   - (b) Microencapsulation technique does not increase the cost of the product
   - (c) Microencapsulation technique cannot produce uniform and continuous film
   - (d) Skill and knowledge are required for microencapsulation

8. To assess the surface chemistry of microspheres
    (a) Density of microspheres is to be measured
    (b) Size distribution of microspheres is to be measured
    (c) Charge of microspheres is to be measured
    (d) Hydrophobicity of microspheres is to be measured

9. In solvent evaporation method for preparing microspheres
    (a) Only a volatile solvent is used
    (b) Both volatile and non-volatile solvents are used
    (c) Only a non-volatile solvent is used
    (d) None of the above

10. Release of drug from biodegradable polymer is influenced by
    (a) Biodegradation
    (b) kinetics of the polymer
    (c) Degradation kinetics of the drug
    (d) Average size of the microcapsules
    (e) Size distribution of the microcapsules

11. Microcapsules are prepared to
    (a) Protect the product          (b)    Only to mask the taste
    (c) Protect the drug             (d)    None of the above

12. pH triggered microparticles are used in
    (a) Gene therapy                 (b)    The treatment of diarrhoea
    (c) Hyperglycaemia               (d)    All of the above

13. Selection of method for microencapsulation depends on
    (a) Coating material             (b)    Release mechanism
    (b) Properties of core           (d)    All of the above

14. Which of the following is spray drying process parameter?
    (a) The size of the dying chamber
    (b) Contact period between core and coating material
    (c) Temperature of the drying air/gas
    (d) All of the above

15. Complex coacervation involves
    (a) Complexation between two oppositely charged polymers
    (b) Complexation between two polymers
    (c) Complexation between core and polymer
    (d) Complexation between two similarly charged polymers

16. In coacervation technique, phase separation is done by
    (a) Changing the pressure        (b)    Changing the temperature
    (c) Adding an insoluble salt      (d)    Diluting with solvent

17. The rate of removal of solvent in emulsification method for preparation of microparticles depends on
    (a) The temperature         (b) The solvent used
    (c) Solubility of polymer      (d) All of the above

18. In-situ polymerization method involves
    (a) Polymerization between suitable polymers
    (b) Polymerization between suitable monomers
    (c) Polymerization between polymer and monomer
    (d) None of the above

19. To encapsulate drug in the core of liposomes, the properties of liposome to be controlled are
    (a) Electrostatic charge      (b) Electromagnetic charge
    (c) Electromotive force       (d) None of the above

20. In general, liposomes are used to deliver
    (a) Vaccines             (b) Hormones
    (c) Enzymes           (d) All of the above

## B. Short Questions

1. Define microencapsulation. Write down the advantages and disadvantages of microencapsulation.

2. Write a note on microsphere.

3. Write down measure parameters of microspheres. What are the advantages and limitations of microspheres?

4. Write down the advantages of microparticles.

5. Name the methods of microencapsulation. How a method of preparation is selected?

6. Write a note on liposome entrapment method of microencapsulation; mention the important properties of liposomes to be controlled.

## C. Long Questions

1. Describe the methods of preparation of microspheres.

2. What is microcapsule and microparticles? Why these are prepared?

3. Describe the spray drying method of microencapsulation; mention the important process parameters of this method.

4. Explain spray chilling and co-crystallization techniques.

5. What is coacervation? Explain the steps involved in coacervation-phase separation technique.

6. Explain the solvent evaporation method and pan coating method used to prepare microparticles.

7. Write down how the microcapsules are prepared by air suspension. Explain the effect of changing temperature on coacervation. What is meant by cross linking?

## CHAPTER 4

# Mucosal Drug Delivery System

*Introduction, Principles of bio-adhesion / muco-adhesion, concepts, advantages and disadvantages, transmucosal permeability and formulation considerations of buccal delivery systems.*

## Introduction

According to physics, the term *adhesion may be defined as the molecular force of attraction in the area of contact between unlike bodies that acts to hold them together.* Bioadhesive refers to adhesion either between two biological bodies or between one biological body and any of the other type. Materials are attached to each other through interfacial forces. When one of the two materials are mucosal surface, the adhesion is called mucoadhesion.

A drug can be administered through a different route to produce a systemic pharmacological effect. The most common route of drug administration is the oral route, the dosage form is swallowed, and the drug enters into the systemic circuplation primarily through the membrane of the small intestine. Absorption of drugs after oral administration may take place at the various body sites from the mouth to rectum. In general, most of the drug is absorbed along the gastrointestinal tract. The more rapid will be its absorption, more would be the therapeutic action of the drug. A drug taken orally must withstand large fluctuation in pH as it travels along the gastrointestinal tract, as well as resist the attack of the enzymes that digest food and metabolized by micro flora that live there. It is estimated that 25% of the population finds it difficult to swallow tablets and capsules and therefore do not take their medication as prescribed by their doctor resulting in high incidence of non-compliance and ineffective therapy. This is usually experienced by pediatrics and geriatric patients, but it also applies to people who are ill bedridden and to those who are busy or traveling, especially those who have no access to water. In these cases, oral mucosal drug delivery is most preferred. Since long, it has been known that buccal and sublingual administration of the drug is rapidly absorbed into the reticulated vein, which lies just below the oral mucosa and transported through the facial veins, internal jugular vein, and brachiocephalic vein and is then drained into the systemic circulation. Therefore, the buccal and sublingual routes of administration can be utilized to bypass the hepatic first-pass elimination of drugs. For systemic drug delivery within the oral mucosal cavity, the buccal region is an attractive route of drug administration. The mucosa has a rich blood supply, and it is relatively permeable. The patients also accept oral cavity.  Since there are no Langerhans cells; the oral mucosa is tolerant to potential allergens.

The **table 4.1** presents some commercially available buccoadhesive drug delivery system along with the polymers.

**Table 4.1:** Commercially available buccal adhesive formulations

| Trade name | Dosage form | Company | Polymer used |
|---|---|---|---|
| Suscard | Tablet | Forest | HPMC |
| Gavisoon | Oral liquid | Rickitt Benckiser | Sodium alginate |
| Orabase | Oral paste | Conva Tech | Pectin, gelatine |
| Corcodyl gel | Oral mucosal gel | Glaxosmithkline | HPMC |
| Corlan pellets | Oral mucosal pellets | Celltech | Acacia |
| Luborant | Artificial saliva | Antigen | Sodium CMC |
| Saliveze | Artificial saliva | Wyvem | Sodium CMC |

There are some whose buccoadhesive formulations are being investigated. **Table 4.2** presents these drugs and the polymer being used.

**Table 4.2:** Polymers used for the design of different bioadhesive dosage forms

| Drug | Dosage form | Polymer |
|---|---|---|
| Ibuprofen | Patch | PVP Carboxymethylcellulose sodium salt (NaCMC) |
| Nystatin | Bi-Layered tablet | Carbomer, Hydroxypropylmethylcellulose |
| Propranolol | Film | Ethyl cellulose, polyvinyl pyrrolidone K-30, hydroxypropyl methyl cellulose-15cps, hydroxyl ethyl cellulose-10cps |
| Clotrimazole | Film | Carbopol-934P, Hydroxypropyl cellulose-M |
| Miconazole nitrate | Slow-Release Tablets | Hydroxypropylmethylcellulose, Sodium carboxymethylcellulose, Carbopol 934P, and sodium alginate |
| Benzocaine | Liquid Gel | Sodium carboxymethylcellulose, Xanthan gum |
| Prednisolone | Ointment | Carbopol 934P, White petrolatum |

## Principles of Bioadhession/Mucoadhesion

Although it is not yet well understood how certain macro-molecules adhere to the surface of mucous tissue, the mucoadhesive must spread over the substrate to initiate close contact for promoting the diffusion of the drug within the mucus. Both attractive and repulsive forces arise. For a successful mucoadhesive delivery system, the attractive forces must dominate. Each step is facilitated by the nature of the dosage form and how it is administered; for example, a partially hydrated polymer can be adsorbed by the substrate because of the attraction by the surface water.

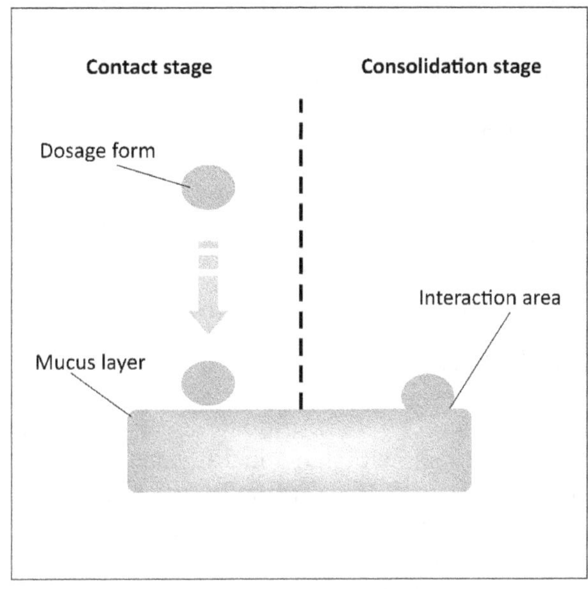


**Fig. 4.1:** Two steps of mucoadhesion.

Thus, the mechanism of mucoadhesion is generally divided into two steps, the contact stage, and the consolidation stage as shown in **fig 4.1**.

The first stage; that is the contact stage is characterized by –

1. The contact between the mucoadhesive and the mucous membrane,
2. Spreading and swelling of the formulation,
3. Initiating its deep contact with the mucus layer. In some cases, the delivery system is mechanically attached over the membrane such as for ocular or vaginal formulations.

In other cases, such as for the nasal route, the deposition is promoted by the aerodynamics of the organ to which the system is administered. On the other hand, in the gastrointestinal tract attachment of direct formulation over the mucous membrane is not feasible.

Peristaltic motions can contribute to this contact, but there is little evidence in the literature showing appropriate adhesion. Additionally, an undesirable adhesion in the oesophagus can occur. In these cases, mucoadhesion can be explained by peristalsis, the motion of organic fluids in the organ cavity, or by Brownian motion. If the particle approaches the mucous surface, it will come into contact with repulsive forces (osmotic pressure, electrostatic repulsion, etc.) and attractive forces (van der Waals forces and electrostatic attraction). Therefore, the particle must overcome this repulsive barrier.

The mucoadhesive materials are activated by the presence of moisture which plasticizes the system, allows the mucoadhesive molecules to break and join by weak van der Waals and hydrogen bonds.

## Diffusion Theory

The mucoadhesive molecules and glycoproteins of the mucus mutually interact using the interpenetration of their chains and the build secondary bonds. In fact, the mucoadhesive device favors both chemical and mechanical interactions. For example, molecules with hydrogen bonds building groups (–OH, –COOH), with an anionic surface charge, high molecular weight, flexible chains, and surface-active properties, spread throughout the mucus layer, and show mucoadhesive properties.

## Dehydration Theory

Some materials can transform into a gel in an aqueous environment. When such materials come in contact with the mucus, can cause its dehydration due to the difference of osmotic pressure. The difference in concentration gradient draws the water into the formulation until the osmotic pressures are balanced. This process leads to the mixture of formulation and mucus, and thus, increases contact time with the mucous membrane. Therefore, it is the motion of water that becomes responsible for the formation of the adhesive bond, and not the interpenetration of macromolecular chains. However, the dehydration theory is not applicable to solid formulations or highly hydrated forms **(fig 4.2)**.

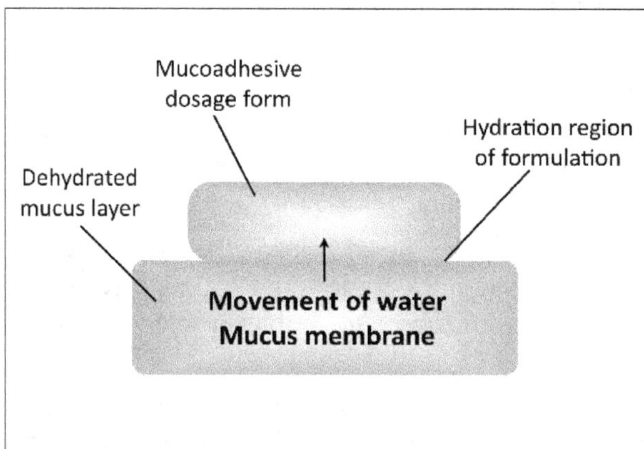


**Fig. 4.2:** Dehydration theory of mucoadhesion.

## Electronic Theory

The electronic theory is based on the principle that both mucoadhesive and biological materials possess opposing electrical charges. When both materials come in contact, they transfer electrons leading to the formation of a double electronic layer at the interface.

The attractive forces present within this electronic double layer determines the mucoadhesive strength.

## Adsorption Theory

According to the adsorption theory, the mucoadhesive device adheres to the mucus by secondary chemical interactions, such as van der Waals and hydrogen bonds, electrostatic attraction or hydrophobic interactions. For example, hydrogen bonds are prevalent in interfacial forces between the polymers containing carboxyl groups. Such forces have been considered the most important in the adhesive interaction phenomenon; because, a great number of interactions can result in an intense adhesion although they are individually weak.

## Wetting Theory

The wetting theory applies to liquid systems. These systems possess affinity towards the surface in order to spread over it. This affinity can be demonstrated when the contact angles are measured. It is generally stated that lower the contact angle, greater is the affinity. To achieve good or adequate spreadability, the contact angles should be equal or close to zero to provide (**fig 4.3**).

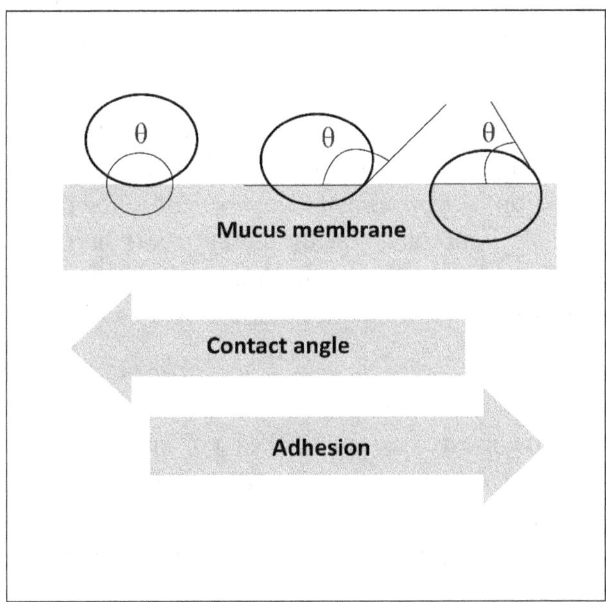


**Fig. 4.3:** Schematic diagram showing influence of contact angle between device and mucus membrane on bioadhesion

The spreadability coefficient, $S_{AB}$, can be calculated from the difference between the surface energies $\gamma_B$ and $\gamma_A$ and the interfacial energy $\gamma_{AB}$, as expressed in the equation.

The greater the individual surface energy of mucus and device about the interfacial energy, the greater the adhesion work, $W_A$, i.e., the greater the energy needed to separate the two phases.

$$W_A = \gamma_A + \gamma_B - \gamma_{AB}$$

## Diffusion Theory

According to the diffusion theory, the interpenetration of both polymer and mucin chains should take place to a sufficient depth so that a semi-permanent adhesive bond can be created. It is believed that the adhesion force increases with the degree of penetration of the polymer chains. Through diffusion the penetration rate depends on;

1. The diffusion coefficient,
2. Flexibility,
3. Nature of the mucoadhesive chains,
4. Mobility and
5. Contact time.

According to the literature, the depth of interpenetration requires to produce an efficient bioadhesive bond with in the range of $0.2 - 0.5\mu m$. This interpenetration depth of polymer and mucin chains, $l$ can be calculated by the equation:

$$l = (t \times D_b)^{1/2}$$

Where, t is the contact time, and $D_b$ is the diffusion coefficient of the mucoadhesive material in the mucus. The adhesion strength for a polymer would be reached a maximum when the depth of penetration is approximately equivalent to the polymer chain size.

For diffusion to occur, it is important that the components involved have good mutual solubility; that is, both the bioadhesive and the mucus have similar chemical structures. The greater the structural similarity, the better the mucoadhesive bond.

## Fracture Theory

This theory is perhaps the most used in studies on the mechanical measurement of mucoadhesion. It analyses the force required to separate two surfaces after adhesion is established. The force, $S_m$, is usually calculated in the tests of resistance to rupture by the ratio of the maximal detachment force, $F_m$, and the total surface area, $A_o$, involved in the adhesive interaction:

$$S_m = \frac{F_m}{A_o}$$

In a single component uniform system, the fracture force, $S_j$, is equivalent to the maximal rupture tensile strength, $S_m$, and is proportional to the fracture energy, $g_c$ for

Young's module ($E$) and to the critical breaking length ($c$) for the fracture site. This is expressed in the following equation:

$$S_f \approx \left( \frac{g_c E}{C} \right)^{1/2}$$

The fracture energy, $g_c$ can be determined from the reversible adhesion work, $W_r$ (energy required to produce newly fractured surfaces), and the irreversible adhesion work, $W_i$ (work of plastic deformation provoked by the removal of a proof tip until the disruption of the adhesive bond). Both the values can be considered as units of fracture surface ($A_f$).

$$g_c = W_r + W_i$$

Since the fracture theory is concerned only with force required to separate the parts; it does not take into account the interpenetration or diffusion of polymer chains (**fig 4.4**). It is appropriate for use in the calculations for rigid or semi-rigid bioadhesive materials, in which the polymer chains do not penetrate into the mucus layer.

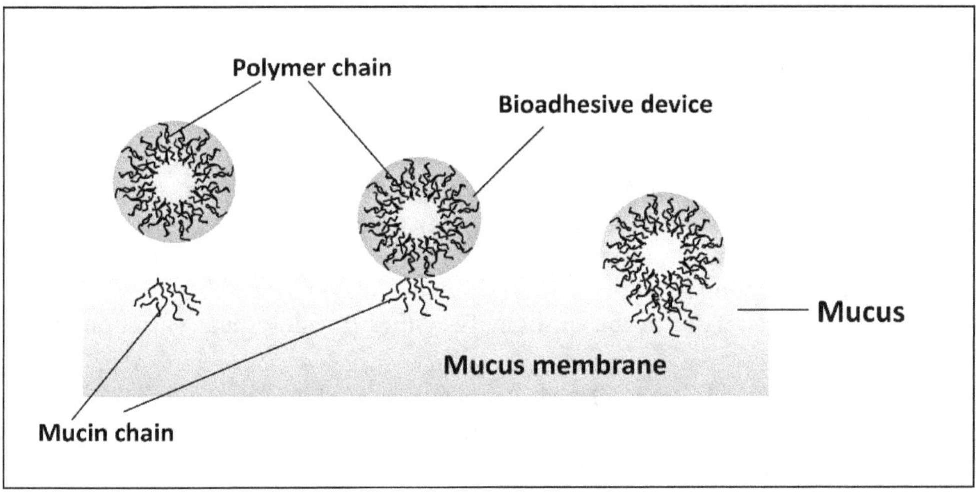


**Fig. 4.4:** Secondary interaction resulting from interdiffusion of polymeric chain of bioadhesive device and mucus membrane.

## Mechanical Theory

According to the mechanical theory, adhesion is due to the filling of the irregularities on a rough surface by a mucoadhesive liquid. Such roughness increases the interfacial area available for interactions; thereby, help dissipating energy. Thus, it can be considered the most important phenomenon in the process. It is doubtful that the mucoadhesion process is the same for all cases; therefore, it cannot be described by a single theory. In fact, all theories are relevant to identify the important process variables.

The mechanisms governing mucoadhesion can also be determined by the intrinsic properties of the formulation and by the environment in which it is applied.

### Factors influencing the rate of penetration

Intrinsic factors of the polymer are related to its –

➢ Molecular weight,
➢ Concentration and
➢ Chain flexibility.

For linear polymers, mucoadhesion increases with molecular weight; but, the same relationship may not be applicable for non-linear polymers. It has been found that more concentrated mucoadhesive dispersions are retained on the mucous membrane for longer periods, as in the case of systems formed by *in situ* gelling. After application, such systems spread easily. Since they possess the rheological properties of a liquid, can gelify as they come into contact with the absorption site, preventing their rapid removal. Chain flexibility is critical to combine the interpenetrations between formulation and mucus.

**Environment-related factors** include,

➢ pH,
➢ Initial contact time,
➢ Swelling, and
➢ Physiological variations.

The pH can influence the formation of ionizable groups in polymers and formation of charges on the mucus surface. Contact time between mucoadhesive and mucus layer controls the extent of chain interpenetration. Super-hydration of the system can build up mucilage without adhesion. The thickness of the mucus layer varies from 50 to 450 μm in the stomach to less than 1μm in the oral cavity. Other physiological variations can also occur with diseases.

None of these mechanisms or theories alone can explain the mucoadhesion which occurs in different situations. However, the understanding of these mechanisms in each instance can help the development of new mucoadhesive products.

## Advantages

The administration of drugs by the buccal route has several advantages over per oral administration such as;

➢ Drug degradation in the harsh gastrointestinal environment can be circumvented by administering the drug via the buccal route.
➢ Therapeutic serum concentration of the drug can be achieved more rapidly.
➢ The drug enters the general circulation without first passing through the liver.
➢ With the right design and formulation of the dosage form, the permeability and the local environment of the mucosa can be controlled and manipulated in order to accommodate drug permeation.

- Delivery can also be terminated relatively easily, if required.
- Significant reduction in dose-related side effects.
- It provides direct entry of the drug into systemic circulation.
- It offers a passive system, which does not require activation.
- Rapid cellular recovery following local stress or damage.
- Ability to withstand environmental extremes like a change in pH, temperature, etc.
- Sustained drug delivery.
- The potential for delivery of peptide molecules unsuitable for the oral route.

## Disadvantages

In general, oral cavity mucosa shows low permeability to drugs. The surface area of the oral cavity is small; it is approximately 214 $cm^2$. Saliva is continually secreted into the oral cavity from major and minor salivary glands. Salivation leads to swallowing which effectively removes the drug from the target site of absorption. The tongue contains taste receptors that may present difficulties to patients and decrease compliance with drugs that are bitter. Some of the oral mucosa (e.g., sublingual and buccal mucosa) is flexible and flexes as a consequence of normal functions of the mouth (e.g., speaking, chewing or swallowing). This may adversely affect the dosage form. Involuntarily swallowing of the delivery system could lead to choking. A buccal delivery system may cause inconvenience to the patient when they are eating or drinking. For some drugs, tissue irritation may arise following the use of an oral mucosal drug delivery system. Numbers of drug administered through this route is less.

- Once placed at the absorption site, the dosage form should not be disturbed.
- Eating and drinking are restricted.
- There is a possibility that the patient may swallow the formulation.
- Drug swallowed with saliva is lost.
- Drugs which are unstable at buccal pH and which irritate the mucosa or have a bitter or unpleasant taste or an obnoxious odor cannot be administered by this route.
- Over hydration may lead to the formation of slippery surface and structural integrity of formulation may get disrupted.

## Transmucosal Permeability

The transcellular and paracellular routes are involved in drug permeation across the epithelial membrane. In general, for skin and gastrointestinal mucosa viewed as lipoidal barriers, so partition coefficient and molecular size are important for diffusion. The same way recent study shows that the absorption of drug increases as the lipophilicity of drug increase in the mucosa. It has been shown that ionic and lipid-soluble compounds rapidly absorbed thorough rat rectal mucosa. The correlation between the rectal absorption and their partition coefficient proves the rectal mucosa as a lipoidal barrier. The studies on human nasal mucosa using propranolol of difference lipophilicity suggest that most lipophilic drugs absorbed highest, but several other works show the presence of aqueous pores along with lipoidal pores — the same way the study on rabbit vaginal barrier suggests that there is the presence of both the pathways lipoidal and aqueous pore.

The study of vaginal absorption of straight chain alkanoic acids in rabbits suggested that permeability coefficient increase as the length of alkyl chain increase but does not correlate linearly with their partition coefficient, indicating neither purely lipophilic nor pure hydrophilic nature.

## Formulation considerations of Buccal Delivery Systems

### Anatomy of the Oral Mucosa

The buccal cavity provides an area of mouth in which lips and cheeks are anteriorly bounded and teeth, gums bounded posteriorly and medially. The buccal glands are positioned between the mucous membrane and buccinator muscle. The surface texture of buccal mucosa is uneven, and its thickness varies from 500-800µm. Due to the rough surface, the buccal mucosa can hold a mucoadhesive drug delivery system. The buccal epithelium is similar to stratified squamous epithelia found in rest of the body. It is about 40–50 cell layers thick.  The non-keratinised stratified squamous epithelium lines the buccal mucosa and having 500-600µ and its surface area of about 50 cm$^2$. Basement membrane, lamina propria is present below the epithelial layer. Lamina propria is rich with blood vessels and capillaries that open to the internal jugular vein.

The oral mucosa consists of three distinctive layers - epithelium, basement membrane, and connective tissues. The buccal cavity is lined with epithelium; supported by a basement membrane which intern is supported by connective tissues. Epithelium, the protective layer is divided into; (a) The surface which is the non-keratinised lining of the soft palate, tongue surface, lips, and vestibule. (b) Hard palate and other non-flexible regions keratinized epithelium present in the oral cavity.

The epithelial cells originate from the basal cells, mature, change their shape, and then increase in size while moving toward the surface. The basement membrane provides mechanical support to the epithelium and forms a distinctive layer between the connective tissues and the epithelium. The underlying connective tissues provide many of the mechanical properties of the oral mucosa. The non-keratinized tissue is a part of buccal epithelium. The connective tissues penetrate the epithelium. These connective tissues are tall and conical in form. These tissues are also referred to as the lamina propria, consisting of collagen fibers, smooth muscles, blood vessels and an underneath film of connective tissues. Lamina propria is followed by the sub mucosa. The external carotid artery supplies blood to the oral mucosa. The main sources of blood supply to the lining of the cheek in the buccal cavity are derived from the buccal artery, some terminal branches of the facial artery, the posterior alveolar artery, and the infra orbital artery.

## Buccal Mucosa

The intercellular ground substance, mucus, surrounds the cells of oral epithelia. The main components of epithelia are proteins and carbohydrates. At physiological pH, the mucus network carries a negative charge (due to sialic acid and sulphate residues) which may play a role in mucoadhesion. At this pH, mucus can form a strongly cohesive gel structure that will bind to the epithelial cell surface as a gelatinous layer.

On the other hand, saliva is the protective fluid for all tissues of the oral cavity. It protects soft tissues from abrasion by rough material and from chemicals. Saliva is an aqueous fluid containing 1% organic and inorganic materials. The major determinant of the salivary composition is its flow rate. It ranges from 0.21 to 1.18 ml/min with a mean of about 0.65 ml/min. The salivary pH ranges from 5.5 to 7 depending on its flow rate. About 0.5 to 2 liters of saliva is formed per day and is available to hydrate oral mucosal dosage forms. The main reason behind the selection of hydrophilic polymeric devices as a vehicle for oral mucosal drug delivery systems is this water-rich environment of the oral cavity.

## Permeability

The oral mucosal epithelium is to some extent leaky. Its characteristics are intermediate between those of the epidermis and intestinal mucosa. The permeability of buccal mucosa is about 4 – 4000 times greater than that of the skin and different regions of the body. Such a difference in permeability of oral cavity is due to its diverse structures and functions. The relative thickness and degree of keratinization of the tissues vary. Both the sublingual mucosa and buccal mucosa are non-keratinized. These differ in thickness. The buccal mucosa is thicker than the sublingual mucosa, and the palatal mucosa is intermediate in thickness but keratinized. The permeability of the oral mucosa is in the decreasing order sublingual >buccal > palatal.

The intercellular ground substance surrounds the oral epithelium known as mucus which envelops the complete oral cavity. Mucus protects the cells under by bounding to the apical cell surface. Primarily mucus consists of about 95–99% water, 0.5– 5% of water-insoluble glycoproteins and several other components in small quantities, such as free proteins (1%), enzymes, electrolytes, and nucleic acids. Mucus behaves like a viscoelastic hydrogel. The composition of mucus varies on the basis of the origin of its secretion in the body. Due to the presence of sialic acid and sulfate residues, the mucus network carries a negative charge at physiological pH. Mucus plays a major role in mucoadhesion by forming a strong cohesive gel structure and is attached to the epithelial cell surface as a gelatinous layer. Depending on the flow rate, the pH of saliva ranges from 5.5 to 7.0. At high flow rates, the pH is proportional to the concentration of sodium and bicarbonate. The daily salivary volume of secretion is between 0.5 to 2 liters and plays a major role in hydrate oral mucosal dosage forms. The main reason behind the selection of hydrophilic polymeric matrices as vehicles for oral transmucosal drug delivery systems is a rich environment of water in the oral cavity.

## Barriers to Penetration Across the Buccal Mucosa

Saliva, mucus, membrane coating granules, basement membrane, etc act as a barrier and retard the rate and extent of drug absorption through the buccal mucosa. The main penetration barrier exists in the outermost quarter to one-third of the epithelium.

- **Saliva:** It moistens the mouth, initiates digestion and protects the teeth from decay. Saliva remains as an unstirred layer. The mucosal surface has a salivary coating about 70 µm thick. Saliva consists of high molecular weight mucin called MG1 which maintains hydration provides lubrication, concentrate protective molecules such as secretory immunoglobulin's and limit the attachment of microorganisms by binding to the surface of the oral cavity. It also controls the bacterial flora of the oral cavity. Because saliva is high in calcium and phosphate, it plays a role in mineralization of new teeth repair and hazardous enamel lesions. It protects the teeth by forming 'protective pellicle'. A constant flow of saliva within the oral cavity makes it very difficult for drugs to be retained for a prolonged period to facilitate absorption at this site. The permeability of different regions of the oral cavity varies greatly due to diverse structures and functions. In general, keratinization of these tissues takes place in the order – sublingual>buccal>palatal. However, the permeability of the buccal mucosa has been found to be 4 – 4000 times greater than that of the skin. The intercellular spaces act as a major source for permeation of hydrophilic compounds. Cell membrane which is lipophilic in nature acts as major transport barrier for lipophilic compounds. Due to a low partition coefficient, it is difficult to permeate through the cell membrane.

- **Basement membrane:** Although the superficial layers of the oral epithelium present the primary barrier to the absorption of substances from the exterior, it is evident that the basement membrane also plays a role in controlling the movement of materials across the junction between epithelium and connective tissue. A similar mechanism appears to operate in the opposite direction. The charge on the constituents of the basal lamina control the rate of penetration of lipophilic compounds. These can cross the superficial epithelial barrier relatively easily.

- **Mucus:** The epithelial cells of buccal mucosa are surrounded by the intercellular ground substance called mucus. The thickness of mucus varies from 40 – 300µm. It acts as an effective delivery vehicle; works as a lubricant allowing cells to move relative to one another. It is believed that it plays a major role in adhesion of bioadhesive drug delivery system. Mucus contains mucins and inorganic salts suspended in water. Mucins are a family of large, heavily glycosylated proteins composed of oligosaccharide chain attached to a protein (core). The composition of mucin is 70–80% carbohydrate, 12–25% protein and 5% ester sulfate About 75% of the protein core are heavily glycosylated and is responsible for a gel-like characteristic of mucus. The water holding capacity of mucins is due to dense sugar coating of mucins. Such dense sugar coating also makes resistant to proteolysis. This may be important for mucosal barrier function.

- **Drug transport mechanisms:** The main mechanisms involved in the penetration of various substances include simple diffusion (paracellular and transcellular), carrier-mediated transport and endocytosis. The passage of drugs across the buccal mucosa follows the mechanism involved in passive diffusion; although it has been reported that carrier-mediated transport plays some role. Depending on the physico chemical properties of the molecule and the type of tissue being traversed, the rate of penetration may vary. The transport of drugs across buccal epithelium may follow different pathways, but their selection depends upon the nature of the permeant, i.e., the overall molecular geometry, lipophilicity, and charge, as well as physiological factors.

## Physiochemical Properties of Drug

- **Molecular size:** For hydrophilic substances, the rate of absorption depends on molecular size. Small molecules (<75 – 100Da) can cross the mucosa rapidly; but, permeability decreases rapidly with an increase in the molecular size of the drug.
- **Lipid solubility:** For any unionizable compound, the relative permeability is a function of its oil-water partition coefficient. The more lipidic compound possesses higher permeability.
- **Ionization:** The degree of ionization of permeant is a function of both its pKa and pH at the mucosal surface. The unionized form of many weak acids and bases show the higher extent of permeabilities for their unionized forms because these possess appreciable lipid solubility. The absorption of many compounds has been found to be maximal at which they are mostly unionized.

## Physiological Factors

- **Inherent permeability of the epithelium:** The permeability of the oral mucosal epithelium is intermediate between that of the skin epithelium and the gut. Skin epithelium is highly specialized for barrier function; while the gut is highly specialized for an adsorptive function. Within the oral cavity, the buccal mucosa is less permeable than the sublingual mucosa.
- **Thickness of epithelium:** The thickness of the oral epithelium varies considerably between sites in the oral cavity. The buccal mucosa measures approximately 500 – 800µm in thickness.
- **Blood supply:** The lamina propria has a rich blood supply and lymphatic network in the oral cavity; thus, drug moieties which traverse the oral epithelium can be readily absorbed into the systemic circulation. The blood flow in the buccal mucosa is 2.4mL per min per cm.
- **Metabolic activity:** Drug substances adsorbed through the oral epithelium can reach directly to the blood. The drugs avoid first-pass metabolism effect at the liver

and gut wall. Thus, oral mucosal delivery may be particularly beneficial for the delivery of enzymatically labile drugs such as therapeutic peptides and proteins.

- **Saliva and mucous:** The main activity of the salivary gland is to wash the oral mucosal surfaces constantly by a stream of saliva, approximately at a rate of 0.5 – 2L per day. The sublingual area is exposed to much saliva which can enhance drug dissolution and therefore, can increase the bioavailability of a drug.

- **Ability to retain the delivery system:** The buccal mucosa comprises smooth and relatively immobile surface; and thus, is ideally suitable for the use of retentive delivery systems.

- **Species differences:** Rodents contain a highly keratinized epithelium; and thus, mucoadhesive drug delivery systems are not very suitable in animal models.

- **Transport routes and mechanism**

  Drug permeation across the epithelium barrier is via two main routes:

  ➤ The paracellular route is between adjacent epithelial cells, and

  ➤ The transcellular route is across the epithelial cells, which can occur by any of the following mechanism – passive diffusion, carrier-mediated transport and via endocytic processes.

## Polymer Properties

The mucoadhesive polymer possesses hydrophilic functional group such as $COOH$, $OH$, $NH_2$, and $SO_4H$, which may be more favorable in formulating targeted drug delivery system. The functional group of polymer interacts with mucus not only through physical entanglement but also through chemical bonding and through cross-linking; for example, urea is well known for disrupting hydrogen bonds. As a result, mucoadhesiveness of mucin/pectin samples decreases the degree of hydration. Hydration is essential for the relaxation and interpenetration of polymer chains. Excess of hydration can lead to decreased mucoadhesion and retention due to the formation of a slippery mucilage. The cross-linked polymers that permit a certain degree of hydration may be beneficial for providing a prolonged mucoadhesive effect. For interpenetration and entanglement with the mucus gel chain length and its flexibility are critical. The properties of polymers are summarized and mentioned below.

1. It must be loaded substantially by the active compound.
2. Swell in the aqueous biological environment of the delivery–absorption site.
3. Interact with mucus or its components for adequate adhesion.
4. When swelled they allow, controlled release of the active compound.
5. Be excreted unaltered or biologically degraded to inactive, non-toxic oligomers.
6. Sufficient quantities of hydrogen bonding chemical groups.
7. Possess high molecular weight.
8. Possess high chain flexibility.
9. Surface tension that will induce spreading into the mucous layer.

- **Molecular weight:** The degree or extent of bioadhesive depends on the type of polymer being used and its molecular weight. For example, polyethylene glycol (PEG) with molecular weight $2\times10^3$ has insignificant adhesive character; but the adhesive character is noticed when its molecular weight is increased to $2\times10^5$ and when the molecular weight increases to $4\times10^5$ appreciable bioadhesive property are observed. Hence, maximum mucoadhesion depends on the type of polymer, its molecular weight and also on the tissue to which the polymer is to adhere.

  Polymers with low molecular weight are suitable for interpenetration; these can penetrate the mucus easily; while high molecular weight polymers exhibit entanglement satisfactorily. Low molecular weight polymers wet easily, form loose gels and can dissolve quickly; while high molecular weight polymers do not moisten easily and their free groups are not exposed for interaction with the substrate.

- **The concentration of active polymer:** To produce desirable adhesion the concentration of a mucoadhesive polymer needs to be optimized. If the concentration of the polymer is increased beyond the optimum level, the adhesive strength reduces significantly; because, the coiled molecules separate from the medium, and availability of chain for penetration becomes limited. Generally, penetration of long-chain polymer into the mucus layer depends on its concentration, particularly when the drug delivery system is liquid and viscous. The concentration of the polymer is important for the development of a strong adhesive bond with mucus. If the concentration of polymer is too less, the number of penetrating polymer chains per unit volume of the volume of mucus becomes less. The effect of polymer concentration depends on the physical state of bioadhesive drug delivery systems.

- **The flexibility of polymer chain:** The mobility and flexibility of polymers are related to their viscosities and diffusion coefficient. If the flexibility of a polymer is high, it can diffuse into mucus. In fact, the interpenetration of chain increases with an increase in structural flexibility of the polymer, even when the polymer is mixed with polyethylene glycol (PEG).

- **Spatial confirmation:** Apart from molecular weight or chain length, the spatial configuration of a polymer molecule is important. For example, dextrans have a molecular weight of 19500 000, but its adhesive strength is similar to that of PEG having a molecular weight of 200 000. The helical configuration of electrons may inactivate many groups active for adhesion unlike PEG polymers. PEG has a linear structure.

- **Hydration:** A mucoadhesive polymer hydrates expand and create a proper 'macromolecular size' to induce mobility in the polymer chain. The mobility of the polymer chain increases interpenetration between polymer and mucins. Swelling is a characteristic property of a polymer and is related to mucoadhesion. Swelling depends on:
  - ➤ The concentration of the polymer,

➢  Its ionic strength, and

➢  The amount of water present.

Maximum bioadhesive requires an optimum amount of water. If the polymer is excessively hydrated (more amount of water is present), the mucilage becomes slippery and loses its adhesive property. During swelling mechanical entanglement due to hydrogen bonding and electrostatic interaction between bioadhesive sites and the polymer (active groups). Thus, when the polymer is adequately hydrated, optimum swelling and bioadhesive occur.

- **Hydrogen bonding capacity:** It has been mentioned earlier that in bioadhesive or mucoadhesion hydrogen bonding plays an important role. For mucoadhesion, the polymer must have functional groups that are capable of forming a hydrogen bond with bioadhesive sites. Hydrogen bonding depends on

  ➢  Presence of capable, functional groups (–COOH, –OH, etc.),

  ➢  The flexibility of the polymer.

  Polymers known for their good hydrogen bonding capacities are poly vinylalcohol, hydroxylated methacrylate, poly methacrylic acid, etc.

- **Cross-linking density:** The structural parameters of a polymer network are –

  ➢  Average pore size,

  ➢  Average molecular weight,

  ➢  Numbers of average cross-linking per mole of the polymer (density of cross-linking).

  These parameters are important as well as interrelated. Thus, water shall diffuse slowly into the polymer network having a higher density of cross-linking. This will result in poor or insufficient swelling of the polymer, and thus, interpenetration between the polymer and mucin shall occur at a slower rate. This has been reported that the degree of swelling of a polymer at equilibrium is inversely related to the degree of cross-linking of the polymer.

- **Charge:** Non-ionic polymers are found to undergo a smaller degree of adhesion than the anionic polymers. The charge on a polymer is important for its bioadhesive property. In fact, for good mucoadhesion, the polymer must have a strong anionic charge. It has also been observed that some cationic polymers demonstrate good bioadhesive; particularly in neutral or slightly alkaline medium. For example, chitosan having a high molecular weight and being cationic demonstrates good adhesive property.

  The strength of mucoadhesion of polymers with carboxylate groups is much stronger than that of polymers having no charge.

# Mucoadhesive Dosage Forms

## Tablets

These are small, flat, and oval, with a diameter of approximately 5–8 mm. Mucoadhesive tablets allow for drinking and speaking without major discomfort. The conventional tablets do not allow the same. The mucoadhesive tablet softens, adheres to the mucosa, and is retained in position until dissolution and release is complete. Generally, these tablets can be used for controlled release drug delivery. Mucoadhesive properties of the tablet have additional advantages; for example, it offers efficient absorption and enhanced bioavailability of the drugs due to a high surface to volume ratio and provides intimate contact with the mucus layer. Mucoadhesive tablets can be tailored to adhere to any mucosal tissue including those found in the stomach, thus offering the possibilities of localized as well as systemic controlled release of drugs. The mucoadhesive tablets capable of being adhered to the mucosal tissues of gastric epithelium is used for administration of drugs for localized action. Mucoadhesive tablets are widely used; because,

- ➢ They release the drug for a prolonged period,
- ➢ Reduce the frequency of drug administration and
- ➢ Improve the patient compliance.

The major drawback of mucoadhesive tablets is their lack of physical flexibility, leading to poor patient compliance for long-term and repeated use.

## Film

Mucoadhesive films may be preferred over adhesive tablets due to their flexibility and comfort. Also, these can avoid the relatively short residence time of oral gels on the mucosa, which are easily washed away and removed by saliva. Moreover, in the case of local delivery for oral diseases, the films also help to protect the wound surface, help to reduce pain, and treat the disease more effectively. An ideal film should be flexible, elastic, and soft, adequately strong to withstand breakage due to stress from mouth movements. It must also possess good mucoadhesive strength so that the film is retained in the mouth for providing prolonged duration of action. Swelling of film, if it occurs, should not be too extensive in order to prevent discomfort.

## Patches

Patches are laminates. These consist of an impermeable backing layer, a drug-containing reservoir layer from which the drug is released in a controlled manner, and a mucoadhesive surface for mucosal attachment. Patches are similar to those used in transdermal drug delivery. Two methods are used to prepare adhesive patches –

- ➢ Solvent casting, and
- ➢ Direct milling.

In the solvent casting method, an intermediate sheet (backing membrane) is prepared first. By punching the membrane, the patches are prepared. After that, by casting the solution of the drug and polymer(s) onto this backing membrane, and subsequently the solvent(s) is allowed to evaporate.

In the direct milling method, constituents of the formulation are homogeneously mixed and compressed to the desired thickness, and patches of predetermined size and shape are then cut or punched out. An impermeable backing layer may also be applied to control the direction of drug release, prevent the drug loss, and minimize deformation and disintegration of the device during the application period.

## Gels and Ointments

Semisolid dosage forms, such as gels and ointments, have the advantage of easy dispersion throughout the oral mucosa. The dose of the drug in semisolid dosage forms may not be as accurate as in tablets, patches, or films. Poor retention of the gels at the site of application has been overcome by using mucoadhesive dosage forms. Certain mucoadhesive polymers, for example, sodium carboxy methylcellulose, carbopol, hyaluronic acid, and xanthan gum, undergo a phase change from liquid to semisolid. This change increases the viscosity, which results in a sustained and controlled release of drugs. Hydrogels are also a promising dosage form for buccal drug delivery. Polymers are used to these formulations that are hydrated in an aqueous environment and physically entrap drug molecules for subsequent slow release by diffusion or erosion. The mucoadhesive gels provide

- ➢ Extended retention time in the oral cavity,
- ➢ Adequate drug penetration, and
- ➢ High efficacy and patient acceptability.

Principally, the adhesive gels are used for the local delivery of medicinal agents during the treatment of periodontitis. This is an inflammatory and infectious disease that causes the formation of pockets between the gum and the tooth, and can eventually cause loss of teeth. The mucoadhesive polymers might be useful for periodontitis therapy when incorporated in antimicrobial formulations that are easily introduced into the periodontal pocket with a syringe. HPMC has been used as an adhesive ingredient in the ointment. Moreover, a highly viscous gel has been developed using carbopol and hydroxypropyl cellulose for ointment dosage forms that could be attached to the tissue for up to 8 hours.

## Common Sites of Application of Mucoadhesive Drug Delivery System

Mucoadhesive formulations have been widely used for targeted and controlled release delivery of drugs. These are applied to many mucosal membrane-based organelles. Such formulations may deliver active ingredient for local or systemic effect. Thereby the enzymatic or hepatic degradation of the drug can be avoided or minimized without compromising the bioavailability.

## Buccal Delivery

For drug delivery, the buccal cavity offers many advantages over many other sites. The most significant advantage is high accessibility and low enzymatic activity. Moreover, the drug delivered through the buccal cavity can be immediately withdrawn in cases of toxicity just by the removal of the dosage form. Thus, this route offers a safe and easy method of drug administration. Various polymers such as sodium carboxy-methyl cellulose, hydroxy propyl cellulose, polycarbophil, etc. have been used for delivery of peptides, protein, and polysaccharides by this route. Although gel and ointments are the most patient favorite; tablets, patches, and films have also been examined. Buccal drug delivery has gained high patient compliance; because of low levels of irritation and significant ease of administration.

## Ophthalmic Delivery

The delivery of drugs to the eye may be achieved using various types of dosage forms including drops, gels, ointments and solid ocular inserts (both degradable and nondegradable). However, delivery through *in-situ* gelling polymer is the most beneficial; because the polymer undergoes a phase transition after application and increases drug-retention time which is most important in case of ophthalmic drug delivery. Mucoadhesive polymers are expected to be the most suitable because they can attach to conjunctival mucus *in vivo*. However, limited bioavailability has been observed *in vivo* for carbomer and polycarbophil, due to their high swelling capacity in the neutral pH environment of the eye. By regulating the pH within the range from 4 – 5 low viscosity can be maintained. However, this low pH is not acceptable, because it may cause patient's unease and mild lacrimation, both of which will have an adverse effect on treatment success.

## Vaginal Delivery

The vagina provides a capable site for systemic drug delivery. There are many advantages of vaginal drug delivery. The important advantages are;
- Hepatic first-pass metabolism can be avoided,
- Hepatic side effects can be decreased, and hence, pain can be avoided,
- Poor tissue damage,
- Large surface area,
- Rich blood supply
- High permeability,

However, it has poor retention due to the self-cleansing action of the vaginal tract is often problematic, residence times within the vagina tend to be much higher than at other absorption sites such as the rectum or intestinal mucosa. Another important consideration is the change in the vaginal membrane during the menstrual cycle and the post-menopausal period. Typical bioadhesive polymers such as polycarbophil, hydroxy propyl cellulose, and polyacrylic acid, have been included in vaginal formulations.

## Nasal Delivery

One of the important advantages provided by intranasal drug delivery is that the nasal cavity provides a large, highly vascularised surface area. Through this route, the first-pass metabolism can be avoided. Blood is drained directly from the nose into the systemic circulation. Effective nasal delivery has been prepared using solutions, powders, gels, and microparticles. The most commonly used intranasal delivery systems are solutions containing sympathomimetic vasoconstrictors for immediate relief of nasal congestion. Local delivery of alpha-adrenergic stimulators is important to the patients with high blood pressure, as vasoconstriction will occur to the greatest degree within the nose. In addition to local effects, the drug administered through the intranasal route has also been used to achieve a distal systemic effect.

## Bibliography


1. A.H. Shojaei, Buccal mucosa as a route for systemic drug delivery: a review, J. Pharm. Pharmaceut. Sci., 1(1) (1998) 15-30.
2. A.H. Shojaei, R.K. Chang, B.A. Burnside, R.A. Couch, Systemic drug delivery via the buccal mucosal route, Pharm. Tech., (2001) 70-81.
3. C.S. Yong, J.H. Jung, J.D. Rhee, C.K. Kim, H.G. Choi, Physiochemical characterization and evaluation of buccal adhesive tablets containing omeprazole, Drug Dev. Ind. Pharm., 27 (5) (2001) 447-455.
4. Duchene, G. Ponchel, Bioadhesion of solid oral dosage forms, why and how? Eur. J. Pharm. Biopharm., 44 (1997) 15-23.
5. Gupta, S. Garg, R.K. Khar, Mucoadhesive buccal drug delivery system-A Review, Indian Drugs, 29 (13) (1992) 586-593.
6. Harris, J.R. Robinson, Drug delivery via mucous membrane of the oral cavity, J. Pharm. Sci., 81(1) (1992) 1-10.
7. L. Martin, C.G. Wilson, F. Koosha, I.F. Uchegbu, Sustained buccal delivery of hydrophobic drug denbufylline using physically cross linked palmitoyl chitosan hydrogels, Eur. J. Pharm. Biopharm., 55 (2003) 35-45.
8. M.S.Wani, S.R. Parakh, M.H. Dehghan, S.A. Polshettiwar, V.V. Pande, V.V. Chopade, Current Status In Buccal Drug Delivery. www.pharmainfo.net as on 28 April (2007).
9. P. Sriamornsak, S. Sungthongjeen, Modification of theophylline release with alginate gel formed in hard capsules, AAPS PharmSciTech.,8(3) (2007) Article 51.
10. R. Khanna, S.P. Agarwal, A. Ahuja, Mucoadhesive buccal drug delivery -A potential to conventional therapy, Ind. J. Pharm. Sci., 60 (1) (1998) 1-11.

11. S.K. Gupta, I.J. Singhavi, M. Shirsat, G. Karwani, A. Agrawal, A. Agrawal, Buccal adhesive drug delivery system: a review, Asian J. Biochemical and pharmaceutical research, 2(1) (2011) 105-114.

12. T.M. Pramodkumar, K.G. Desai, H.G. Shivakumar, Mechanism of buccal permeation enhancers, Ind. J. Pharm. Edu., 36 (3) (2002) 147-152.

13. V.H.K. Li, J.R. Robinson, V.H.L. Lee, Influence of drug properties and routes of drug administration on the design of sustained and controlled release system. In: Robinson J R and Lee VHL (Eds.), Controlled drug delivery: fundamental and applications, 2nd ed. Marcel Dekker, Inc. New York, 1987: 42-43.

14. V.M. Patel, B.G. Prajapati, M.M. Patel, Design and characterization of chitosan-containing mucoadhesive buccal patches of propranolol hydrochloride, Acta Pharm., 57 (2007) 61-72.

15. V.M. Patel, B.G. Prajapati, M.M. Patel, Effect of hydrophilic polymers on buccoadhesive Eudragit patches of propranolol hydrochloride using factorial design, AAPS Pharm. Sci. Tech., 8(2) (2007) Article 45.

16. Vijayraghavan, T.K. Ravi, Buccal delivery of Nifedepine using novel natural mucoadhesive polymer as an excipient in buccal tablets, Indian Drugs, 41(3) (2004) 143-148.

17. Y. Kohda, et.al., Controlled release of lidocaine hydrochloride from buccal mucosa-adhesive films with solid dispersion, Int. J. Pharm., 158(2) (1997) 147-155.

18. Y. Sudhakar, K. Kuotsu, A.K. Bandyopadhyay, Buccal bioadhesive drug delivery - A promising option for orally less efficient drugs, J. Contr. Rel., 114 (2006) 15–40.

19. Y.V. Vishnu, K. Chandrasekhar, G. Ramesh, Y.M. Rao, Development of mucoadhesive patches for buccal administration of carvedilol, Current Drug Delivery, 4 (2007) 27-39.

# Exercise

## A. Multiple Choice Questions

1. Adhesion refers to
   (a) The molecular force of attraction in the area of contact between unlike bodies that acts to hold them together.
   (b) The molecular force of attraction in the area of contact between like bodies that acts to hold them together.
   (c) The molecular force of attraction in the area of contact between unlike bodies that acts to keep them away.
   (d) None of the above

2. Bioadhesion refers only to the
   (a) Adhesion between two biological bodies.
   (b) Adhesion between one biological body and any of the other type.
   (c) Adhesion either between two biological bodies or between one biological body and any of the other type.
   (d) Adhesion between two bodies.

3. Mucoadhesion refers only to
    (a) Adhesion between two biological bodies.
    (b) Adhesion between one biological body and any of the other type.
    (c) Adhesion either between two biological bodies or between one biological body and any of the other type.
    (d) Adhesion between one biological membrane and any of the other type.

4. Materials are attached to each other through
    (a) Intermolecular force
    (b) Interfacial forces
    (c) Chemical forces
    (d) All of the above

5. Mucoadhesive materials are activated for adhesion by
    (a) Moisture present in mucous membrane
    (b) Enzyme present in the environment
    (c) van der Waals forces
    (d) Hydrogen bonding

6. The consolidation stage of mucoadhesion involves
    (a) Spreading of the formulation
    (b) Swelling of the formulation
    (c) Initiating its deep contact with the mucus layer.
    (d) None of the above

7. Through diffusion the rate of permeation depends on
    (a) Flexibility of the mucoadhesive system
    (b) Nature of the mucoadhesive chains
    (c) Contact time
    (d) All of the above

8. Environmental factor influences the rate of permeation of drug through membrane is
    (a) pH
    (b) Molecular weight
    (c) Chain flexibility
    (d) Concentration of drug

9. Intrinsic factor of the polymer that influences the rate of permeation of drug through membrane is
    (a) Swelling
    (b) Physiological variation
    (c) Chain flexibility
    (d) pH

10. Which of the following does not influence rate of permeation of drug through membrane
    (a) Molecular weight of the polymer
    (b) Adhesive strength
    (c) Contact time
    (d) Swelling

11. Which of the following statements is correct?
    (a) Mucoadhesive drug delivery system can reduce the dose related side effects.
    (b) Mucoadhesive drug delivery system cannot be used as sustained drug delivery system.
    (c) Mucoadhesive drug delivery system can be used to deliver peptides.
    (d) Mucoadhesive drug delivery system cannot withstand change of pH, temperature, etc.

12. Which of the following statements is correct?
    (a) Oral mucosa consists of only one layer – epithelium
    (b) Oral mucosa consists of only one layer – lamina propria
    (c) Oral mucosa consists of three layers – epithelium, lamina propria and connective tissues.
    (d) Oral mucosa consists of only one layer – connective tissues.

13. Under normal conditions the flow rate of saliva is
    (a) 0.65*l*ts/hr
    (b) 0.65ml/min
    (c) 0.65m*l*/sec
    (d) 0.65lt/min

14. Which of the following statements is correct?
    (a) Permeability of oral mucosa in various areas of oral cavity is buccal >sublingual >palatal
    (b) Permeability of oral mucosa in various areas of oral cavity is buccal <sublingual <palatal
    (c) Permeability of oral mucosa in various areas of oral cavity is buccal >sublingual >palatal<buccal
    (d) Permeability of oral mucosa in various areas of oral cavity is sublingual >buccal >palatal

15. Which of the following statements is correct?
    (a) Under normal condition the pH of saliva ranges from 5.5 to 7.0 and depends on its flow rate.
    (b) Under normal condition the pH of saliva ranges from 3.5 to 5.0 and is independent on its flow rate.
    (c) Under normal condition the pH of saliva ranges from 3.5 to 10.0 and depends on its flow rate.
    (d) None of the above.

16. Which of the following statements is correct?
    (a) The permeability of the buccal mucosa is greater than that of the skin.
    (b) The permeability of the buccal mucosa is equal to that of the skin.
    (c) The permeability of the buccal mucosa is less than that of the skin.
    (d) None of the above

17. Which of the following statements is correct?
    - (a) A mucoadhesive polymer should have high drug loading capacity, low swelling capacity, high chain flexibility and a large number of hydrogen bonding groups.
    - (b) A mucoadhesive polymer should have high drug loading capacity, low swelling capacity, less chain flexibility and a large number of hydrogen bonding groups.
    - (c) A mucoadhesive polymer should have high drug loading capacity, high swelling capacity, high chain flexibility and a large number of hydrogen bonding groups.
    - (d) A mucoadhesive polymer should have high drug loading capacity, low swelling capacity, high chain flexibility and a smaller number of hydrogen bonding groups.

18. Which of the following statements is correct?
    - (a) Swelling of a polymer depends on concentration of polymer
    - (b) Swelling of a polymer depends on ionic strength of the polymer
    - (c) Swelling of a polymer depends on the amount of water present
    - (d) All of the above

19. Which of the following statements is correct?
    - (a) Non-ionic polymers exhibit good adhesion property
    - (b) Non-ionic polymers exhibit poor adhesion property
    - (c) Cationic polymers exhibit poor adhesion property
    - (d) Anionic polymers exhibit poor adhesion property

20. Which of the following statements is correct?
    - (a) Mucins contain large amount of carbohydrate
    - (b) Mucins contain small amount of carbohydrate
    - (c) Mucins contain large amount of proteins
    - (d) Mucins contain large amount of lipids

## B. Short Questions

1. What is the difference between the term bioadhesion and mucoadhesion?
2. Briefly discuss the pros and cons of buccal drug delivery system over the oral and parenteral route.
3. Discuss the wetting theory of bioadhesion with a labeled diagram.
4. Write a brief note on polymers used for the preparation of buccoadhesive dosage form.
5. What are the approaches to enhance drug permeation across biological membranes.

## C. Long Questions

1. Define the term bioadhesion. Write a detailed note on different theories of mucoadhesion.

2. Explain in detail about the anatomy of the oral mucosa.

3. Write in detail about various mucoadhesive dosage form with suitable example. Write the name of any 5 commercially available bioadhesive product.

4. Write a detail note on drug permeation along with the barriers of drug permeation across buccal mucosa.

5. Enlist various factor influencing the rate of drug permeation across the buccal mucosa and development of buccal drug delivery system with a suitable description of each.

## CHAPTER 5

# Implantable Drug Delivery Systems

---

*Introduction, advantages and disadvantages, concept of implants and osmotic pump.*

---

## Introduction

The orally administered drug must be protected from degradation in the gastrointestinal tract, and the drug should be absorbed across the wall of the stomach or the intestine. After absorption and reaching the portal circulation, it must resist the hepatic enzymes. The rate of drug absorption and elimination should ensure the blood levels within the therapeutic window. Moreover, the amount of intact drug that reaches the site of action should be sufficiently large to obtain the desired therapeutic effect; but, should not cause any untoward side effects.

Effective plasma concentration of drug the can be maintained for an extended period by the technique such as continuous intravenous infusion or repeated injections. The patients are regularly required to visit the hospital for administration of the drug and continuous medical monitoring. A short-acting medicine deteriorates the condition; since the number of injections or the infusion needs to be administered to maintain a therapeutically effective level of the drug is more.

It was accidentally discovered that silicone elastomers permeate at a controlled rate. It is reported that in 1961 silicone capsules containing pyrimethamine were used to protect the chicks from malaria. After that, the concept of controlled drug delivery became the point of attention and researches went on. A controlled drug action may be achieved by either chemical modification of the drug or by modification of formulation in a specific way to control its release. There are some oral controlled- release dosage forms can provide efficacy for about 24 hours. The main limitation of such oral dosage form is the long transit time, approximately 12 hours through the gastrointestinal tract (GIT). If a drug cannot be administered orally, an alternative route is a parenteral route. Many proteins or peptides and other drugs are susceptible to the adverse conditions of GIT, and these are administered intravenously. Unfortunately, most of the drugs administered intravenously show the short duration of action; and therefore, frequent injections are required. The development of injectable controlled-release dosage forms is more likely to succeed commercially than other routes; although it is assumed that these dosage forms provide the desired efficacy and safety. In case of topical drug administration, most drugs show limited percutaneous absorption due to physiological characteristics of the drugs and presence of highly impermeable stratum corneum. Such limitations are not seen in case of implantable drug delivery devices as associated with oral, intravenous, topical drug administration. Implantable drug delivery devices offer one unique advantage of a retrievable mechanism. For the integration of various therapeutic agents with different physicochemical characteristics and the improved mechanism of drug release, some additives are used. Thus, more current implantable formulations generally are prepared with the therapeutic agent in a rate controlling systems. Implantable formulations are available in various sizes and shapes. Although oral delivery is considered the preferred method of administration of most drugs, additional methods are being employed. Pulmonary, infusion, and implantable systems have been developed to overcome drug delivery constraints; for example, many macromolecules are either digested in the gastrointestinal tract or are not well absorbed into the bloodstream. Oral administration may also not be appropriate for drugs that require rapid onset of action. Similarly, drugs that are readily absorbed into the blood from the lungs can be administered through pulmonary route; such as inhalers. Drug delivery by injection has other disadvantages. Patients cannot receive an injection while traveling; either he/she has to be at home or a treatment site. Moreover, the discomfort of frequent injections leads to poor patient compliance. Finally, a multiple, timed drug-injection regimen is complicated to administer and may require a clinician's help. Portable infusion system allows unassisted intravenous administration; however, these systems can only be used to deliver drugs in liquid form and needs both a transcutaneous catheter and an external pump. Completely implantable drug delivery devices are required where alternate forms of delivery are not preferred or not feasible. These devices allow drugs to be delivered at efficacious locations without the issue of patient compliance. An advanced implantable system can be used to precisely control the rate of drug delivery. Some drugs exert therapeutic action when administered in a pulsatile pattern, similar to the way they are produced in the body. Alternatively, some therapies require drugs to be released continuously to maintain a constant therapeutic level for an extended period. Pulmonary, transdermal, intravenous or subcutaneous injection or infusion, and implantable systems have been developed; because oral drug delivery is not feasible. Implantable drug delivery devices are desirable when compliance with a prescribed drug regimen is critical. Such tools allow a drug to be delivered at a specific rate without regular physician or patient intervention. Currently available implants for drug delivery can be divided into two main categories, based on whether they deliver the drug passively or actively. (1) Polymer depots are the most common passive drug delivery systems. These are designed to maintain a constant rate of diffusion of the drug from the polymer, or (2) they degrade in the body at a particular rate, thereby releasing drug at that rate. Conventional programmable implantable drug delivery systems (DDD) are provided 25-50% of the volume of implanted device for a battery that is intended to work during 5-10 years (life of the implant). Typical IDDDs medication is typically refilled every 10 weeks by transdermal injection into a subcutaneous refill port.

The implantable therapeutic systems are mainly developed for;

- Long-term,
- Continuous drug administration, and
- Controlled release.

Ideal requirements of implantable drug delivery systems are;

- Environmentally stable.
- Biocompatible.
- Sterile.
- Biostable.
- Improve patient compliance by reducing the frequency of drug administration over the entire period of treatment.
- Release the drug in a rate-controlled manner that leads to enhanced effectiveness and reduction in side effects.
- Readily retrievable by medical personnel to terminate medication. Easy to manufacture and relatively inexpensive.

## Advantages

During the selection of materials, the methods of manufacture, the degree of drug loading, drug release rate, etc. should be considered. From a regulatory view point, it is regarded as a new product and can lengthen the market protection of the drug for an additional 5 years (for a new drug entry) or 3 years (for existing drugs).

The **advantages** of the implantable drug-delivery system are summarized below:

- Improved efficiency,
- Very effective,
- A small dose is sufficient to elicit the action. For example, progesterone 2–8 mg
- Reduced side effects,
- On-spot delivery,
- Convenient therapy,
- Provide linear delivery for long periods, from a few weeks to many months,
- Plasma drug levels are continuously maintained in a therapeutically desirable range,
- Harmful side effects from systemic administration can be reduced or eliminated by local administration from a controlled release system,
- Drug administration may be improved and facilitated in underprivileged areas where proper medical supervision is not available,
- Administration of drugs having short in vivo half-lives may be significantly facilitated,
- Continuous small amounts of drug may be less painful than several large doses.

- ➤ Patient compliance may be improved,
- ➤ Relatively less expensive and less wasteful of the drug.

Implantation treatment permits the patients to get medication outside the hospital with marginal medical observation. In comparison to an in dwelling catheter-based infusion system, the treatment with implantation is characterized by a lower chance of infection and associated problems. The drug is distributed locally or in systemic circulation with minimum interference by metabolic or biological barriers. The drug can bypass the GIT and the liver, the major sites of drug metabolism. The by-passing effect is beneficial to drugs, which are either easily inactivated or absorbed poorly in the GIT and the liver before systemic distribution. The patient can forget to take a medicine, but continuous drug release can be maintained from an implant and is not dependent on patient input. Periodical refilling is required in some implants; but, despite this limitation, the patient has less involvement in delivering the required medication. Ideal implants should follow zero-order controlled release kinetics. The advantages of zero-order controlled release are:

(a) Peaks (toxicity) and troughs (ineffectiveness) of conventional therapy can be avoided,

(b) Dosing frequency can be reduced,

(c) Patient compliance would be increased.

Bio-responsive release from implants is an area of on-going research. Intermittent release can be facilitated by externally programmable pumps. The periodic release can promote drug release, but the release depends on:

(a) Circadian rhythms,

(b) Fluctuating metabolic requirements,

(c) Pulsatile release of many peptides and proteins.

## Disadvantages

- ➤ Invasive. The therapy requires either a minor or a major surgical procedure. Thus, trained surgical personnel would be necessary for this, and may be time-consuming, traumatic.
- ➤ Chance of adverse reactions. May cause some scar formation at the site of implantation, and in a minimal number of patients, surgery-related complications may be observed.
- ➤ Uncomfortable feeling for the patients wearing the device.
- ➤ Risk of device failure. There is no associated danger with this treatment when the device may fail to work for some reason. This again requires surgical involvement to rectify.
- ➤ Termination. Osmotic pumps and non-biodegradable polymeric implants also are surgically removed at the end of therapy. The surgical recovery is not required in case of biodegradable polymeric implants. Its on-going biodegradation makes it

difficult to end drug delivery, or to maintain the accurate dose at the end of its lifetime.

➤ Limited to potent drugs. To minimize the patient's discomfort, the size of an implant is usually kept small. Therefore, most implants have a limited loading capacity; hence, for the delivery of potent medicines such as hormones may be appropriate for delivery through implantable devices.

➤ Biocompatibility. Body reactions to a foreign substance often increase the issues of biocompatibility and safety of an implant.

➤ Unsuitable for all drugs. A high concentration of the drug cannot be delivered by an implantable device; because at the implantation site, it may produce adverse reactions.

## Concept of Implants

A variety of dosage forms and dosage levels of a particular drug are being manufactured and marketed by pharmaceutical industries. The purpose of this activity is to make the physician enable to control the onset and duration of action of a drug during treatment therapy by changing the dose and mode of administration. Sometimes, the drug-drug interaction that can affect the disposition of another drug is used to control the therapy; for example, inhibition of the elimination of penicillin by probenecid can be used to prolong the therapeutic effect of penicillin. Moreover, there are examples where one drug can potentiate, synergize, or antagonize the other drug, if administered simultaneously. Similarly, a drug can be formulated in such a way that the rate and extent of drug-absorption is modified as per requirement. Implants come under this category. The advantages of implants and limitations of conventional dosage forms have been mentioned earlier. The purpose of developing implants in simple words is to control the rate of drug release in such a way that the drug can exert its therapeutic action over a long period may be for few months or year. This type of products includes inserts (implants) which are placed inside the body.

Ideally, implants should have specific characteristics such as

- A high ratio of drug to polymer,
- Good mechanical strength
- Free from drug leakage,
- Easily sterilizable,
- Easy to manufacture,
- Zero-order drug release,
- Biocompatible,
- Non-toxic,
- Non-immunogenic,
- Non-mutagenic,
- Non-carcinogenic and

- Economic.

Based on these characteristics the design of IDDSs depend on

- The properties of drug,
- A side effect of drugs,
- Targeted site, and
- The type of disease.

The rate of drug release from an implant can be regulated by its shape and size, and on the selection of polymer(s) materials for its manufacture. In the case of all dynamic systems, internal packaging of components, as well as the design of drug storage volumes, may be critically examined. The concept of implantable drug delivery system lies on modification of release characteristics of the drug from the dosage form. There are two concepts based on which implantable therapeutic systems are developed.

1. Diffusion controlled-release

2. Activated controlled-release

1. **Diffusion controlled-release system:** This type of systems may be prepared by following release characteristics. By modifying the release characteristics, three types of products may be developed.

(a) *Membrane permeation-controlled system*: In this system, the reservoir of drug is entirely enclosed by a polymeric membrane which can control the rate of release of the drug. In the reservoir, the drug may remain as solid particles, or in the form of a solid

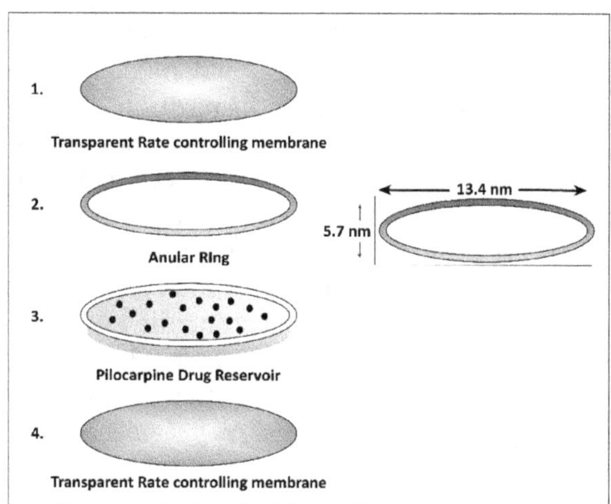


**Fig. 5.1:** Schematic representation of pilocarpine occusert.

or liquid dispersion or solution. The membrane can be fabricated from a homogeneous or heterogeneous non-porous polymer. However, this membrane may be microporous or a semipermeable type. Encapsulation of drug-reservoir can be done by molding, or encapsulation, or microencapsulation, or any other suitable method. The device may be of different sizes and shapes. This system is composed of any of the three types of membranes. The drug released, diffuses out of the membrane and is absorbed. Based on the kind of release of the drug, membranes may be classified as;

- Nonporous membrane
- Microporous membrane
- Semipermeable membrane

**Occusert** system is a device containing solid drug reservoir in a thin disc of pilocarpine alginate. The disc is placed in between two transparent sheets of the microporous membrane of ethylene-vinyl acetate copolymer. Such a system is designed for management of glaucoma. At a constant rate of $20 - 40$ µg/hr the drug, pilocarpine can penetrate the microporous membrane.

Similarly, **Progestasert IUD** (intrauterine device) shown in figure 5.2, is a device containing a suspension of progesterone in liquid silicone polymer. It can release about 65µg of progesterone per hour locally in the uterine cavity.

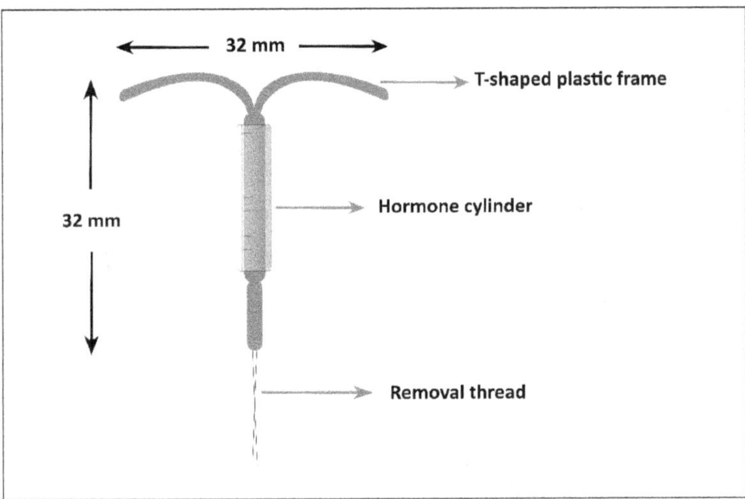


**Fig. 5.2:** Schematic representation of progestasert.

(b) **Matrix diffusion-controlled system:** This type of implantable therapeutic system is prepared using a suitable polymer. The polymers used in matrix diffusion-controlled systems can be classified into three categories;

- Lipophilic polymers
- Hydrophilic or swellable polymer
- Porous polymer

This type of device is designed to deliver drug at a controlled rate. The drug reservoir contains a homogeneous dispersion of solid drug particles in a hydrophilic or lipophilic polymer matrix.

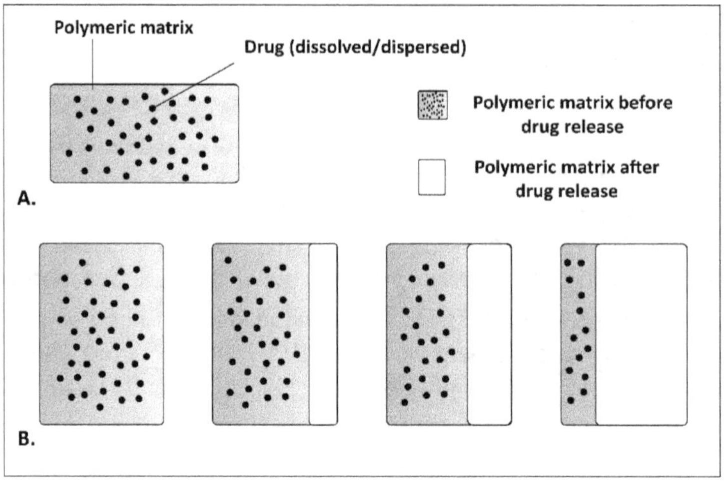

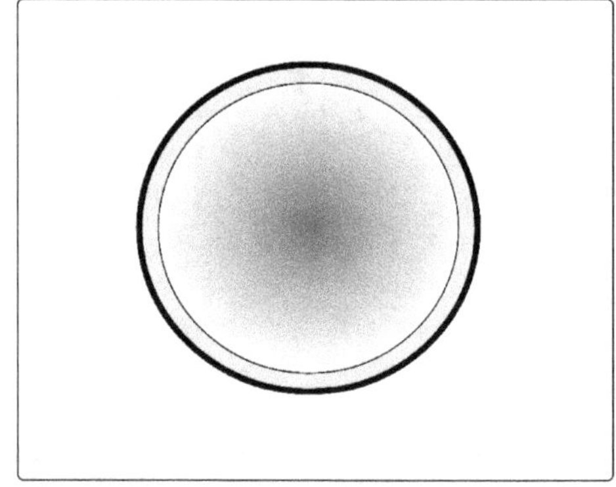

**Fig. 5.3:** Schematic representation of matrix type implant; (A) Implant and (B) Release of drug with time.

The dispersion can be made by any one of the following ways - (1) by mixing the solids (drug) with a suitable polymer which is viscous liquid, (2) by mixing with a semisolid polymer at room temperature, (3) mixing with a melted polymer at higher temperature (4) by combining with polymer solution in organic solvent; the solvent is then removed by evaporation. The drug-polymer blend is then extruded to form a drug delivery device. The size and shape of the devices may vary. Some common examples are;

**Fig. 5.4:** Schematic diagram of contraceptive vaginal ring.

**The contraceptive vaginal ring** is used to administer contraceptive steroid into the vagina. It contains a dispersion of micronized solid drug particles are homogeneously dispersed in a viscous mixture of silicone elastomer and catalyst. The dispersion is then filled into a donut-shaped vaginal ring. The ring is inserted into the vagina and placed around the cervix; so that a constant plasma progestin level and cyclic intravaginal contraception can be maintained for 21 days. There are other implants of this category such as Syncro-Mate-B implant, Compudose implant.

**(c)** **Micro-reservoir dissolution-controlled system:** As the name implies, this type of implantable therapeutic system may be prepared using two forms of the reservoir system.

- Hydrophilic reservoir/lipophilic matrix
- Lipophilic reservoir/hydrophilic matrix

This type of implant is used for controlled delivery of drug from the drug reservoir. Fine crystals or particles of the drug is dispersed in aqueous solution of a polymer or polymer solution in a water miscible solvent. Thus, homogeneous dispersion of minute drug particles is obtained in the polymer matrix as shown in figure 5.5. The micro-dispersion of drug particles is prepared by high-energy dispersion technique. Different shapes and sizes of drug delivery devices of this micro-reservoir can be made by molding or extrusion technique. The device can be coated with a layer biocompatible polymer to modify the mechanism and rate of drug release. However, this depends on the physicochemical properties of the drug and the desired rate of drug release.

Syncro-Mate-C implant, Dual-release vaginal contraceptive ring, etc. are of this type of implantable drug delivery system.

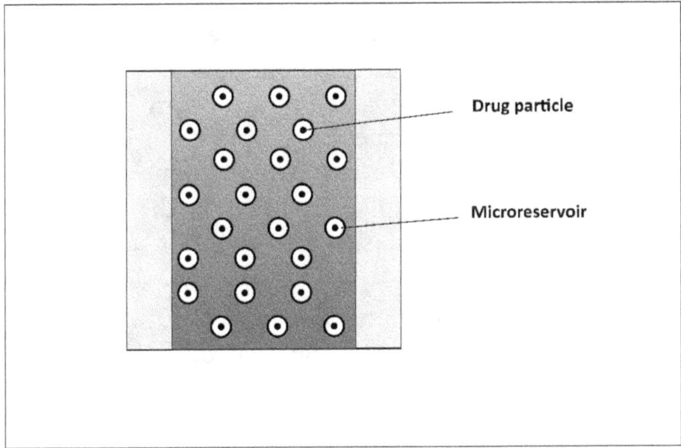


**Fig. 5.5:** Schematic diagram of Microreservoir type drug delivery system.

### Syncro-Mate-C Implant

This is a cylindrical type of implant. This provides a better release rate of the drug and relatively inexpensive than a Syncro-Mate-B implant. The drug such as norgestomet is dispersed homogeneously in an aqueous solution of polyethylene glycol 400 (PEG 400). This dispersion is further dispersed in a viscous mixture of silicone elastomers using a high-energy dispersion technique. Then, a suitable catalyst is mixed with the dispersion. The homogeneous mixture is filled into silicone tubing of medical grade. This serves as the mold and also as the coating membrane by an extrusion technique.

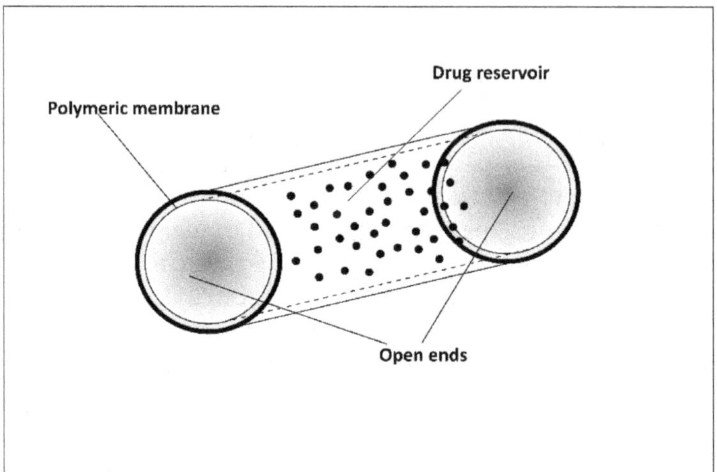


**Fig. 5.6:** Schematic diagram of Microreservoir type - Syncro-Mate-C Implant.

This polymerized solid drug-polymer mixture is then cut into small cylindrical shaped drug delivery devices as shown in figure 5.6. The device has two open ends. Such tiny cylinder is implanted into subdermal tissue to deliver the drug (e.g., norgestomet) by a special implanter. Usually, the implant is administered into the animal's ear flap for control and synchronization of estrus and ovulation. The implant remains at the site of administration for about 20 days; so that stable plasma concentration and better therapeutic effect is obtained.

2. **Activated controlled-release system:** This type of formulation is designed by the particular mechanism which activates the system for release of drug from the system.

There are various devices of this category are available to deliver the drug at a controlled rate. There are five systems which work on activated controlled-release concept.

   (a)   Osmotic pressure activated system

   (b)   Vapour pressure activated system

   (c)   Magnetically activated system

   (d)   Hydrolysis activated system

   (e)   Ultrasound activated system.

   (a)   **Osmotic pressure activated system:** The drug reservoir is a solution contained within a semipermeable housing. The drug is released in solution form at a controlled and constant rate under an osmotic pressure gradient.

### Alzet osmotic pump

This device works under the osmotic pressure gradient. Inside a collapsible, impermeable polyester bag the drug is kept. The external surface of the bag is coated with a layer of an osmotically active salt. The drug reservoir compartment is sealed within a rigid housing made of the semipermeable polymer membrane. When the device is implanted, at the implantation site the water from the tissue migrates through the semipermeable membrane and dissolve the osmotically active salt. As a result, osmotic pressure is created at the narrow space in between flexible reservoir wall and the rigid semipermeable housing. Under this osmotic pressure gradient, the volume of the reservoir compartment gets reduced, and the drug in a solution state is forced to be released at a controlled rate through the flow moderator. The amount of drug released can be varied by varying the concentration of the drug solution. The schematic diagram of the Alzet osmotic pump is shown in figure 5.7.

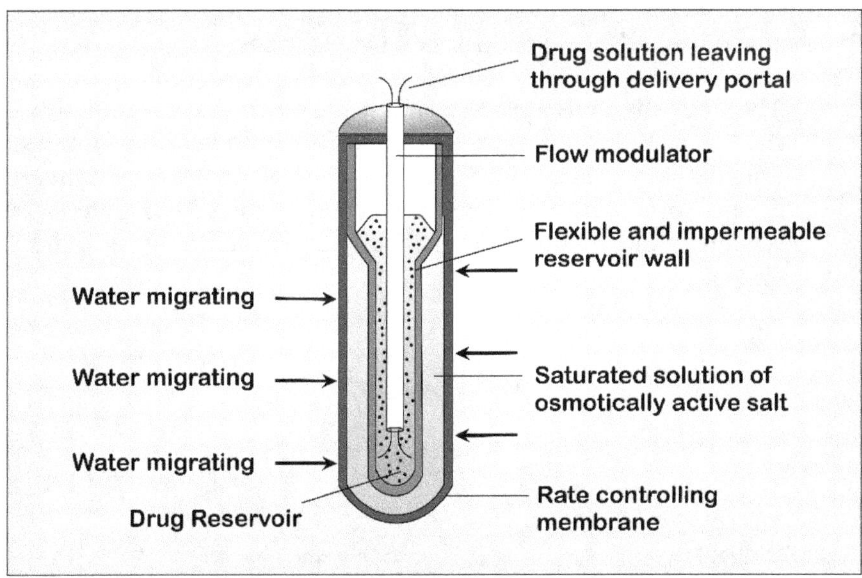


**Fig. 5.7:** Schematic diagram of Alzet osmotic pump.

**(b) Vapour pressure activated system:** In this type of system, the drug reservoir in the form of the solution remains inside an Infusate chamber. The chamber is separated from the vapor chamber by freely moveable bellows. A volatile liquid such as fluorocarbon is placed in the vapor chamber. The liquid vaporizes at the body temperature and creates vapor pressure. There is a series of flow regulator and a delivery cannula attached to the device. When the device is implanted into the body tissues and vapor pressure increases, the bellows move upwards and imparts force the drug solution present in the Infusate to release. The drug releases through the flow regulator and cannula into the bloodstream at a constant rate. Infusaid is a marketed product used to administer insulin, or heparin, or morphine. A schematic diagram of such a system is shown in figure 5.8.

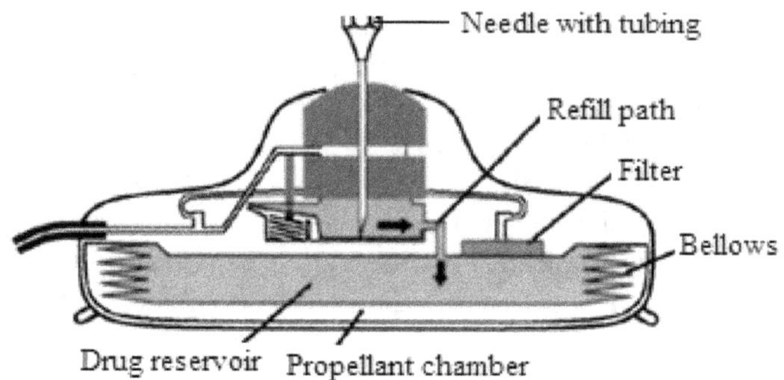


**Fig. 5.8:** Schematic diagram of vapour activated implant device.

**(c) Magnetically activated system:** It is known that macromolecular drugs such as peptides are released at a relatively lower rate from a polymeric drug delivery system. By using tiny magnets in the drug delivery system, a zero- order drug release rate can be achieved. Figure 5.9 shows a schematic diagram of a magnetically controlled polymeric drug delivery system.

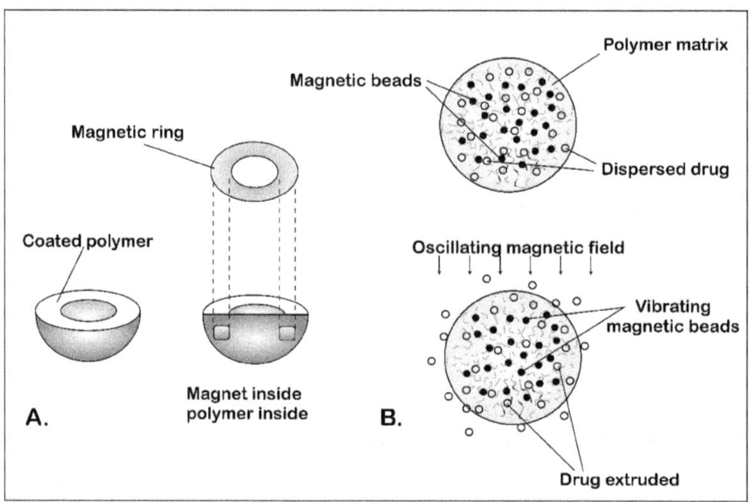


**Fig. 5.9:** Schematic diagram of a magnetically controlled polymeric drug delivery system; (A) Single unit and (B) Drug delivery system.

Such a device is fabricated by placing a donut-shaped magnet at the center of a biocompatible polymer matrix. The system contains a homogeneous dispersion of a macromolecular drug. The drug: polymer ratio is relatively high. The polymeric matrix forms a hemispheric magnetic pellet. The pellet is then coated with a suitable polymer such as ethylene-vinyl acetate (EVA) copolymers or silicone elastomers. Except for a cavity at the center of the flat surface, all surfaces of the pellet are coated. From the central cavity, the macromolecular drug is released at a controlled basal rate by diffusion process under non-triggered condition. When the system is activated by an external magnetic field, the drug is released at a much higher rate.

**(d)**    **Hydrolysis activated system:** This type of drug delivery system is prepared by dispersing a loading dose of solid micronized drug particles in a biodegradable or bioerodible polymer matrix. The homogeneous mixture of drug and polymer is then molded into pellet or beads shaped implants: the embedded drug particles released at a controlled rate due to hydrolysis and erosion of the polymer, and subsequent diffusion of the drug through the polymer matrix.

The rate of drug release depends on –

   (i)   the rate of bioerosion or biodegradation,

   (ii)   polymer composition,

   (iii)   molecular weight,

   (iv)   drug loading, and

   (v)   the interaction between drug and polymer.

Naltrexone pellets have been prepared following this principle and using poly (lactide/glycolide) copolymer for the treatment of opioid-dependent addiction. Other biodegradable or bioerodible polymers can be used for the same purpose. The polymers are a polysaccharide, polypeptide, and homopolymer of polylactide and polyglycolide.

A new biodegradable polymer – poly (ortho esters) has been synthesized and used to prepare a controlled release contraceptive (device) for the release of levonorgestrel (steroid).

The erosion rate of such polymer depends on the pH of the medium; hence, a suitable buffering agent such as calcium chloride is mixed with the polymer. In contact with water, calcium chloride or the buffer present solubilizes in water and produce the desired pH. If the polymer used is very hydrophobic, the buffering agent present at the surface layer of the pellet would be eroded first, and then the polymer will hydrolyze. As a result, the drug will be released at a constant zero order. Such a system has been depicted in figure 5.10.

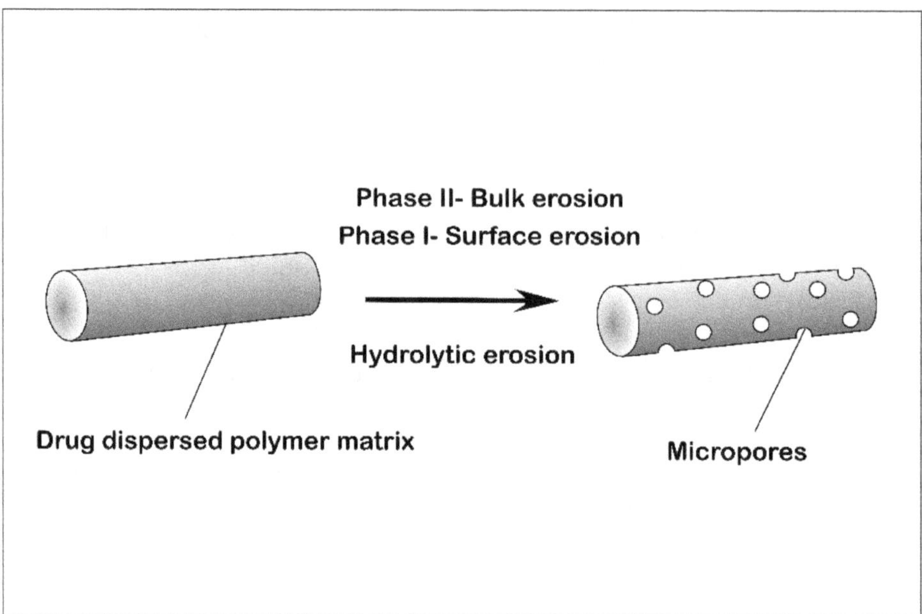


**Fig. 5.10:** Schematic diagram of hydrolysis activated implant system.

(e)    **Ultrasound activated system:** This type of system utilizes ultrasonic wave as the source of energy. Hence, such system can release the drug at a relatively higher rate from the polymeric matrix. The device contains a bioerodible polymer matrix such as poly [bis (þ-carboxyphenoxy) alkane anhydride]. The rate and extent of drug release can be controlled by ultrasonic wave.

# Mechanisms of Drug Release from Implantable Drug Delivery Systems

Generally, the drug to polymer ratio is high in implants. The implants should have excellent mechanical strength and no drug-leakage. These should be efficiently and economically manufactured. The drug release from implants is expected to follow zero-order kinetics. Most importantly, the implants must be biocompatible, non-toxic, non-immunogenic, non-mutagenic and non-carcinogenic. The rate of drug release from an implant depends on its shape and size, and the polymer(s) used to manufacture an implant. Primarily, the drug particles diffuse the polymer membrane or from the polymer matrix and are released. The diffusion of drug particles may be expressed as Fickian or non-Fickian diffusion.

The device or system may contain either a solution or dispersion of drug substances.

## Classification of Implants

Based on the route of administration implants can be classified as;

1. Subdermal implants
2. Intraocular implant/Occusert
3. Intravaginal insert
4. Intrauterine implant
5. Brain implant
6. Gliadel implant
7. Cochlear implant
8. Fetal Tissue implant
9. Harrington implant
10. Dental implant
11. Extraocular implant
12. Scrotal implant
13. Transdermal implant

## Concept of Osmotic Pump

Osmotic pressure is one of the colligative properties, and it has been extensively used for the development of controlled drug delivery systems.

Osmosis is a process of movement of a solvent through a semipermeable membrane from a lower concentration of solute to a higher concentration of solute at a particular temperature until the concentrations become equal. In other words, it is a process of movement of solvent from a solution having a higher concentration of solvent through a semipermeable membrane towards a solution having a lower concentration of solvent at a particular temperature until the concentration of the two solutions become equal.

According to Van't Hoff law, the osmotic pressure P depends on the molar concentration of the solute and the temperature. The law can be expressed as;

$$P = \frac{RTC}{M}$$

Where, C is the concentration of solute (g/lt), M is the molecular weight of the solute, R is the gas constant, and T is the temperature.

The equation applies to very dilute solutions in which the molecules do not interact (association).

Various drugs require to be externally controlled for their delivery at the desired rate and volume. The magnetic-type delivery systems can be used for this purpose. Pump systems can be used to provide the control required in these cases. With the help of advanced microtechnology, it is now possible to make small pump systems which can be implanted subcutaneously for delivery of the drug. As a result, it becomes possible to maintain the controlled drug release without any external pump system. For example, insulin implantable pump systems have been recently developed and used for the control of type-1 diabetes.

Because of their mechanism of drug delivery pump systems differ from other implantable systems. Pump systems release drugs through a pressure difference generated a gradient that results in the bulk flow of a drug at controllable rates.

The permeability of water varies on a wide range of pressures. To develop formulation using osmotic pressure, water-permeable membranes of cellulosic polymers such as cellulose acetate is commonly used.

Osmotic pumps are unique and dynamic. The rate of drug release from an osmotic pump is directly proportional to osmotic pressure developed due to inhibition of fluid movement by osmogene. An osmotic pump is composed of a semipermeable membrane on one side to allow water is permeating towards the drug reservoir. The factors to be considered while designing an osmotic pump are;

- The surface area of the semipermeable membrane available for osmosis,
- Nature of the semipermeable membrane,
- The diameter of the drug delivery device,
- Nature and concentration of osmogene, and
- pH and concentration of electrolyte present in the external fluid.

## Advantages

Osmotic pump is used as a controlled drug delivery system. It provides various advantages apart from the common advantages related to controlled drug delivery system. Most important advantages of this system are;

- It follows zero-order release kinetics,
- The rate of drug delivery does not depend on pH and outside agitation,
- The drug is delivered in the form of a solution; hence immediately is absorbed.
- Delivery rate can be readily determined *in vitro*,
- If the dose is large, the delivery rate can be increased by using a suitable osmotic pump,
- It can be designed for drugs with a wide range of solubility in water.

## Disadvantages

- For making an orifice in the system, special equipment is required,
- May cause irritation or abscess due to high residence time in the body,
- It may offer a stability problem,
- Additional patient education and counseling is needed,
- The device may be expensive

## Excipients and Formulation Considerations

An osmotic pump essentially contains a drug and a semipermeable membrane. When the drug possesses excellent aqueous solubility, it behaves as an osmogene; but if the drug is not soluble in water or poorly soluble, a suitable osmogenic substance such as soluble inorganic salt, sucrose, etc. is added to the formulation. In general, an osmotic pump contains the following components;

1. Semipermeable membrane
2. Wicking agent
3. Polymeric matrix
4. Osmogen
5. Surfactant, and
6. Flux regulator

1. **Semipermeable membrane:** It helps the movement of solute/solvent from the implant towards the biological environment. Thus, selection of suitable and efficient semipermeable membrane is the most important activity during the development of an osmotic pump. Cellulose acetate is widely used as the polymer for making an osmotic pump. Various grades of cellulose acetate based on their acetyl content are available. Cellulose acetate with acetyl content within 30 – 36 is generally used.

2. **Wicking agent:** Wicking agent is a material which can attract water into the osmotic device from the surroundings through the porous network of the device. These may be swellable or non-swellable when the wicking agent draws water through the channels, the surface area of the channels increases. The materials which are used as a wicking agent are sodium lauryl sulfate, colloidal silicon dioxide, bentonite, alumina, titanium dioxide, niacinamide, kaolin, and polyvinylpyrrolidone of low molecular weight, etc.

3. **Polymeric matrix:** To prepare a drug-polymer matrix for an osmotic pump suitable polymer should be used. Generally, a mixture of hydrophilic and hydrophobic polymers is used when the drug is water soluble. Selection of polymer depends on
   - the solubility of the drug,
   - the rate of drug release required, and
   - the amount of drug to be released from the pump.

   Polymers are of two types – swellable and non-swellable. When the drug is moderately soluble in water, a swellable polymer such as sodium carboxymethyl cellulose (sodium CMC) is suitable. If the drug is highly soluble in water non-swellable polymer is used.

4. **Osmogen:** These play a significant role in osmotic pump formulations. Generally soluble inorganic salts such as sodium chloride, sodium phosphate monobasic, potassium chloride, potassium sulfate, calcium chloride, etc. and carbohydrates

such as dextrose, fructose, mannitol, etc. are used as osmogen in osmotic pump formulations.

5. **Surfactant:** The surfactant is used in a formulation to regulate the surface energy of the material, to improve the wettability of an active constituent by reducing the surface tension; so that the mixing of the elements is improved and the integrity of the formulation is maintained during drug release. Sodium oleate, sodium dioleate, sodium trioleate, glyceryl laurate, etc. are commonly used as the surfactant.

6. **Flux regulator:** To regulate the fluid permeability of the wall inside an osmotic pump, a flux regulator is mixed with the materials used to form the wall. The flux may be increased or decreased depending on the particular situation; accordingly, a suitable material is to be used as a flux regulator. The flux regulator can improve the flexibility and porosity of the lamina. Low molecular weight glycols such as polypropylene, polybutylene, and polyhydric alcohols such as poly alkylene glycols are used as flux regulator.

## Factors Influencing the Drug Release from the Oral Osmotic Pump

The solubility of the drug:

1. Solubility of a drug present in the core is directly proportional to the rate of release of the drug from the implant.
2. For osmotic drug delivery, neither highly nor poorly soluble drugs are suitable.
3. For highly and poorly soluble drugs there are various techniques available to prepare osmotic pump.

Coating membrane:

1. On the type and nature of the polymer used to prepare membrane, the drug release rate depends.
2. The rate of drug release depends on the thickness of the membrane.
3. The drug release rate depends on the permeability of the membrane.
4. The drug release rate depends on other excipients present in the formulation.
5. The drug release rate depends on the type and nature of plasticizer and flux regulator used in the formulation.

Orifice for drug delivery:

1. Various techniques are available to create orifice within the membrane.
2. The drug release rate depends on the diameter of the orifice in the membrane.

Osmotic pressure:

1. The rate of drug release is directly proportional to the osmotic pressure of the core of the osmotic pump.
2. The rate of drug release from the osmotic pump can be modified by adding suitable osmogen.

## Selection of Implant Material

Before the development of formulation, it is the primary responsibility of the development scientist to design the formulation. Before or at the time of designing certain factors related to the drug and other necessary excipients should be considered — for example, solubility, pKa, partition coefficient, stability data, etc.

The rate of degradation of the polymer in the body depends on the factors; such as a change in pH of the body fluids, change of temperature due to inflammation, other reasons. These can cause fluctuation in the degradation rate. Similarly, the surface area of the implant is a key variable that can affect degradation. If the erosion of the system occurs not only through the surface but also throughout its volume, the overall ratio of surface area to volume of the implantable system typically increases. This may accelerate the degradation rate; the monolithic implant degrades into smaller sub-units. However, the total surface area available for erosion will gradually decrease, if the erosion takes place only at the surface of the implant without any non homogeneous decomposition or break down into smaller units. As a result, the degradation rate reduces. Consequently, the transformation in shape of the implant due to *in vivo* degradation should be considered at the time of design. The geometric shape of implants whose surface area does not change substantially as a function of time during erosion should be regarded as for uniform and constant release. A flat, slab-like shape implant which does not show edge-erosion, is expected to exhibit approximate a zero-order release kinetic profile. Alternatively, an inert, biodegradable core, coated with the active drug matrix, is used to improve the change in surface area problem encountered during erosion. Slow diffusion of the drug from the polymer matrix is another limitation of bioerodible systems. The rate of drug diffusion is usually slower than the bioerosion of the system and depends on the physicochemical properties of the polymeric matrix utilized in the formulation of the IDDS. This becomes a significant challenge for extended-release applications particularly for drugs with a narrow therapeutic index.

## Classification of Osmotic Pumps

There are various types of osmotic pumps used to administer at different sites of the body.

1. Oral osmotic pump
   - Elementary osmotic pump
   - Push-pull osmotic pump
   - Controlled porosity osmotic pump
   - Bursting osmotic pump
   - Osmotic pump containing effervescent agent and drug
   - A pump comprising an insoluble drug

2. Implantable osmotic pump
   - Rose Nelson pump
   - Higuchi-Leeper pump
   - Higuchi-Theeuwes pump
   - Alzet osmotic pump

## Biodegradable Systems

Among these, osmotic pump and diffusion-release based formulations have been found to be the most successful in delivering the drug in a linear process; wherein the drug dosage released is proportional to square root of the release time. There are two types – biodegradable and non-degradable systems. The popularity of biodegradable systems has become much popular over nondegradable delivery systems. The major advantages of biodegradable systems are - (1) the inert polymers are used for the fabrication of the delivery system, and (2) the polymer is absorbed or excreted by the body. This requires surgical removal of the implant after the end of therapy; as a result, patient acceptance is increased.

Development of biodegradable systems is more complicated and challenging activity than formulating nondegradable systems. When fabricating new biodegradable systems, these variables should be considered. For example, *in vivo* degradation kinetics of the polymer or rate of degradation must remain constant to maintain a sustained release of the drug. Many factors can affect the rate of degradation of the polymer in the body. Change in body pH or temperature can cause a temporary increase or decrease in the degradation rate of the system. The surface area of the delivery system also plays an essential role in its degradation. As erosion of the system starts, the surface area of the implantable system decreases. Thus, the change in shape of the drug delivery system occurs after administration of an implant. To achieve a uniform and constant release, it is necessary to use an implant of such a geometrical shape whose surface area does not change with time during erosion.

A flat slab-type shape having no edge erosion would provide approximately a zero-order release kinetics. Some manufacturers have also designed systems that contain a bioerodable inert core coated with the active drug matrix to improve the change in surface area problem generally found during erosion. Slow diffusion of the drug from the polymer matrix is another problem that happens with bioerodible systems. Diffusion of the drug usually takes place at a slower rate than the bioerosion of the system. It depends on the chemical nature of the polymer used in the formulation of the drug delivery system. This is a significant challenge while developing bioerodible systems to overcome. Such a system is designed to extend the release of drug which may have a narrow therapeutic index (fig. 5.11).

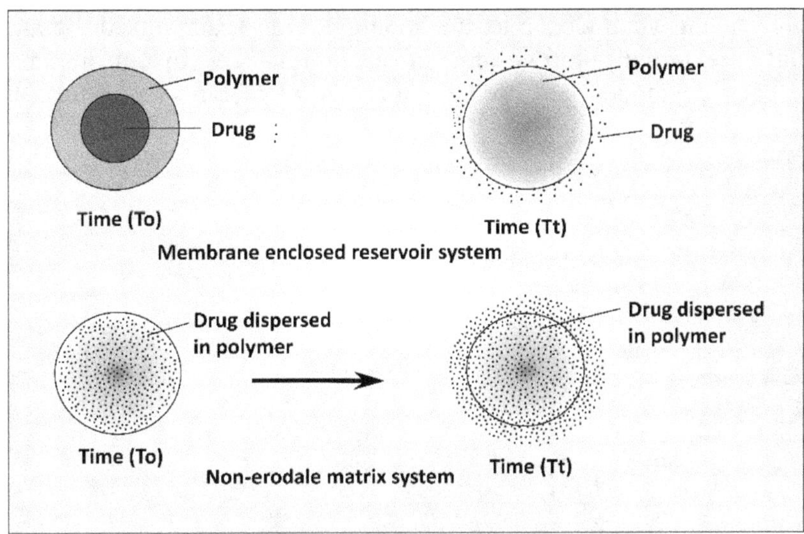



**Fig. 5.11:** Cross section view of idealized non-erodible reservoir and matrix system, showing diffusion of the drug across the polymer.

In recent times two different types of biodegradable delivery systems are available - (1) a reservoir system which has similarity in structure of the nondegradable reservoir type. From both systems, the mechanism of drug release is almost similar. However, these biodegradable systems contain an exterior polymeric membrane that degrades at a slower rate than the expected rate of drug diffusion through the membrane. Thus, the membrane remains intact while the drug is released completely. Ultimately, the outer polymeric membrane degrades in a biological system (*in vivo*) and is eventually eliminated. (2) In this system, the drug remains dispersed in a polymer (monolithic type) which is slowly eroded in a biological system (*in vivo*) by biological processes at a controlled rate. Currently, the most popular biodegradable polymers being investigated include polyglycolic acid, polylactic acid, polyglycolic-lactic acid, polyaspartic acid, and polycaprolactone. For the delivery of macromolecular drugs such as insulin, ethyl vinyl acetate copolymer matrices have been studied extensively. A new form of lactic acid/lysine copolymer has been developed as a matrix for the mammalian cells and tested. This copolymer can be chemically attached to a biologically active peptide. This new copolymer can effectively promote the cell adhesion and for a nonadherent surface. Such a system will play a significant role in the development of implantable polymers in the future.

## Implantable Pump Systems

There are many drugs that require external control of delivery rate and volume. Such control cannot be achieved by using biodegradable or nondegradable delivery systems except the magnetic-type delivery systems. In such situations pump systems have been used to control release. Recently, it has been possible to develop small pump systems to implant drug by using advanced microtechnology. This maintains the controlled drug release without an external pump system. In recent advances, insulin implantable pump systems have been developed and used for the control of type-1 diabetes, as shown in figure 5.12.

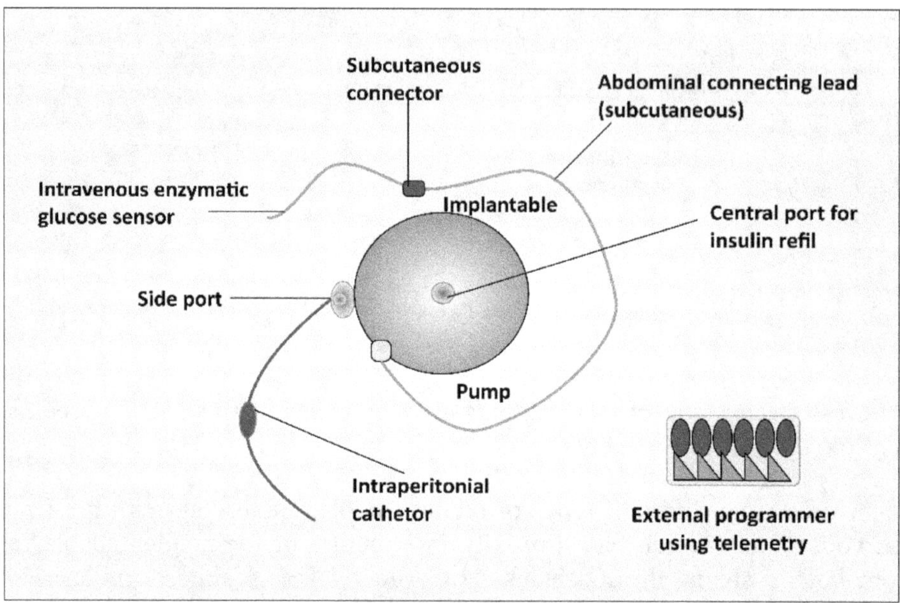


**Fig. 5.12:** Cross section view of idealized non-erodible reservoir and matrix system, showing diffusion of the drug across the polymer.

Because of the mechanism of drug, delivery pump systems differ from other implantable systems. Pump systems release drugs through a pressure difference generated that results in bulk flow of a drug at controllable rates. Recently, five different types of implantable pump systems have been developed and tested such as;

1. Infusion pumps,
2. Peristaltic pumps,
3. Osmotic pumps,
4. Positive displacement pumps, and
5. Controlled release micropumps.

1. **Infusion Pumps:** Infusion pumps are of a mechanical type, implantable systems. These utilize a fluorocarbon propellant to administer the drug in the biological system. Such pumps had been initially developed for the administration of insulin to diabetic patients. For example, Infusaid (Infusaid Corp. Sharon, MA, USA) was one of the first commercially available pumps. Generally, insulin-dependent diabetics require injections once or twice daily.

   This type of dosing results in abnormal peaks and valleys in blood glucose levels. It is believed that if blood glucose level is poorly controlled, heart and kidney disease may be affected. It is also thought that continuous infusion of insulin using such pumps may help the elimination of such risk factors in the diabetic population.

The pump contains a canister, disc-shaped, made of light-weight biocompatible titanium. The canister consists of a collapsible welded bellow. The bellow separates the canister interior into two separate chambers. The first chamber contains the fluorocarbon propellant and the second includes the insulin formulation.

At a particular temperature, the propellant (gas) pushes the drug through a filter and a flow regulator. As a result, the drug is administered at a constant rate. The delivery rate can be changed by changing the drug concentration in the pump reservoir. The advantage of this system is that no external energy is required to operate the pump. The pump reservoir can be refilled by injecting drug through a membrane consisting of self-sealing silicone rubber and Teflon septum. The force of the injection recompresses the fluorocarbon propellant. This pump system can be used to administer anticoagulant and chemotherapeutic agents, besides insulin.

2. **Peristaltic pump:** The peristaltic pump consists of a rotary solenoid-driven system that runs via an external power source which is usually a battery. Like the infusion pump, the peristaltic system is filled through a silicone rubber septum, and it can be used for several years depending on the life of the battery-powered system. The advantage of this type of system is that the rate of drug administration can be controlled by an external remote-control system. The peristaltic systems have been very costly; thus, could not gain market acceptance.

3. **Osmotic pumps:** The most popular type of implantable drug delivery system is the osmotic pump. Theeuwes and Yum first developed the osmotic pump. This is also known as Oros or the gastrointestinal therapeutic system. The pump consists of a drug reservoir which is surrounded by a semipermeable membrane. The membrane allows a steady influx of water and biological fluid into the reservoir through osmosis. The hydrostatic pressure developed from this influx results in a steady, constant or zero order release of the drug from an opening in the membrane called the *drug portal* until the drug in the reservoir is completely released. By changing the structure of the semipermeable membrane, the rate of drug administration of these systems can be improved. This requires removal of the system. Osmotic pump systems containing hydromorphone are implanted subcutaneously for the management of pain.

Results have shown that Alzet's osmotic pumps can release the drug, hydromorphone at a rate of 262 mg/h and can produce stable plasma concentrations of about 30–40 mg/mL over 2 weeks. This type of delivery system is advantageous over other systems; because, the 'initial burst effect,' observed in other forms of degradable or nondegradable matrix systems, does not occur. The prolonged release of a drug at a constant rate has been found to be effective in the treatment and management of chronic pain.

4. **Positive displacement pumps:** To provide continual insulin delivery in diabetic patients, positive displacement pumps have been developed. Flexible tubing is attached to most of these systems utilizing piezoelectric disk benders. Such pumps are activated initially by exposing the disks to specific voltages. They form spherical surfaces. The bellow-type system is connected to a drug reservoir via a three-way solenoid driven valve when exposed to electrical pulses, the valves in the pump open or close depending on the direction of the pulse. This causes the release of drug in a controlled manner by the rate of the electrical pulse. For delivery of insulin other types of positive displacement pumps using similar designs are currently being developed.

5. **Implantable rods:** Implantable rods have been prepared with the help of a different types of biodegradable and nonbiodegradable polymers. The implantable rods release the drug in a controlled manner.

## Mechanism of Drug Release from Biodegradable Implants

From biodegradable polymeric systems, the drug is released in a controlled manner by diffusion, degradation or a combination of both. The degradation-controlled release takes place when the rate of diffusion of a drug is less than the degradation or erosion rate of the polymer carrier. The drug release and polymer degradation happen simultaneously; in such case, sigmoidal release profiles are usually observed. Both polymer erosion mechanism and drug release based on the degradation-controlled mechanism can also be divided into two approaches –

1. Surface-erosion/degradation, and

2. Bulk-degradation

When the drug is released from implants is controlled by the surface-erosion, the factors that control the release are the surface-to-volume ratio and the geometry of implants. In this case, polymer degradation takes place at the outer surface of the device.

On the other hand, the degradation may occur almost homogeneously throughout the implant through bulk-degradation of the polymer. In both the cases, hydrolytic degradation of the polymer the water needs to enter into the implant. Hence, water plays a critical role in controlling degradation as well as release kinetics. Semi-crystalline polymers degrade in two stages;

1. The water is infused into the amorphous regions, resulting in random hydrolytic cleavage of labile ester bonds at the boundaries.

2. The degradation of polymer throughout entire areas of the implant; particularly when the polymer is amorphous.

Generally, the fragments of the polymer chain broken down are significantly shorter than the original string. This resultant decrease in the average molecular weight of the polymer may be used as a metric to quantify the extent of degradation. PLGA or PLA polymer undergoes bulk degradation. Drug-release from such carriers is controlled only by a bulk degradation-controlled release mechanism. However, the physicochemical properties of the drug also play a role in drug-release from hydrolytically degraded PLGA- or PLA-based products. Implants containing highly water-soluble drugs showed a significant initial burst release; after that, a rapid release. Finally, the drug loading has also an effect on the release rates. For example, implants formulated with high drug-loading shows fast release.

## Bibliography


1.  Alekha KD, Greggrey CC. Therapeutic applications of implantable drug delivery systems. J Pharmacol Toxicol Methods 1998; 40:1-12. Available from: http://www.pharmainfo.net/pppc06/implantable-drugdelivery-system. [Last accessed on 2010 Nov 1].

2.  Baker R. Controlled Release of Biologically Active Agents. New York: John Wiley; 1987. p. 40-56.

3.  Barrera D, Zylstra E, Lansbury PT, Langer R. Synthesis and RGD peptide modification of a new biodegradable copolymer: Poly(lactic acid-colysine). J Am Chem Soc 1993;115:11010-1.

4.  Blackshear PJ, Rhode TII. Artificial devices for insulin infusion in the treatment of patients with diabetes mellitus. In: Burk SD, editor. Controlled Drug Delivery, Clinical Applications. Vol 2. Boca Raton, FL: CRC Press; 1983. p. 11.

5.  Brown LR, Wei CL, Langer R. *In vivo* and *in vitro* release of macromolecules form polymeric drug delivery systems. J Pharm Sci 1983; 72:1181-5.

6.  Cao L, Mentell S, Polla D. Design and simulation of an implantable medical drug delivery system using microelectromechanical systems technology. Sens Actuators A Phys 2001; 94:117-25.

7.  Costantini LC, Kleppner SR, McDonough J, Azar MR, Patel R. Implantable technology for long-term delivery of nalmefene for treatment of alcoholism. Int J Pharm 2004; 283:35-44.

8.  Dagani R. Biodegradable copolymer eyed as tissue matrix. Chem Eng News 1993; 22:5-8.

9.  Danckwerts M, Fassihi A. Implantable controlled release drug delivery systems: A Review. Drug Dev Ind Pharm 1991; 17:1465-502.

10. Dash AK, Suryanarayanan R. An implantable dosage form for the treatment of bone infections. Pharm Res 1992; 9:993-1002.

11. Graham NB. Polymeric inserts and implants for the controlled release of drugs. Br Polymer J. 1978; 10:260-6.

12. Higuchi T. Rate of release of medicaments from ointment base containing drugs in suspension. J Pharm Sci 1961; 50:874-879.

13. Juni K, Ogata J, Nakano M, Ichihara T, Mori K, Akagi M. Preparation and evaluation *in vitro* and *in vivo* of polylactic acid microspheres containing doxorubicin. Chem Pharm Bull 1985; 33:313-8.

14. Kimura H, Ogura Y, Hashizoe M, Nishiwaki H, Honda Y, Ikada Y. A new vitreal drug delivery system using an implantable biodegradable polymeric device. Invest Ophthalmol Vis Sci 1994; 35:2815-9.

15. Langer R. Implantable controlled release systems. In: Ihler GM, editor. Methods of Drug Delivery. New York: Pergamon Press; 1986. p. 121-37.

16.    Lewis DH. Controlled release of bioactive agents from lactide/glycolide polymers. In: Chasin M, Langer R, editors. Biodegradable Polymers as Drug Delivery Systems. New York: Marcel Dekker; 190. p. 1-41.

17.    Ranade V. Drug delivery systems Implants in drug delivery. J Clin Pharm 1990; 30:871-89.

18.    Renard E. Implantable closed-loop glucose-sensing and insulin delivery: The future for insulin pump therapy. Curr Opin Pharmacol 2002; 2:708-16.

19.    Rhine W, Hsieh DS, Langer R. Polymers for sustained macromolecule release: Procedures to fabricate reproducible delivery systems and control release kinetics. J Pharm Sci 1980; 69:265-70.

20.    Sefton MV. Implantable pumps. CRC Crit Rev Bioeng 1987; 14:201-40. News 1993; 22:5-8.

21.    Sershen1 S, West J. Implantable, polymeric systems for modulated drug delivery. Adv Drug Deliv Rev 2002; 54:1225-35.

22.    Wang X, Chen T, Yang Z, Wang W. Study on structural optimum design of implantable drug delivery micro-system. Simul Modelling Pract Theory 2007; 15:47-56.

23.    Wood DA. Biodegradable drug delivery systems. Int J Pharm 1980; 7: 1-18.

24.    Zaheer S, Lehman J, Stevenson G. Capsular contracture around silicone implants: The role of intraluminal antibiotics. Plast Reconstr Surg 1982; 69:809-12.

## Exercise

## A. Multiple Choice Questions

1. Which of the following statement is correct?
   - (a) Drugs can be orally administered for their rapid onset of action.
   - (b) Drugs cannot be orally administered for their rapid onset of action.
   - (c) Drugs can be transdermally administered for their rapid onset of action.
   - (d) Drugs can be rectally administered for their rapid onset of action.

2. Drugs that are readily absorbed into the bloodstream from the lung can be administered through
   - (a) Pulmonary route
   - (b) Oral route
   - (c) Topical route
   - (d) Injection

3. Implantable therapeutic are mainly developed for
   - (a) Short term therapy
   - (b) Conventional release of drug
   - (c) Long term therapy
   - (d) Interrupted therapy

4. Which of the following statements is not correct?
   - (a) Implantable drug delivery system should be biostable.
   - (b) Implantable drug delivery system should be environmentally stable.
   - (c) Implantable drug delivery system should be sterile
   - (d) None of the above

5. Which of the following statements is correct?
    (a)  Implantable drug delivery system provides improved therapeutic efficacy.
    (b)  Implantable drug delivery systems are easy to manufacture.
    (c)  Implantable drug delivery system fails to reduce side effect.
    (d)  None of the above.

6. Implantable drug delivery systems
    (a)  Are non-invasive.
    (b)  Are independent of fluctuating metabolic requirement.
    (c)  Do not show any risk of failure.
    (d)  Provide uncomfortable feeling for the patients wearing the device.

7. Which of the following statements is correct?
    (a)  Implantable drug delivery systems are limited to potent drugs.
    (b)  Implantable drug delivery systems can be prepared for all drugs.
    (c)  Implantable drug delivery systems have a risk of drug leakage.
    (d)  All of the above.

8. The rate of drug release from an implant can be regulated by
    (a)  It's shaped                        (b)  It's size,
    (c)  On the polymer(s) used             (d)  All of the above

9. The concept of developing implantable therapeutic systems is
    (a)  Diffusion controlled-release
    (b)  The rate of release of drug
    (c)  The rate of elimination of the drug
    (d)  The rate of metabolism of the drug

10. Membrane permeation-controlled release implantable drug delivery system consists of
    (a)  Nonporous membrane only
    (b)  Microporous membrane only
    (c)  Semipermeable membrane only
    (d)  Anyone of the above three membranes

11. Which of the following systems work on activated controlled-release concept?
    (a)  Membrane permeation-controlled system
    (b)  Osmotic pressure activated the system
    (c)  Matrix diffusion-controlled system
    (d)  Micro-reservoir dissolution-controlled system

12. Which of the following systems work on diffusion controlled-release concept?
    (a)  Magnetically activated system
    (b)  Membrane permeation-controlled system
    (c)  Hydrolysis activated system
    (d)  Ultrasound activated the system

13. Osmotic pump releases drug under
    (a) Osmotic pressure gradient          (b)  Concentration gradient
    (c) Vapour pressure gradient           (d)  None of the above

14. The driving force in an activated, controlled release IDDS is
    (a) Osmotic pressure                   (b)  Vapour pressure
    (c) Ultrasound                         (d)  Anyone of the above

15. Diffusion of drug particles from an implantable drug delivery system can be expressed as
    (a) Only Fickian diffusion             (b)  Only non-Fickian diffusion
    (c) Anyone of the above                (d)  None of the above

16. Implants can be classified by
    (a) Route of administration only       (b)  Mechanism of drug release only
    (c) Both of the above                  (d)  Anyone of the above

17. Osmotic pressure depends on
    (a) The molecular weight of wicking agent
    (b) The molecular weight of the drug
    (c) The molecular weight of surfactant
    (d) The molecular weight of osmogen

18. For osmotic drug delivery, the drug may be
    (a) Highly soluble in water            (b)  Soluble in water
    (c) Sparingly soluble in water         (d)  All of the above

19. Drug release from osmotic pump follows
    (a) Zero-order                         (b)  First-order
    (c) Second-order                       (d)  Complex-order

20. Which of the following statements is correct?
    (a) The rate of drug release from an osmotic pump depends on pH of the surroundings
    (b) The rate of drug release from an osmotic pump independent of pH of the surroundings
    (c) The rate of drug release from an osmotic pump depends on agitation of the surroundings
    (d) None of the above

## B. Short Questions

1. What is the implantable drug delivery system? Why are the implantable drug delivery systems developed?
2. Explain the advantages of an implantable drug delivery system.
3. Explain the micro-reservoir dissolution-controlled system.
4. What is hydrolysis activated system?

5. What are the factors that influence the drug release from an oral osmotic pump?

6. Write a note on Infusion pump and osmotic pump.

## C. Long Questions

1. Discuss the concept of the implant.
2. Explain the advantages and disadvantages of the implant.
3. Write down the implantable systems that are based on diffusion controlled-release concept.
4. Explain the concept of the osmotic pump with its advantages and disadvantages.
5. Discuss activated controlled-release systems.
6. Describe the excipients used to formulate osmotic pump.
7. Explain the biodegradable IDDS.

# CHAPTER 6

# Transdermal Drug Delivery Systems

*Introduction, Permeation through skin, factors affecting permeation, permeation enhancers, basic components of TDDS, formulation approaches.*

## Introduction

Since long for topical administration of drug skin has been used as the site of administration. Its use for systemic drug delivery has been considered during last 3 – 4 decades. Such delivery is called transdermal drug delivery (TDD). But, is known for its barrier function. It resists the loss of water from the body and entrance of external agents into the body. There are some drug substances which can penetrate the skin in sufficient amounts and produce systemic effects. Drugs having short elimination half-lives or face extensive first-pass metabolism, should be administered through this route.

The concept of TDDS first introduced in the early 1950s and a commercial product, transdermal patch, first came in USA market in early 1980s. These transdermal patches were designed to control nausea, vomiting, and angina. But these products could not sustain in the market for long. However, for the cessation of smoking habit, this technology was considered suitable and started designing nicotine patches. Nowadays, many transdermal patches are available in the market mostly for the administration of hormones and analgesics (painkiller). The primary purpose of development and application of TDDS is percutaneous or transdermal absorption.

Novel TDDS such as iontophoresis, thermophoresis, and phonophoresis have been used to improve transdermal drug delivery. The drug can penetrate through the skin via three pathways-through hair follicles, through sebaceous glands, through sweat duct. Transdermal drug delivery systems are used in various skin disorders, also in the management of angina pectoris, pains, smoking cessation & neurological disorders such as Parkinson's disease.

*A transdermal patch or skin patch is a medicated adhesive patch that is placed on the skin to deliver a specific dose of medication through the skin and into the bloodstream.*

Transdermal absorption or bioavailability of drug depends primarily on:

- Physicochemical properties of drug,
- The ability of the drug to penetrate the skin, and
- Physiology of the skin.

Hence, before proceeding further, it is necessary to know the fundamentals of anatomy and physiology of the skin.

## Advantages of Transdermal Drug Delivery System

1. First pass metabolisms of drug get avoided.
2. Gastrointestinal incompatibilities get avoided.
3. Self-medication is possible.
4. Duration of action gets extended & predictable.
5. Unwanted side effects get minimized.
6. Drug plasma concentration gets maintained.
7. The number of doses gets which improve patient compliance.
8. The therapeutic value of many drugs get increased by avoiding problems associated with drug like-lower absorption, irritation, decomposition due to hepatic first pass metabolism.

## Disadvantages of Transdermal Drug Delivery System

1. Chances of allergic reactions at the site of application such as itching, rashes, local edema, etc.
2. The larger molecular size of drug (above 1000) faces difficulty in absorption.
3. The barrier function of skin varies from site to site on the same or different person.
4. A drug with hydrophilic character is less suitable as compared to a drug with the lipophilic nature because of their low permeability.

## Anatomy & Physiology of Skin

The mucosal linings of the urogenital, digestive, respiratory tracts combine with the skin to protect the internal body structures from the hostile external environment. Skin is the largest organ of the body. It contains fat. Without fat, the skin of an average adult weighs about 4kg, and its surface area is more than 20, $000cm^2$.

The human skin is a multi-layered organ composed of many histological layers. Skin is the most accessible organ in the body. The primary functions of the skin are;

- Protection of major or vital internal organs from the external influences,
- Protection from ultraviolet rays,

- Temperature regulations,
- Control of water output and sensation.
- Regulation of blood pressure.

Human skin is composed of three tissue layers as mentioned below:

(A)  The stratified, vascular, cellular epidermis,

(B)  Underlying dermis of connective tissues,

(C)  Hypodermis.

## Epidermis

The epidermis is a stratified, squamous, keratinizing epithelium. The multi-layered epidermis varies in thickness, depending on cell size and number of cell layers of epidermis. The thickness of epidermis varies from 0.8 mm on palms and soles to 0.06 mm on the eyelids. The cells of basal layer (stratum germinativum) divide and migrate upwards and produce stratum corneum or horny layer. This layer is composed of dead cells. This dead and dense layer is impermeable to most of the chemical and other substances. For this reason, a human being can survive in a non-aqueous environment. In dry condition, the thickness of the stratum corneum is the only 10μm; but in water, it swells several times. About 90% of epidermal cells are keratinocytes arranged in layers and produce keratin protein. Melanocytes produce melanin a yellow or brown-black pigment that contributes to skin color and absorbs damaging UV light. A Langerhans cell arises from red bone marrow and migrates to the epidermis, where they constitute a small fraction of epidermis cells. Markel cells are least numerous of epidermal cells. There are two main types of horny layers – (1) the pads of palms and soles, adapted for bearing weights, protecting the skin from friction; (2) remaining part of this layer (epidermis) is a flexible and impermeable membranous layer. Stratum corneum is the rate-limiting barrier for inward and outward movement of chemicals. Stratum corneum is structurally heterogeneous. The outer layer is less densely packed than the adjacent to underlying granular layer. The chemical composition of this barrier is not known. The main cellular components are protein, fat, and water. These are combined into a structured form. It contains 75 – 85% of protein, 15 – 20% of lipid and about 15% of water on the dried basis.

Five layers of the epidermis

(a)  Stratum basale

(b)  Spinosum

(c)  Granulosum

(d)  Lucidum

(e)  Corneum

## Dermis

The dermis or corneum is about 3 – 5mm thick.  It consists of a (mixture) matrix of connective tissue, made up of fibrous proteins, such as collagen, elastin, and reticulin. These proteins are embedded in an amorphous ground substance of mucopolysaccharides. Through it, the nerves, blood vessels, lymphatics move across the matrix and skin appendages such as eccrine sweat glands, apocrine glands, and pilosebaceous units. The dermis consists of about 80% of proteins. This layer requires an efficient blood supply to transport nutrients, remove waste products regulate pressure and temperature, mobilize defense forces and contributes color to the skin. Branches from the arterial plexus supply blood to sweat glands, hair follicles, subcutaneous fat, and dermis. The supply of blood reaches to within 0.2mm of the skin surface. As a result, the blood can absorb and systemically dilute the compounds transported passed through the epidermis. Thus, the blood can absorb and dilute the materials diffused in-ward through the epidermis. Once the diffusing materials or penetrants reach to the capillaries, the concentration of the penetrant in the dermis is reduced greatly, and the concentration gradient in the epidermis is increased; so that the percutaneous absorption is facilitated.

The boundary between dermis and epidermis layer is called Dermal- Epidermal junction which provides a physical barrier for the large molecules of drug and cells. The dermis incorporates blood and lymphatic vesicles and nerve endings. The dermis is divided into the papillary & reticular region.

**Papillary region:** It makes up one-fifth of the thickness of the total layer, contains areolar connective tissue containing fine elastic fibers.

**Reticular region:** It is attached to the subcutaneous layer; consist of dense irregular coactive tissue containing fibroblast, a bundle of collagen and some coarse elastic fibers (fig. 6.1).

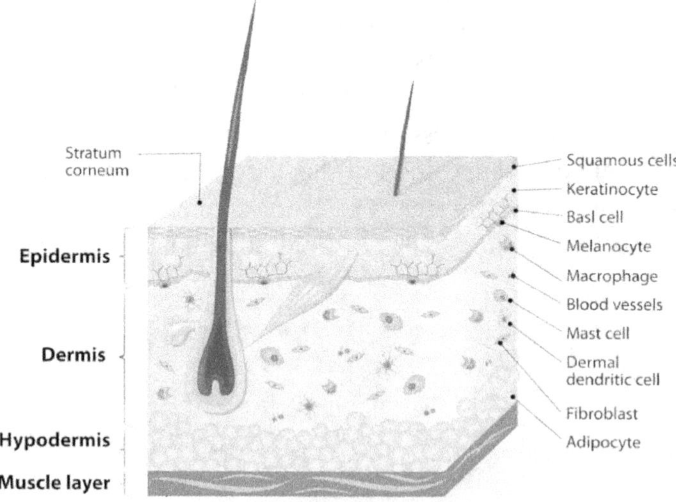


**Fig. 6.1:** Structure of skin.

## Hypodermis

The hypodermis or subcutaneous fat tissue supports the dermis and epidermis. It serves as a fat storage area. This layer helps to regulate temperature, provides nutritional support and mechanical protection. It carries major blood vessels and nerves to skin and may contain sensory pressure organs. The hypodermis layer is composed of loose connective tissues, and its thickness varies according to the surface of the body.

## Subcutaneous Tissue

Subcutaneous fat also called as subcutis, hypoderm provides a mechanical cushioning effect and acts as a thermal barrier. It synthesizes and stores high energy chemicals. These chemicals are readily available.

## Skin Appendages

The number of **eccrine sweat glands** in the body is about 2.5million ($2.5 \times 10^6$), and pH of the sweat varies from 4.6 to 6.8. The eccrine sweat glands produce sweat and may secrete drugs, protein, antibiotics, and antigens. The primary function of these glands is to regulate the heat of the body. Sweating also can be increased by emotional stress.

**Apocrine sweat glands** develop at the pilosebaceous follicle and provide the characteristics of adult distributions in the armpit (axilla), the breast areola and perianal region. The milky or oily secretions may be colored. It contains proteins, lipids, lipoproteins, and saccharides. Bacteria present in the body surface metabolize this odorless secretion and produce characteristic body smell.

**Hair follicle** grows throughout the skin except at the red part of lips, palms, soles, and certain parts of the sex organs. In some regions of the body an apocrine gland and one or more sebaceous open into the follicle above the muscle that links the follicle to the dermo-epidermal junction.

Numbers of sebaceous glands are many and mostly present on the face, forehead, ear, on the midline of the back, and anogenital surfaces. Usually, palms and soles lack them. The holocrine glands produce sebum from the disintegration of cells. The principal components of sebum are glycerides, free fatty acids, cholesterol, and esters of cholesterol, esters of wax and squalene. Abnormal sebaceous activity may produce seborrhoea (excess sebum), gland hyperplasia without clinical seborrhoea, obstruction of the pilosebaceous canal (acne and comedones –whiteheads or blackheads) and other types of dysfunction – the dyssebacias.

Like hair, nails consist of 'hard' keratin with a relatively higher amount of sulfur; mainly a cysteine. The nail behaves as a hydrophilic matrix concerning its permeability. This is not found with stratum corneum.

# Functions of the Skin

The skin has various functions. Here we shall be limited to those which are relevant to drug absorption from TDDS. Mainly mechanical and protective functions are related to this delivery system.

## Mechanical Function

The mechanical properties of skin are provided by dermis. However, epidermis plays although minor role. Skin is elastic; but, once it takes up its initial slack, it extends further with difficulty. Skin wrinkles with an edge, and it becomes more rigid. Thin horny layer is reasonably strong, and its liability depends on a correct balance of lipids, water-soluble hygroscopic substances, called natural moisturizing factor (NMF) – mainly water. To maintain its suppleness, the tissue requires about 10-20% of moisture to act as a plasticizer.

## Protective Function

The barrier function of the skin can be classified as:
- Microbiological barrier
- Chemical barrier
- Radiation barrier
- Heat barrier
- Electrical barrier
- Mechanical barrier

**The microbiological barrier** is provided by the stratum corneum. Sloughing of corneocytes groups (squames), with adhering microorganism helps to protect the skin. Microorganism can penetrate through superficial cracks and injured/damaged tissues, where infection may develop. Sebaceous and eccrine secretions, at pH 4.2 – 5.6, called acid mantle probably cannot protect the skin against bacteria. Skin glands also secrete short-chain fatty acids which inhibit the growth of bacteria and fungus. Nitric oxide produced from nitrates of sweat, helps to prevent infection from skin pathogens. Acidified nitric oxide possesses antimicrobial activity in the oral and gastrointestinal tract. The opening of inner duct of the eccrine gland is so small that the bacteria cannot enter; while the bacteria can enter into the duct of the apocrine gland and hair follicle because the openings of these ducts are relatively much wider. For this reason, these appendages are susceptible to bacterial or fungal infections.

**A chemical barrier** is another vital function of the skin. This has been mentioned already that skin does not allow any foreign or unwanted molecule to enter into the skin from outside. The also controls the loss of water, electrolytes and other endogenous constituents. Most of the chemicals cannot penetrate the body through a horny layer of the skin. Their penetration is usually rate-limiting step in transdermal absorption. Intact skin functions as an effective barrier because large diffusional resistance is offered by the horny layer. The permeable route is the appendageal route which provides an only a tiny area of about 0.1%.

**Radiation barrier** refers to protection from UV-radiation. When skin is exposed to sunlight, ultraviolet light of 290 – 400nm (wavelength) damage the skin greatly, usually called as sunburn. Most important skin reactions are – erythema, pigmentation and epidermal thickening. Ultraviolet light stimulates melanocytes and melanin is produced. Melanin protects the skin partially. In case of a severe photosensitive disease such as xeroderma pigmentosum, sunlight induces changes in patients even with intense racial pigmentation. Intense racial pigmentation makes people less susceptible to sunburn. Chronic interaction with sunlight may cause 'aging effect,' pre-malignancy and malignancy. Prolong exposure to sunlight may produce solar keratosis, particularly in sun-damaged skin. This may further lead to squamous cell carcinoma.

**The heat barrier** function of the skin refers to the regulation of body temperature. The thickness of stratum corneum is very less. It cannot protect effectively underlying living tissues from extreme cold or heat. Thus, skin is not an efficient heat insulator. However, skin is the organ primarily responsible for maintaining the body temperature at 37°C. Therefore, to conserve heat, the peripheral circulation shuts down to reduce heat loss from the body surface. Again, in severe cold or chilling weather, shivering takes place. Because through this shivering body generates energy. On the other hand, to lose heat blood vessels dilate to emit heat to surroundings, eccrine sweat glands pour out their dilute saline secretions, and water starts evaporating. As a result, the heat is removed in the form of heat of vaporization, and the body becomes cool.

**Electrical barrier** refers to a situation when the skin is dry, resistance and impedance are much higher than in other biological tissues.

**The mechanical barrier** means resistance to mechanical shock. An acute, violent blow bruises and blisters the skin; friction may blister or thicken the epidermis, producing callosities and corns. Accidental minor trauma to the patients on corticosteroids may severely damage the skin. This happens when the collagen is thinned by overuse of drug.

## Permeation through Skin

Usually, the primary objective of topical drug therapy is to produce a desired therapeutic action at a specific site or sites on epidermal tissue. However, certain topical preparations such as emollient, deodorant, antibacterial, etc. are applied for their action on skin surface only. For most of the topical preparations, the target area lies in the viable epidermis or upper dermis.

It is, therefore, necessary to understand how a drug penetrates the skin, an insert member, and then, proceed towards the special situation of skin transport. There is two penetrations of the drug through the skin:

- Ways of penetration, and
- Principle involved.

## Ways of Penetration

There are three ways of percutaneous penetration (shown in fig. 6.2):

- Transepidermal absorption
- Transfollicular absorption
- Sebum and Surface material

Through sweat gland, and unbroken stratum corneum between the appendages. No or little convincing evidence is there that the penetration takes place through eccrine sweat glands. Substances may enter into the ducts or the glands; but the substances cannot move further since the openings of these ducts are too small.

The substances absorbed by the transepidermal route can penetrate more or less rapidly. However, this rate of absorption is slower than that in gastrointestinal absorption. In most cases, with this type of absorption some extent of pilosebaceous penetration

- **Transepidermal absorption:** The epidermal barrier function rests upon the stratum corneum. Similar to 'brick wall' stratum corneum has 'brick and mortar' structure. The brick structure is contributed by corneocytes which are composed of hydrated keratins. The corneocytes (bricks) are embedded in the complex lipid mixture of ceramides, fatty acids, cholesterol, and cholesterol esters (mortar). This mixture remains in the form of the bilayer (multiple layers). Such 'brick and mortar' structure provides an intercellular micro route. Through this route, most of the molecules penetrate the skin.

Since stratum corneum is formed by dead tissue layer, it is logically accepted that no active transport can take place in penetration through stratum corneum. Simultaneously, there shall be no difference between *in-vivo* and *in-vitro* penetration/permeation processes.

But, there are some differences between the amounts of drug penetrate through intact skin (*in-vivo*) and excised skin (*in-vitro*). Most probably the reason lies in the preparation of the skin for in-vitro determination. The skin is partially damaged during its preparation. The drugs such as hexachlorophene, steroids, griseofulvin, etc. are topically administered.  These drugs can form a depot or reservoir by binding within the stratum corneum. Some diseases such as exfoliative dermatitis, eczema can disrupt the residence time of a drug on the dermal papillary layer depends on the number of capillaries present. The number of capillaries in the papillary layer is so huge that the drug can reside not more than a minute and washed away. The usually deeper dermal layer does not have any effect on transdermal absorption; however, the drugs such as nonsteroidal anti-inflammatory drugs reach maximum up to the muscle. Hormones such as testosterone may be bound by dermis, and its systemic elimination is decreased. Principally it is believed that the horny layer of the skin. As a result, the drugs can easily penetrate the skin. A drug can be inactivated, or a prodrug can be activated through metabolization in the viable layers (mostly the epidermis) of the skin.

Transdermal penetration takes place due to diffusion of the drug across the skin. Stratum corneum resists the passage of the drug;

> ➤ Before diffusion the drug is first partitioned in the stratum corneum. Then, the drug is diffused across the tissue.
>
> ➤ It is believed that the drug is diffused across the stratum corneum through the intercellular lipoidal route.
>
> ➤ Completely polar compounds and ions pass across the stratum corneum through microscopic route.
>
> ➤ Lipophilic molecules accumulate in and diffuse relatively easily through the horny layers' intercellular region.
>
> ➤ When a penetrating drug exits at the stratum corneum, it enters the wet cell of the epidermis. Since there is no direct blood supply to epidermis; the drug is forced to diffuse across the epidermis and to move below the epidermis. The viable epidermis is permeable and functions as a viscid watery region.
>
> ➤ It appears that ions and polar non-electrolyte molecules can pass through the hydrophilic ions and lipophilic non-electrolytes through the hydrophobic zone of the epidermis.
>
> ➤ The cell membranes of the epidermis are tightly joined, and little or no intercellular space is left for movement of ions and polar non-electrolytes.
>
> ➤ For permeation of water-soluble compounds frequent crossing of cell membranes is required. But, these crossings are thermodynamically unsuitable for movement of such molecules. On the other hand, extremely lipophilic molecules cannot be dissolved in watery regions of the cell (cytoplasm); hence, thermodynamically such movement/passage is restricted.
>
> ➤ For diffusion/passage of nonpolar molecules, the viable tissue is the rate-limiting. For systemic absorption, passage through the dermal region becomes the final problem. Permeation through dermis takes place through the interlocking channel of the ground substance since the gaps between the collagen fibers are wide enough so that the molecules of any type (polar or nonpolar) can penetrate.

- **Transfollicular absorption:** Area available for absorption through the skin appendages is small, about 0.1% and this is a secondary route for permeation. This route contributes slightly to the steady-state flux of a drug. For ions and polar molecules, this route is essential because these molecules and ions cross intact stratum corneum with difficulty. Sebaceous and eccrine glands are considered as the shunts for bypassing stratum corneum, and these appendages are distributed throughout the body. Out of these two types of glands the number of eccrine glands is more, but their orifices are relatively less. Skin appendages can function as shunts and are important for short times before steady-state diffusion.

For example, in bioassays using pharmacological reactions. Hence, may be a very little number of corticosteroids penetrate rapidly down the shunt; the route can quickly trigger erythema or blanching, respectively. Therefore, these are not considered as the main route for percutaneous absorption.

In general, we do not consider hair follicle for percutaneous absorption under steady-state conditions. But, the follicular route functions as an important route for percutaneous absorption of large molecules and even the particles of colloidal dimensions.

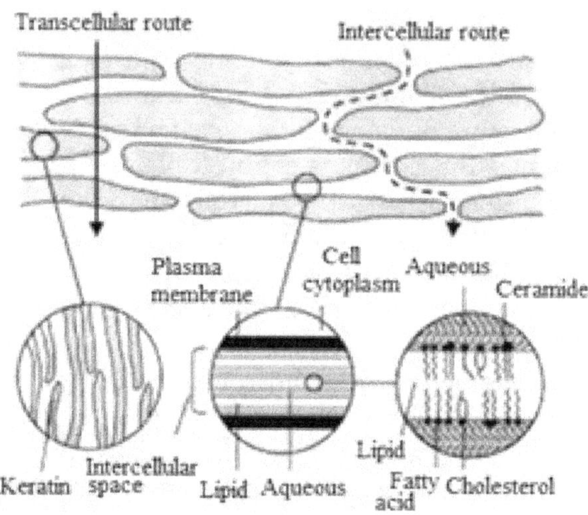


**Fig. 6.2:** Mechanism of drug permeation through skin.

Because, the openings of follicular pores, where the hair shaft exits the skin, are relatively large and sebum helps in the diffusion of penetrants (molecules/particles penetrating). The 'naked' DNA has been applied over the skin for immunization. It has been observed that normal follicles have effectively induced the immune response to the proteins in the follicle. This indicates that the follicles have an efficient mechanism of percutaneous absorption of large molecules. Partitioning of molecules in sebum and diffusion through the sebum into deeper layer of the epidermis are the possible mechanisms of permeation by this route.

Hair-loss is a common side effect of toxic chemotherapeutic agents used in the treatment of cancer. If a preparation made out of antibodies from transgenic plants is rubbed over the scalp, it stops/reduces hair-loss. Similarly, colloidal particles such as liposomes and small crystals have been found beneficial for targeting the hair follicle. Generally, particles bigger than 10µm cannot penetrate the skin surface; but, the particles smaller than 10µm and up to 3µm concentrate in the hair follicle, and the particles smaller than 3µm penetrate the follicles and stratum corneum too.

- **Sebum and Surface material:** Sweat, bacteria and dead cells together form a thin layer over the skin. The thickness of such layer varies from 0.4 to 10µm at various places of the body. The layer is irregular and discontinuous and has hardly any effect on percutaneous absorption. But, more than 300 volatile compounds and many non-volatile compounds have been identified on the skin surface.

## The Principle involved in Transdermal Penetration

To understand percutaneous absorption properly, it is necessary to know first how molecules penetrate an inert membrane and the mathematics involved therein.

### Diffusion process

In the process of passive diffusion, the molecules of a substance move from one region of a system to another. During this movement, the molecules move randomly. The mathematical concept behind this process for the substances having identical structure and diffusion characteristics (isotropic) in all directions assumes that the rate of transfer of a diffusing substance is proportional to the concentration gradient of that substance. This can be expressed as Fick's first law of diffusion:

$$J = -D\,\frac{dC}{dx} \qquad\qquad .....(6.1)$$

Where  J is the rate of transfer per unit area of the surface (flux),

C is the concentration of diffusing substance ($g/cm^3$),

D is the diffusion coefficient of the penetrant (also called diffusant),

$X$ is the distance (cm) of movement perpendicular to the surface of the barrier, and t is the time. The negative sign indicates that the flux is in the direction of decreasing concentration. In most of the cases D is constant; but in some cases, particularly for more complex substances D depends on concentration. The dimension of the diffusion coefficient is $cm^2/sec$.

According to the Fick's first law, there are three variables, J, C, and $x$. If the amount m transfers in time, t; then the rate of transfer would be $\dfrac{dm}{dt}$; where 'm' is the amount of drug transferred in time 't.' Under this circumstance, Fick's second law is employed. Accordingly,

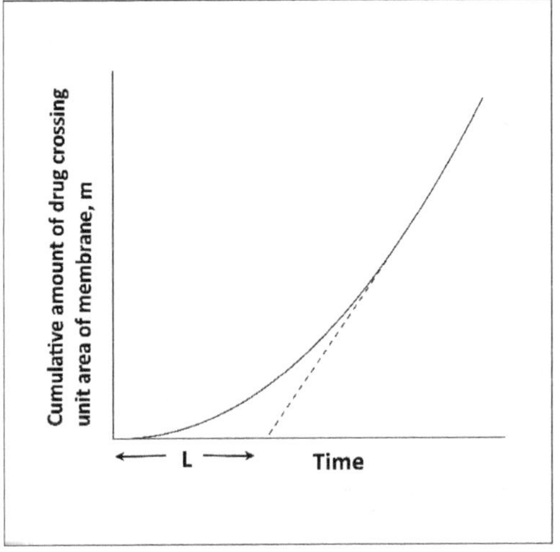


**Fig. 6.3:** Plot of m Vs time for simple zero order.

$$\frac{dC}{dt} = D\frac{d^2C}{dx^2} \qquad\qquad .....(6.2)$$

In many experiments where the solute (drug) moves a membrane separating two compartments. At both 'sink' and operating conditions, the movement of solute is governed by the concentration gradient as happens in case of receptor compartment. If the cumulative amount of solute (drug) diffused, m, per unit area through the membrane during a particular period, t, is measured and is plotted against time, a graph as shown in fig. 6.3 would be obtained. At a longer period when the plot becomes straight, its slope provides steady-state flux $\dfrac{dm}{dt}$ ;

$$\frac{dm}{dt} = \frac{DC_oK}{h} \qquad\qquad .....(6.3)$$

Where, $C_o$ is the constant concentration of the drug in the donor compartment, K is the partition coefficient of the drug between the bathing solution and membrane, and h is the thickness of the membrane.

When a steady-state plot is extrapolated to X-axis (time-axis) as shown in fig 6.3, an intercept L is obtained at m = 0. This intercept, L is called lag time and

$$L = \frac{h^2}{6D} \qquad\qquad .....(6.4)$$

From equation 4, the value of D can be calculated if the value of h is known; L is known from the plot.

If the value of D is known, the value of $C_o$ can be calculated easily from equation 3; because of the values of K and $\dfrac{dm}{it}$ can be determined experimentally.

Sometimes, the value of D cannot be separated from K, particularly with a biological membrane such as skin. In such cases a parameter P, known as the permeability coefficient is used; where,

$$P = KD$$

Or, $\qquad\qquad P = \dfrac{KD}{h}$ .

When h is uncertain for example in case of penetration through the skin, the second equation, $\qquad\qquad P = \dfrac{KD}{h}$ is used.

## Complex Barriers for Diffusion

The above discussion is limited to a simple and single barrier system, where diffusion takes place in a single isotropic medium. But skin is not a simple and single barrier system; it is a heterogeneous multi-layer tissue.

## Barrier in Series

Skin being a heterogeneous multilayer tissue and hence, in percutaneous absorption, the concentration gradient occurs in several strata. Let us assume that skin may is a laminate of multiple layers in which each layer has diffusional resistance, R. This resistance, R is directly proportional to the layer's thickness, h and indirectly proportional to KD; where D is the diffusivity of the layer and K is the partition coefficient with respect to the external phase.

Then, the total diffusional resistance, $R_T$ for a three-layered skin (stratum corneum, epidermis, and dermis) can be expressed as;

$$RT = \frac{1}{P_T} = \frac{h_1}{D_1 K_1} = + \frac{h_2}{D_2 K_2} + \frac{h_3}{D_3 K_3} \qquad \text{.....(6.5)}$$

Where $P_T$ is the thickness-weighted permeability coefficient. If the resistance offered by a particular layer such as stratum corneum (first layer) is much greater and the resistance offered by other layers such as epidermis and dermis are insignificant; then, the equation 5 would be reduced to

$$RT = \frac{1}{P_T} = \frac{h_1}{D_1 K_1}$$

And the overall permeability of the skin can be expressed the s;

$$P_T = \frac{D_1 K_1}{h_1}$$

## Barrier in Parallel

The hair follicles and sweat glands pierce the human skin through shunts and pores. This complex situation may be considered as a simple situation wherein diffusional medium consists of two or more diffusional pathways connected parallelly. Hence, the total diffusional flux per unit area of the composite, $J_T$ would be the sum of individual fluxes through separate routes. This can be expressed as;

$$J_T = f_1 J_1 + f_2 J_2 + \ldots\ldots\ldots\ldots +$$

Where, $f_1$, $f_2$, etc. are the fractional area for each diffusional route and $J_1$, $J_2$, etc. represent the fluxes per unit area of individual routes.

Generally, the total diffusional flux per unit area of the composite, for independent linear parallel pathways during steady-state diffusion is written as;

$$J_T = Co \ (f_1 P_1 + f_2 P_2 + \ldots\ldots\ldots\ldots +)$$

Where, $P_1$, $P_2$, etc. represent the thickness-weighted permeability coefficients.

If diffusion through only one route takes place and other routes do not allow the diffusant to pass, then the situation becomes diffusion through simple membrane model. The steady-state flux can be determined by the fractional area and the permeation rate through the open channel.

The mechanism involved in percutaneous drug delivery is mentioned below;

| Sl No | Skin Region | Thickness (μm) | Permeation rate (mg/cm$^2$/hr) | Diffusivity (cm$^2$/sec×10$^{10}$) |
|---|---|---|---|---|
| 1. | Abdomen | 15 | 0.34 | 6.0 |
| 2. | Volar forearm | 16 | 031 | 5.9 |
| 3. | Back | 10.5 | 0.29 | 3.5 |
| 4. | Fore head | 13 | 0.85 | 12.9 |
| 5. | Scrotum | 5 | 0.17 | 7.4 |
| 6. | Back of hand | 49 | 1.56 | 32.3 |
| 7. | Palm | 400 | 1.14 | 535 |
| 8. | Plantar | 600 | 3.90 | 930 |

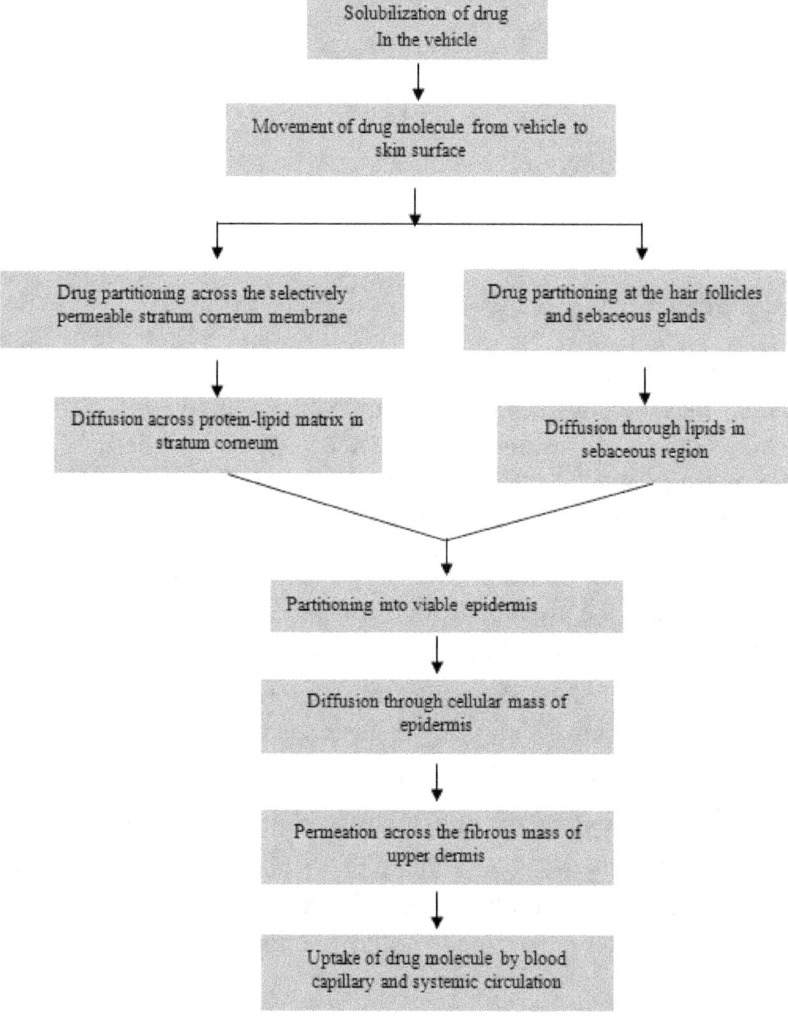

# Factors Affecting Permeation

(A)  Physicochemical properties of permeate:
1. Partition coefficient
2. Molecular size
3. Solubility/melting point
4. Ionization

(B)  Physiological & pathological conditions of skin:
1. Reservoir effect of horny layer
2. Lipid film
3. Skin hydration
4. Skin temperature
5. Regional variation
6. Pathological injuries to the skin
7. Cutaneous self-metabolism
8. Skin barrier properties in the neonate and young infant
9. Skin barrier properties in aged skin
10. Race
11. Body site
12. Penetration enhancers used

## (A)  Physicochemical properties of permeate

1. **Partition coefficient:** Water & lipid soluble drugs favorably absorbed through the skin. The intercellular route is applicable for drugs with an intermediate partition coefficient (log K 1 to 3) & having high lipophilicity. The transcellular route probably predominates for more hydrophilic molecules (logK < 1).

2. **Molecular size:** There is an inverse relationship existed between transdermal flux and molecular weight of the molecule. The drug molecule selected as candidates for transdermal delivery tend to lie within the narrow range of molecular weight (100-500 Dalton).

3. **Solubility/melting point:** Lipophilicity is a desired property of transdermal candidates as lipophilic molecules tend to permeate through the skin faster than more hydrophilic molecules. Drugs with high melting points have relatively low aqueous solubility at normal temperature and pressure.

4. **Ionization:** According to the pH-partition hypothesis, only the unionized form of the drug can permeate through the lipid barrier in significant amounts.

**(B) Physiological and pathological conditions of the skin**

1. ***Reservoir effect of horny layer***: The horny layer is a deeper layer. The drug can bind with the skin. This binding may be reversible or irreversible. The reservoir effect of the horny layer is due to the irreversible binding of a part of the applied drug with the skin.

2. ***Lipid film***: This has been mentioned earlier that there is a lipid film on the skin surface and this film acts as a protective layer.

   Being lipid in nature, the film prevents the removal of moisture from the skin; hence, helps in maintaining the barrier function of stratum corneum.

3. ***Skin hydration***: Hydration of skin can be achieved simply by covering or occluding the skin with a plastic sheet. This will not allow the sweat to evaporate and will accumulate. The accumulated sweat will increase the opening of the dense, closely packed cells in the skin. Due to the increased porosity of the skin, the penetration by the drug would enhance.

4. ***Skin temperature***: It is observed that the rate of skin permeation increases with an increase in skin temperature. Probably, this happens due to the availability of energy required for diffusivity.

5. ***Regional variation***: The variation in color, nature, and thickness of skin depends on various factors; climatic conditions of the region is one of these factors. Due to such differences in nature and thickness of skin, the barrier function of the skin varies and cause variation in permeability.

6. ***Pathological injuries to the skin***: Injuries to the skin disrupt the continuity of the stratum corneum and in some areas the barrier layer; stratum corneum is removed; hence, vasodilatation takes place. Due to vasodilation, the skin permeability is increased.

7. ***Cutaneous self-metabolism***: Catabolic enzymes present in the epidermis may make the drug inactive. Because the drug may be metabolized by these enzymes and thus the topical bioavailability of the drug is affected.

8. ***Skin barrier properties in the neonate and young infant***: The pH of the skin surface of newly born is higher than those in adult skin. The skin surface of the new-born is slightly hydrophobic and relatively dry and rough when compared to that of older infants. Stratum corneum hydration stabilizes by the age of 3 months.

9. ***Skin barrier properties in aged skin***: The physiology of aged skin changes with age, particularly after 65 years. The corneocytes are shown to increase in surface area which may have implications for stratum corneum function due to the resulting decreased volume of inter-corneocyte space per unit volume of stratum corneum. The moisture content of human skin decreases with age.

10. ***Race***: Racial differences between black and white skins have been observed in some anatomical and physiological functions of the skin. In black skin, increased intracellular cohesion, higher lipid content and higher electrical skin resistance levels compared to whites have been demonstrated.

11. ***Body site***: Skin structure varies at different sites of the body. Generally, genital tissues usually provide the most permeable site for transdermal drug delivery. The skin of the head and neck is also relatively permeable compared to other sites of the body such as the arms and legs. Intermediate permeability for most drugs is found on the trunk of the body.

# Permeation Enhancers

## Chemical Permeation Enhancers

In the last 50 years, a large number of chemical permeation enhancers (CPEs) which are defined as substances that interact with the major constituents of the skin barrier, stratum corneum, to promote penetration of drugs into the skin.

The ideal enhancer should have the following characteristics:

1. Non-pharmacological activities.
2. Nontoxic, non-allergenic, and non-irritating.
3. Rapid-acting with predictable and reproducible activity.
4. When removed from the skin surface, the penetrability of the skin should recover immediately.
5. Cosmetically acceptable with suitable skin feel.

The part of penetration enhancer in topical formulations has been becoming significantly and undoubtedly, and they would permit the delivery of broader classes of drugs through the stratum corneum in the future.

## The Classification of Chemical Permeation Enhancers

From the above mentioned, we can know that the skin provides such a formidable obstacle to the delivery of most drugs, a variety of different chemical permeation enhancers have been tested to enhance transdermal penetration. Immense amounts of research during the past two decades has led to the formulation of some different classes of penetration enhancers, including surfactants (for example, sorbitan trioleate), fatty acids/esters (for example, lauric acid), terpenes (for example, menthone), azone-like compounds (for example, azone), and solvents (for example, ethanol and dimethyl sulphoxide). These have been summarized in the table below;

**Table 6.1:** Types of excipients commonly used in TDDS

| Types | Example |
|---|---|
| Surfactants | Sorbitan monopalmitate, Sorbitan trioleate, Cetyl trimethyl ammonium bromide |
| Fatty acids/esters | Alkanoic acids, oleic acid, lauric acid, capric acid, Cetyl lactate, butyl acetate, isopropyl myristate |
| Terpenes | Nerolidol, Farnesol, Carvone, Menthone |
| Azone-like compounds | Azone (Laurocapram, 1-dodecylazacycloheptan-2-one), 1-alkyl- or 1-alkenylaza cycloalkanones |
| Solvents | DMSO, ethanol, 1-octanol, 1-hexanol |

## Fatty Acids, the Skin Permeation Enhancers

Fatty acids are composed of an aliphatic hydrocarbon chain with a terminal carboxylic acid group. The number, position, and configuration of double bonds of their aliphatic chain are visibly different. The aliphatic chain may be saturated or unsaturated and may have branching and other substituents. Fatty acids have different characteristics and enhancing effects.

A study of Florence *et al.* indicates that with increasing of the carbon chain length, the lipophilicity of fatty acids can be improved. Hence, long-chain fatty acids have a much higher affinity to lipids in the stratum corneum. The short-chain fatty acids have insufficient lipophilicity which fails to penetrate the skin. The stratum corneum of the human skin is lipophilic, and the compounds of low lipophilicity tend to remain in the stratum corneum; thus, prevents drugs to penetrate the deeper tissues. Evidence from many studies has confirmed that fatty acids having a chain length from C10 to C12 can enhance penetration significantly.

Moreover, the penetration enhancing the effect of fatty acid depends on bond saturation. Studies have shown that the unsaturated long-chain fatty acids have a greater penetration enhancing activity when compared to saturated fatty acids of the same chain length. This is principally due to the higher lipid disrupting nature of the unsaturated long-chain of the fatty acids.

The effects of fatty acids on penetration through the stratum corneum also depends on the concentrations of fatty acids. Studies have shown that the permeation of meloxicam through human skin increased when the concentration of oleic acid is increased from 0.4 to 1 %.

## Terpenes, the Skin Permeation Enhancers

Terpenes belong to a series of volatile oil from natural sources. As per the basic chemical structure, terpenes consist of repeated isoprene ($C_5H_8$) units, in a head-to-tail orientation to form linear chains or rings. Terpenes are clinically acceptable penetration enhancers. These have the following advantages:

1. Compared to other synthetic skin penetration enhancers, terpenes are generally less toxic and less irritant. Few terpenes have been considered as generally regarded as safe by the Food and Drug Administration (FDA).

2. Terpenes can increase skin permeation by interacting with stratum corneum lipids and keratin, and by increasing the solubility of the drug into stratum corneum lipids. Some factors play an essential role in the permeation enhancing activity of terpenes:

   (a)  The chemical structures of terpenes: It has been observed that stereoisomers of terpene can affect their enhancing activity. The (-) enantiomer of a terpene is more effective than the corresponding (+) isomer or (±) racemate. Some terpenes with a minimal degree of saturation are more effective enhancers and can deliver the hydrophilic drugs.

   (b)  High lipophilicity is an essential structural feature for terpenes. Accordingly, hydrocarbon, nonpolar terpenes, such as limonene, are more useful to promote the transdermal absorption of lipophilic drugs than oxygen-containing polar terpenes and vice versa.

   (c)  Some studies indicate that the liquid terpenes have a greater ability to form hydrogen bonds with intercellular lipids of stratum corneum; hence, liquid terpenes can produce better-enhancing effects than the solid ones.

## Azone-like Compounds, the Skin Permeation Enhancers

Azone is a highly lipophilic substance with a logP, around 6.2. It is compatible with many organic solvents, such as alcohols and propylene glycol. Besides, azone has low irritancy and very low toxicity. It is more effective for hydrophilic drugs than lipophilic drugs. The efficacy of azone depends on its concentration. It is more effective at lower concentrations, and is used between 0.1 to 5%. However, the lag time of azone was very high, from 2h to 10h. But, its effects can last for many days.

Azone increases the ability of drugs to penetrate the skin by interacting with the lipid compounds of the stratum corneum, disordering lipid bilayers, disrupting their packing arrangement, and increasing lipid solubilization.

**Table 6.2:** Various classes of penetration enhancers commonly used are summarized below;

| Sl. No | Class of penetration enhancer | Examples |
|---|---|---|
| 1 | Solvent | |
| | Universal solvent | Water |
| | Short-chain alcohols | Ethanol, Isopropyl alcohol (IPA) |
| | Long-chain alcohols | Decanol, hexanol, Lauro alcohol, myristyl alcohol, octanol, etc. |
| | Ether alcohols | Trascutol |
| | Glycols | Polyethylene glycol, Propylene glycol, 1,2 butylene glycol, etc. Dipropylene glycol. |

**Table 6.2:** *Contd...*

| Sl. No | Class of penetration enhancer | Examples |
|---|---|---|
| 2 | Terpenes and terpenoids<br>Monoterpenes<br><br>Sesquiterpenes | Geraniol, menthol, menthone, D-lemonene, etc.<br><br>Farnesol, nerolidol, etc. |
| 3 | Esters<br>Alkyl esters<br>Benzoic acid esters<br>Fatty acid ester | <br>Ethyl acetate<br>Octyl salicylate, Padimate-O<br>Ethyl oleate, Glyceryl mono-oleate, Isopropyl Myristate, Isopropyl Palmitate, |
| 4 | Amides<br>Cyclamides | <br>Azone |
| 5 | Fatty acids<br>Long chain fatty acids | Lauric acid, linoleic acid, linolenic acid, myristic acid, oleic acid, stearic acid etc. |
| 6 | Sulphoxides<br>alkyl methyl sulfoxides | Dimethyl sulfoxide (DMSO), Decylmethyl sulphoxide. |
| 7 | Surfactants<br>Anionic surfactants<br><br>Cationic surfactants<br><br><br>Non-ionic surfactants | <br>Dioctyl -sulphosuccinate, Sodium lauryl-sulfate, Decodecyl dimethylsulphoxide.<br>Alkyl dimethyl benzyl ammonium halides, Alkyl trimethyl ammonium halides, Alkyl pyridinium halides.<br>Brij 36T, Tween 80 |
| 8 | Bile salts | Sodium deoxycholate, Sodium Tauroglyco- cholate, Sodium taurocholate. |
| 9 | Binary systems | Propylene glycol-oleic acid and 1,4-butane diol-linoleic acid. |
| 10 | Miscellaneous chemicals | N, N-dimethyl-m-toluamide, Urea, Calcium thioglycolate, Anticholinergic agents. |

## Basic Components of TDDS

Usually, the following components are used to manufacture the transdermal drug delivery system (TDDS):

1. Polymer matrix/drug reservoir
2. Drug
3. Penetration enhancer

4.  Pressure sensitive adhesive (PSA)
5.  Backing membrane
6.  Release Liner
7.  Other excipients.

1. **Polymer matrix/Drug reservoir:** The release of drug from the formulation/device is controlled by the polymer. The polymer should have the following characteristics;

    ➢ Molecular weight, glass transition temperature and chemical properties of the polymer should be such that the drug is released from the formulation and can diffuse through the membrane.

    ➢ It should be stable, inert, readily available/manufactured/fabricated, and also economical.

    ➢ It should not be antagonistic to the drug.

    ➢ It or its degradation product should be non-toxic.

    ➢ If a large amount of drug is present in the formulation, the mechanical properties of the polymer used or of the product is not affected or degraded.

The polymer used for making TDDS may be of three types:

Natural polymers such as cellulose derivatives, zeins, gelatine, shellac, proteins, waxes, gums and their derivatives, natural rubber, starch, etc.

Synthetic elastomers such as polybutadiene, hydrin rubber, polysiloxane, silicone rubber, nitrile, acrylonitrile, butyl rubber, styrene butadiene rubber, neoprene, etc.

Synthetic polymers such as polyvinyl alcohol, polyvinyl pyrrolidone, polyvinyl chloride, polyamide, polyethylene, polypropylene, polyacrylate, polyurea, polymethylmethacrylate, epoxy, etc.

Different types of polymers which are commonly used to prepare TDDS are given below;

| Class | Example |
| --- | --- |
| Amides | N,N-dimethyl-m-toluamide |
| Fatty acid | Oleic acid, Undecanoic acid |
| Fatty alcohol | Nonanol, Octanol |
| Lactam | Laurocapram |
| Polyol | Polyethylene glycol, Propylene glycol |
| Sulphoxide | Dimethyl sulphoxide, Dodecyl methyl sulphoxide |
| Surfactant (anionic) | Sodium lauryl sulphate |
| Surfactant (cationic) | N,N-bis(2hydroxy ethyl) oleyl amine |
| Surfactant (non-ionic) | Polyoxymethylene (20) sorbitan mono oleate |
| Surfactant (zwitter ionic) | Dodecyl dimethyl ammonium propane sulfate |
| Sugar | Cyclodextrins |
| Terpene | Menthol, Thymol, Limonene |
| Urea | Urea |

2. **Drug:** Selection of an appropriate drug is the most important for the development of transdermal drug delivery system (TDDS). For use in TDDS a drug should have the following properties:

Physicochemical properties

> The molecular weight of the drug should be less than 1000 Daltons.
> The drug should have an affinity towards both hydrophilic and lipophilic phases.
> Extreme lipophilic or extreme hydrophilic drugs are not suitable.
> The melting point of the drug should not be high.

Biological properties

> The daily dose of the drug should be less; that is, about a few milligrams per day.
> The biological half-life of the drug should be short.
> The drug should be non-irritant to the skin and should not produce an allergic reaction.
> A drug which degrades in the gastrointestinal tract or which are inactivated by hepatic first-pass effect is suitable for TDDS.
> Under zero-order or nearly zero-order release for TDDS, the tolerance to the drug should not be developed.
> Drugs which are administered for an extended period, are suitable for TDDS.
> Drugs which produce adverse effects on non-target tissues can be administered through TDDS.

3. **Permeation enhancers:** The compounds or substances which temporarily reduce the impermeability of the skin are called permeation enhancer, sorption promoter, an accelerant. These should be non-toxic and safe. An ideal penetration enhancer should have the following characteristics;

> Should be pharmacologically inert.
> Should be non-toxic, non-irritating and non-allergic.
> It should exert an immediate action, and the effect should be suitable and predictable.
> On removal of penetrant enhancer, the skin should regain its normal barrier property.
> Should not cause the loss of body fluids, electrolytes, or other endogenous materials.
> Should be compatible with all drug and excipients used in the formulation.
> Should be a suitable solvent for drugs.
> Should be cosmetically acceptable (good spreadability and skin 'feel').
> Should formulate into all types of topical preparations.
> Should be odorless, tasteless, colorless and inexpensive.

No material can have all these properties; some can have many of these. The substances having most of these properties have been investigated clinically or in the laboratory. Usually, the type of substances which have been either used or examined for the development of TDDSs are;

- Water,
- Alcohols and glycols,
- Essential oils, terpenes, and their derivatives,
- Fatty acids and alcohols,
- Surfactants (anionic, cationic, and non-ionic)
- Sulphoxides (dimethyl sulphoxide) and their analogs,
- Urea and its derivatives,
- Azone and its derivatives,
- Pyrrolidones,
- Synergistic mixtures.

Among all these compounds, water is the best penetration enhancer because it is the safest and also effective. Most of these compounds are more effective when the stratum corneum is hydrated than when the skin is dry. Hence, any compound which is pharmacologically inert, non-toxic, and can hydrate the hard layer, can be used as a penetration enhancer; for example, urea.

The enhancer interacts with organized intercellular lipid structure of stratum corneum; the structure is disrupted. As a result, the skin becomes more permeable to drug molecules. Many penetration enhancers work in this way. There are some solvents which can extract the lipid components of the stratum corneum and can make the horny layer of the skin more permeable.

Ionic surface-active agents interact with the keratin in the corneocytes, the dense keratin structure is opened up, and make the skin more permeable. The intracellular route is not such a common route that the drug can penetrate through the skin; however, if the resistance of the skin is reduced excessively, it becomes an alternative route for permeation of drugs.

There are many solvents which can enter into the stratum corneum and change the solvent-property of stratum corneum. As a result, partitioning of other molecules is increased into the horny layer. Other molecules include drug, co-enhancer or co-solvent. For example, ethanol is used to increase the permeation of drug molecules such as nitro-glycerine and oestradiol. Propylene glycol has commonly been used along with azone, oleic acid, terpene, etc. to provide synergistic permeation enhancing effect, and the concentration of these enhancers increases in the horny layer of the skin.

4. **Pressure sensitive adhesive (PSA):** PSA is a material that adheres to a substrate; here it is the skin. When it is removed by applying light (energy), no residue is left. The PSAs are bound by interatomic and intermolecular attractive forces at the interface if they are in intimate contact with skin. To measure the degree of contact, the material used must be able to be deformed even when slight pressure is applied; for this reason, it is called 'pressure sensitive.' Adhesion is resulting in a liquid-like flow, due to wetting of the skin surface and application of pressure.

When the pressure is withdrawn or removed, the adhesive sets in that state. A PSA wets and spreads over the skin when its surface energy is less than that of the skin. After initial adhesion, the bond between PSA and skin can be formed by stronger interactions such as hydrogen bonding. This depends on skin characteristics and other parameters. Polyisobutylene-based adhesives, acrylics, and silicone-based PSAs, hydrocarbon resin, etc. are widely used as PSA polymers in TDDS. The PSA can be used around the edge of the TDDS or can be used as a continuous adhesive laminated layer on the TDDS surface. However, the PSA must be compatible with the drug and other excipients, because their presence can modify the mechanical properties of the product and the rate of drug delivery.

5.  **Backing membrane:** Selection of the backing membrane is made by appearance, flexibility, and need for occlusion; hence, while designing a backing layer, the chemical resistance of the material is most importantly considered. Compatibility between the excipients should also be considered; because the prolonged contact between the backing layer and the excipients may cause the additives which may itself leach out of the backing layer or may lead to diffusion of excipients including drug or penetration enhancer through the layer. The most satisfactory and suitable backing layer would be the one that exhibits the lowest modulus or high flexibility, good oxygen transmission, and a high moisture vapor transmission rate. Polymers generally used for making backing materials are vinyl, polyethylene, polyester films, aluminum, and polyolefin films.

6.  **Release Liner:** During storage, the patch should be covered by a protective liner, and before the application of the patch to the skin this liner should be removed and discarded. Since the liner remains in intimate contact with the TDDS for a long period, the liner should be chemically inert. Generally, a release liner is composed of a base layer and a release coating layer. The base layer may be nonocclusive such as paper fabric, or occlusive. The occlusive layer is made up of polyethylene, polyvinyl chloride, etc. For the release of drug silicon or Teflon may be used. Other materials used for TDDS release liner are polyester foil and metalized laminates.

7.  **Other excipients:** Pressure sensitive adhesive is used to fasten the transdermal devices to the skin. The position of the pressure sensitive adhesive is kept either facing the device towards the skin or in the back of the device extending peripherally. Whatever may be the type of adhesive system used, it should fulfill the following requirements:
    - It should not irritate or sensitize the skin,
    - During its contact with the skin, normal skin flora should not be disturbed,
    - It should be adhered to the skin firmly, should not be disturbed or should not change its position during bathing, exercise, etc.,
    - Should be easily removed from the skin,
    - Should be washed away completely, no residue should be left,
    - Should provide intimate contact with the skin at the macroscopic and microscopic level.

The peripheral adhesive contains several layers, is larger. Compared to a peripheral adhesive system intended for application over the face, it is difficult to manufacture such a system. The peripheral adhesive system is less elegant. When the peripheral systems are used, it is not necessary to further pack the reservoir layer. The face adhesive systems are packed in an aluminum foil pouch because these are not usually hermetically contained. Poly isobutylene, acrylics, and silicones are widely used in pressure sensitive systems.

The adhesive system applied over the face should fulfill the following requirements:

> ➤ All the components including adhesive, drug, permeation enhancer and other excipients should be physicochemically compatible,

> ➤ Whether simple or blended enhancer is used, penetration should not be affected,

> ➤ The drug should penetrate the skin without any hindrance,

## Formulation Approaches

The transdermal dosage form is composed of a few layers; each has a specific function. When a transdermal patch is placed over the skin the first layer, the backing layer prevents the system from wetting during its use. Second layer functions as a reservoir. It supplies the drug to the skin for exerting its therapeutic action for a predetermined period. Next, to this layer, there is the third layer of polymer. This layer regulates or controls the rate of drug release during the predetermined time interval. The drug delivered diffuses through the skin and enters into the systemic circulation. Usually, the rate of drug release from the transdermal systems is much greater than the rate of absorption by the skin. Although the permeability of the skin varies, a constant supply of the drug to the systemic circulation is required to be maintained.

There are four approaches to prepare a transdermal drug delivery system.

1. **Membrane permeation-controlled TDDS:** In this type of system, the drug reservoir layer remains encapsulated as shown in fig. 6.4. The encapsulating compartment is molded from a drug-impermeable metallic membrane (foil) which is laminated with plastic. The compartment is covered with a microporous or non-porous copolymer such as ethylene vinyl acetate (EVA). The polymeric membrane possesses a defined drug-permeable porosity. The drug molecules are released through the rate-controlling membrane.

   The drug (solid) is either dispersed uniformly in a solid polymer matrix or uniformly suspended in a viscous liquid medium such as silicone fluid. The suspending medium should be unreachable, and its consistency should be such that a paste-like the suspension is produced. Whether it is solid dispersion or paste, the drug mixture in the form of a membrane is put in the drug reservoir compartment. At the outer side of the rate-controlling membrane, an adhesive polymeric coating is applied so that the system can firmly adhere to the skin to ensure intimate contact between the system and skin when it is applied. Silicone or polyacrylate is used as the adhesive polymer. The polymer used as adhesive should be compatible with the drug and should not cause any type of allergic reaction. The permeability of the rate-controlling membrane can be varied by varying the composition of polymers.

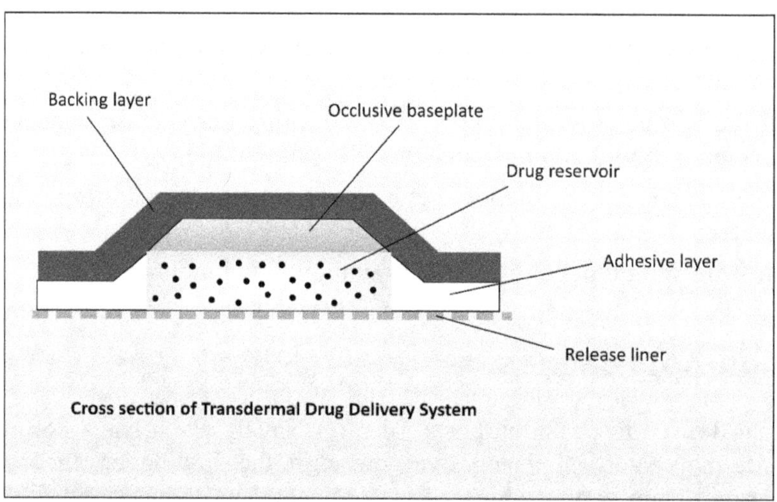


**Fig. 6.4:** Membrane permeation-controlled TDDS.

Generally, the drug is released from the transdermal system at a constant rate. If the rate-controlling membrane is broken accidentally, dose dumping or rapid release of the drug may take place. The drugs commonly administered through this route are nitroglycerin, scopolamine, clonidine, estradiol, etc.

The intrinsic rate of drug release from this type of transdermal system can be expressed as;

$$\frac{dQ}{dt} = \frac{C_R}{\dfrac{P_m + P_a}{P_m P_a}} = \frac{C_R}{\dfrac{1}{P_a} + \dfrac{1}{P_m}} \qquad \qquad .....(6.6)$$

Where, $C_R$ = concentration of drug in the reservoir,

$P_a$ = permeability coefficient of the adhesive layer,

$P_m$ = permeability coefficient of rate-controlling membrane.

In the case of the microporous membrane, $P_m$ is the sum of permeability coefficients of polymeric materials for simultaneous penetration across the pores. $P_m$ and $P_a$ can be defined as follows;

$$P_m = \frac{K_{m/r} \cdot D_m}{h_m} \qquad \qquad .....(6.7)$$

$$P_a = \frac{K_{a/m} \cdot D_m}{h_a} \qquad \qquad .....(6.8)$$

Where, $K_{m/r}$ and $K_{a/r}$ are the partition coefficients for the interfacial partitioning of the drug from the reservoir to the membrane and from the membrane to the adhesive layer respectively. $D_m$ and $D_a$ are the diffusion coefficients in the rate-controlling membrane and adhesive layer respectively; hm and ha are thicknesses of rate-controlling membrane and adhesive layer respectively.

By substituting the equation 2 and 3 for $P_a$ and $P_m$ in equation 3, we get

$$\frac{dQ}{dt} = \frac{K_{m/r} \cdot K_{a/r} \cdot D_m \cdot D_a}{K_{m/r} \cdot D_m \cdot h_a + K_{a/m} \cdot D_a \cdot h_m} C_R \qquad \qquad .....(6.9)$$

Equation 4 expresses the intrinsic rate of drug-release from a membrane permeation-controlled transdermal system.

Such product consists of three substrates held together by two layers containing the drug. The drug is processed into the physical or chemical form necessary for making the formulation. The drug, excipients, and polymers (adhesive) are mixed thoroughly with a solvent to produce a uniform mixture (solution or dispersion). This is an essential and critical step; should be carried out carefully; because the composition of the product depends on it.  The solvent is removed by drying the mixture.

The dried adhesive layer and other layers are then five layers are laminated. The five layers are: release linear, contact adhesive, a control membrane, the drug reservoir, and backing membrane. All the layers are cut into required size using a die and printed. Lamination and coating of films are also important and critical steps; because laminated films must be wrinkle free and thickness of coating must be uniform throughout. Hence, the process variables are to be controlled accurately. The products thus prepared are packed individually in an aluminum foil pouch.

2. **The adhesive dispersion type system:** This is a simple form of the membrane permeation-controlled system. The drug is dispersed in an adhesive polymer such as poly (isobutylene) or poly (acrylate) to prepare drug reservoir. This type of system is prepared by solvent casting or hot melt method and put over a flat, metallic plastic membrane. The metallic membrane (foil) is coated with a plastic material which is impermeable to drug. The whole of metallic-plastic membrane forms a thin casing for holding the drug dispersed in the adhesive polymer (drug-reservoir). Thin layers of nonmedicated, rate-controlling adhesive polymer are applied over the top of the drug-reservoir layer. The adhesive layer should have a specific permeability and should provide uniform thickness throughout the layer;

so that an adhesive diffusion-controlled delivery of the drug is possible. Isosorbide dinitrate is administered for angina pectoris through this type of delivery system. However, verapamil can be delivered through this route using the same delivery system.

The rate of drug-release, $\dfrac{dQ}{dt}$ through the membrane can be expressed as;

$$\dfrac{dQ}{dt} = \dfrac{K_a/_r \cdot D_a}{h_a} C_R \qquad \qquad .....(6.10)$$

Where, $K_a/_r$ = permeation coefficient for the interfacial partitioning of the drug from the reservoir layer to adhesive layer, $D_a$, $C_R$, and $h_a$ have the same meaning as given earlier. This type of drug delivery system can be modified to achieve a gradient of drug reservoir along the multi-laminate adhesive layers. This is possible by loading the drug at increments. From such a drug reservoir gradient-controlled system the rate of drug release can be expressed as;

$$\dfrac{dQ}{dt} = \dfrac{K_a/_r \cdot D_a}{h_a(t)} A(h_a) \qquad \qquad .....(6.11)$$

In equation 6, the thickness of the adhesive layer for drug molecules to diffuse through the membrane increases with time, $h_a$ (t). The drug loading level is enhanced with the thickness of the diffusional path, $A(h_a)$.

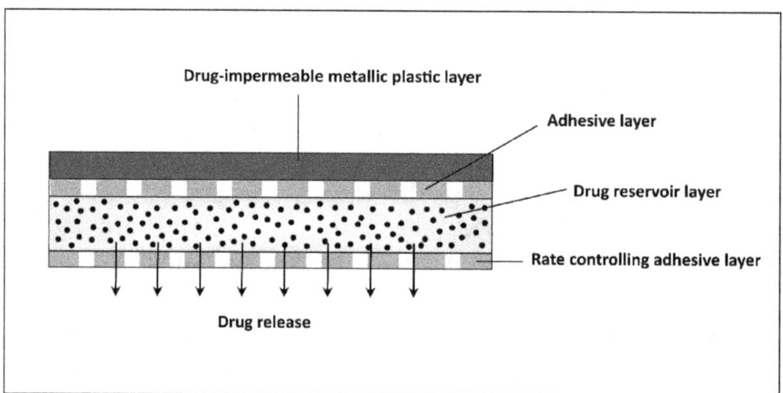


**Fig. 6.5:** Schematic representation of adhesive dispersed type TDD system.

The manufacture of this system comprises the following steps, and the schematic representation of this type of system is shown in Fig 6.5.

> ➤ ***Preparation of individual matrix solution:*** Each of the polymer, tackifier, softening agent is dissolved in an organic solvent. The solid content and other parameters are measured. These solutions are mixed to prepare a matrix

solution. To this matrix solution drug and other insoluble excipients as per the formula are added and mixed thoroughly. Similarly, as per the Master Formula, other matrix solutions are prepared. However, all these may be solution or dispersion. Each of the solutions or dispersions is poured on a smooth paper and dried to remove the solvent and to obtain a smooth film.

> ➤ ***Coating of the individual matrix layer:*** The particular layer is coated with a polymer using a suitable coating machine such as roll coater, coating heads, knife system, etc. The coating unit is hermetically closed; so that air cannot enter into the coating chamber from outside. The coating machine is directly connected to a drying unit. As a result, the solvent is evaporated out from the layer. Both drying and coating processes influence the quality of the layers. In case of large-scale or continuous production, jumbo rolls of the layered materials are prepared and used for uninterrupted production.

> ➤ ***Multilayer lamination:*** To prepare a multilayer matrix system, lamination of the layer is necessary. For example, lamination of two matrix layers is made by putting one layer over the other one and then, by pressing. The up-side of the pressed layer remains coated. Similarly, to prepare a three-layered laminate, a third layer is put over a two-layer laminate with the laminated side of two-layered to the laminated side of the third layer and pressed. In this way, the multi-layer laminate is prepared. During lamination pressure applied is important; because it must ensure proper adhesion of one layer over the other and there should be no void space (air entrapment). The wide rolls thus obtained are stored properly for further processing.

> ➤ ***Punching of laminated roll/making unit dose:*** The rolls prepared in the earlier step is cut into small pieces of required size; so that each piece can provide the desired dose of the drug and can be dispensed as a single unit-dose. This is done using a suitable punching machine. In this step, liner with required release aids is applied to the system.

> ➤ ***Packaging:*** This refers to the packing of an individual unit in the sealed, rectangular pouch and then, a specified number of units are packed in a cardboard box. Further, a specified number of cardboard boxes are packed in a corrugated box for shipment.

3. **Matrix diffusion-controlled system:** The drug reservoir is a dispersion of drug particles within a polymer matrix. This is done by homogeneously dispersing finely powdered drug in a liquid polymer or rubbery polymer at a higher temperature. The dispersion is thoroughly mixed by continuous stirring. This can be alternatively done by dissolving the drug and polymer in a particular solvent. The mixture is mixed thoroughly. The solvent is then evaporated in a mold at a higher temperature or under vacuum. The drug reservoir discs are pasted onto an occlusive base plate in a compartment fabricated from a drug impermeable plastic backing. The adhesive polymer is then spread along the circumference to form a strip of adhesive rim around the medicated disc (fig. 6.6).

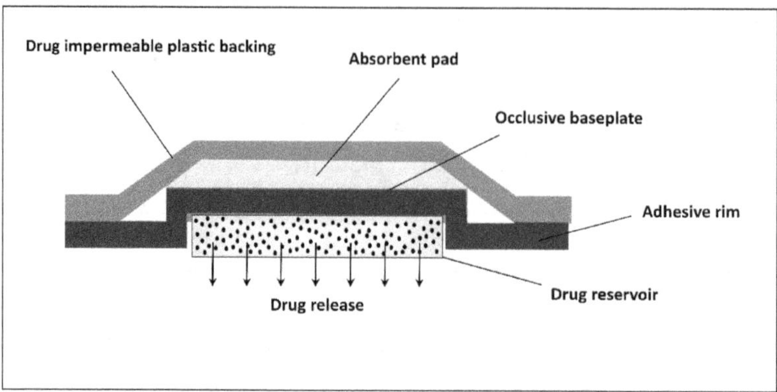


**Fig. 6.6:** Matrix diffusion-controlled TDDS.

This type of transdermal system is commonly used to administer nitroglycerin. The rate of drug release from this type of transdermal system can be expressed as;

$$\frac{dQ}{dt} = \left[\frac{AC_pC_p}{2t}\right]^{1/2}$$

Where A is the dose of drug dispersed in the polymer matrix, Cp and Dp are solubility and diffusivity of the drug in the polymer respectively. Since the polymer can release the drug only, Cp is essentially equal to $C_R$; where $C_R$ is the concentration of drug in the reservoir compartment.

$$\frac{Q}{t_{1/2}} = [(2A - C_p)C_pD_p]^{1/2}$$

When this type of transdermal system is used, dose dumping does not occur; because the polymer used does not rupture.

4. **Microreservoir/micro sealed dissolution-controlled system:** This appears to be a combination of reservoir and matrix diffusion type drug delivery system. In this system, the drug reservoir is made by two steps – (1) dispersion of solid drug particles in an aqueous solution of water-soluble liquid polymer, (2) homogeneous dispersion or suspension of drug in a lipophilic polymer by high energy dispersion technique. As a result, numbers of separate, microscopic spheres of drug reservoirs are formed which do not leach the drug. This is a thermodynamically unstable system; hence requires stabilization. It is stabilized by immediate in-situ cross-linking the polymer chains. Thus, medicated polymer discs having a definite or constant surface area and of fixed thickness are obtained (fig. 6.7). The device so obtained may be further coated with a layer of biocompatible polymer to modify the mechanism and rate of release of the drug. However, this depends on the physicochemical properties of the drug and the desired rate of release of the drug.

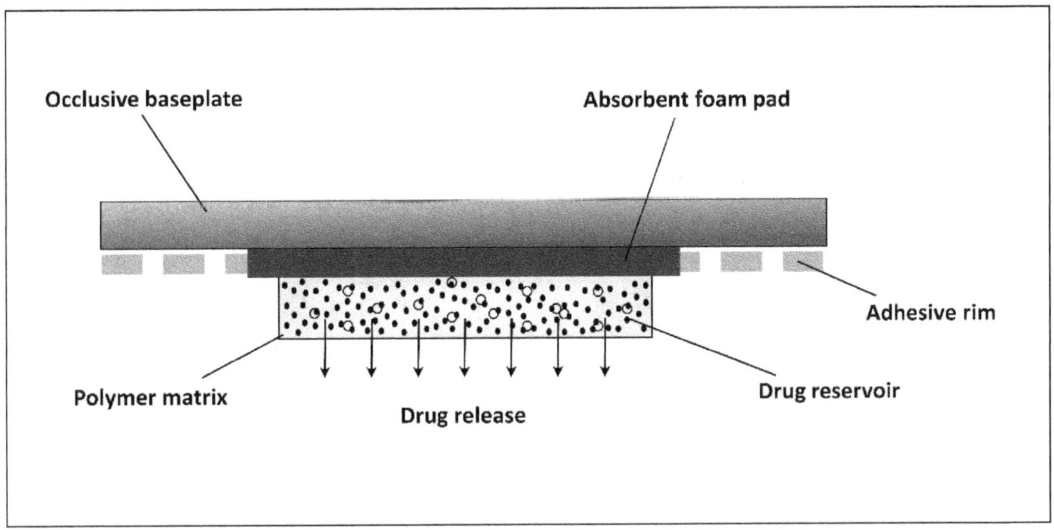


**Fig. 6.7:** Microreservoir dissolution-controlled TDDS.

By placing the medicated disc at the center and by surrounding disc with an adhesive film, a transdermal drug delivery system is produced.

For the preparation of nitroglycerin, this technique has been utilized which can release 0.5 mg of nitroglycerin per sq.cm, once daily to treat angina pectoris. Micro reservoir system can release the drug following zero-order kinetics without the chance of dose dumping. The rate of release of the drug from this system can be expressed as;

$$\frac{dQ}{dt} = \frac{D_p \times D_d \times m \times K_p}{D_p \times h_d + D_d \times h_p \times m \times K_p} \left[ n \times S_p \frac{D_l S_l (1-n)}{h_l} \left( \frac{1}{K_l} + \frac{1}{K_m} \right) \right]$$

Where, m = a/b;

$$a = \frac{\text{The concentration of drug in the bulk of elution medium}}{\text{The solubility of the drug in the same elution medium}}$$

$$b = \frac{\text{The concentration of the drug at the outer edge of the polymer coating}}{\text{The solubility of the drug in the same polymer composition}}$$

$D_l$ = Diffusivity of the drug in the liquid layer surrounding the drug particle,

$D_p$ = Diffusivity of drug in polymer coating membrane surrounding polymer matrix,

$D_d$ = Diffusivity of drug in the hydrodynamic diffusion layer surrounding polymer coating with a respective thickness of $h_l$, $h_p$, $h_d$.

$K_l$ = Partition coefficient for the interfacial partitioning of the drug from the liquid compartment to the polymer matrix,

$K_m$ = Partition coefficient for the interfacial partitioning of the drug from the polymer matrix to the polymer coating membrane,

$K_p$ = Partition coefficient for the interfacial partitioning of the drug from the polymer coating membrane to the elution solution (skin),

$S_l$ = Solubility of the drug in the liquid compartment,

$S_p$ = Solubility of the drug in the polymer matrix,

$$n = \frac{\text{The concentration of drug at the inner edge of the interfacial barrier}}{\text{The solubility of the drug in the polymer matrix}}$$

Depending on the relative values of $S_l$ and $S_p$ the release of drug from this system can follow either a partition control or matrix diffusion-control process.

## Bibliography


1. Al- Khamis K, Davis S.S and Hadgraft J. Microviscosity and drug release from topical gel formulations. Pharm. Res. 1986; 3: 214-217.

2. Anon.  Transdermal delivery systems-general drug release standards.  Pharmacopeial Forum, 1980; 14: 3860-3865.

3. Baker W and Heller J." Material Selection for Transdermal Delivery Systems", In Transdermal

4. Berner B and John V.A.  Pharmacokinetic characterization of Transdermal delivery systems. Jour. Clinical pharmacokinetics 1994; 26 (2): 121-34.

5. Brown M.B and Jones S.A.  Hyaluronic acid:  a unique topical vehicle for localized drug delivery  of drugs to the skin. JEDV 2000; 19:308-318.

6. Chein Y.W. Transdermal drug delivery and delivery system.  In, Novel drug delivery system, Vol.  50, Marcel Dekker, Inc., New York, 1992 pp.301-381.

7. Crawford R.R and Esmerian O.K.  Effect of plasticizers on some physical properties of cellulose acetate phthalate films. J. Pharm. Sci. 1997;60: 312-314.

8. Deo M.R, Sant V.P, Parekh S.R, Khopade A.J and Banakar U.V.   Proliposome-based Transdermal delivery of levonorgestrel. Jour. Biomat. Appl. 1997; 12: 77-88.

9. Drug Delivery: Developmental Issues and Research Initiatives, J. Hadgraft and R.H. Guys, Eds. Marcel Dekker, Inc., New York 1989 pp. 293-311.

10. Jain NK.  Advances in controlled and novel drug delivery, 1$^{st}$ Ed., CBS Publishers and distributors, New Delhi, 2001 pp.108-110.

11. Loyd V. Allen Jr, Nicholas G. Popovich, Howard C. Ansel.  Pharmaceutical dosage forms and drug delivery systems, 8$^{th}$  Edition., Wolter Kluwer Publishers, New Delhi, 2005 pp. 298-299.

12. Mayorga P, Puisieux F and Couarraze G. Formulation study of a Transdermal delivery system of primaquine. Int. J. pharm. 1996; 132: 71-79.

13. Pellet M, Raghavan S.L, Had graft J and DavisA.F.  "The application of supersaturated systems to percutaneous drug delivery" In:  Guy R.H and Hadgraft J.  Transdermal drug delivery, Marcel Dekker, Inc., New York 2003pp. 305-326.

14. Singh J, Tripathi K.T and SakiaT.R.  Effect of penetration enhancers on the invitro transport of ephedrine through rate skin and human epidermis from matrix based Transdermal formulations. Drug Dev. Ind. Pharm. 1993; 19: 1623-1628.

15. Tsai J.C, Guy R.H, Thornfeldt C.R, GaoW.N, Feingold K.R and Elias P.M. "Metabolic Approaches to Enchance Transdermal drug delivery". Jour. pharm. Sci., 1998; 85:643-648.

16. Wade A, Weller P.J.  Handbook of pharmaceutical Excipients. Washington, DC: American Pharmaceutical Publishing Association; 1994:  362-366.

17. Wiechers J.   Use of chemical penetration enhancers in Transdermal drug delivery-possibilities and difficulties. Acta pharm. 1992: 4: 123.

18. Willams, A.C.  and  barry  B.  W., "Penetration Enhancers," Adv.  Drug Del.Rev.2004;56: 603-618.

19. Yamamoto T, Katakabe k, Akiyoshi K, Kan K and Asano T.  Topical application of glibenclamide lowers blood glucose levels in rats.  Diabetes  res. Clin. Pract. 1990; 8: 19-22.

20. Yan-yu X, Yun- mei S, Zhi-Peng C and Qi-nerg P. Preparation of silymarin proliposomes; A new   way to increase oral bioavailability of silymarin in beagle dogs. Int. pharm. 2006; 319: 162-168.

# Exercise

## A. Multiple Choice Questions

1. Which of the following statements is correct?
    (a) Drugs having long elimination half-life is suitable for TDDS.
    (b) Drugs having short elimination half-life is suitable for TDDS.
    (c) There is no relation between the elimination half-half of the drug and formulation of TDDS.
    (d) None of the above.

2. Which of the following statements is correct?
    (a) Drugs can penetrate the skin through hair-follicle.
    (b) Drugs can penetrate the skin through the sebaceous gland.
    (c) Drugs can penetrate the skin through sweat gland.
    (d) All of the above.

3. Bioavailability of drug from TDDS depends on
    (a) Physicochemical properties of the drug.
    (b) Therapeutic efficacy of the drug.
    (c) Anatomy of the patient.
    (d) The short biological half-life of the drug.

4. Which of the following statements is correct?
    (a) Physicochemical properties of the drug.
    (b) Physiology of the skin.

(c) All of the above.

(d) None of the above.

5. Which of the following statements is correct?

    (a) Percutaneous absorption of a drug having larger molecular size is more.

    (b) Percutaneous absorption of a drug having larger molecular size is less.

    (c) Percutaneous absorption of the drug with hydrophilic character is more.

    (d) All of the above.

6. The temperature of the body is regulated by

    (a) Protein layer of the skin

    (b) Regulating the blood circulation within the underlying living tissues

    (c) All of the above

    (d) None of the above

7. The thickness of the layer containing sebum and surface material is

    (a) Irregular and discontinuous throughout the body

    (b) Irregular but continuous throughout the body

    (c) Regular and discontinuous throughout the body

    (d) Regular and continuous throughout the body

8. When a plot of the cumulative amount of drug crossed unit area of membrane is plotted against time, the plot becomes straight after some time with a steady-state flux which is expressed as; $\dfrac{dm}{dt} = \dfrac{DC_0K}{h}$ where $C_o$ is

    (a) the concentration of drug in the donor compartment

    (b) the constant concentration of drug in the donor compartment

    (c) the concentration of drug in the receiver compartment

    (d) the constant concentration of drug in the receiver compartment

9. Permeation rates at different areas of the body can be expressed as

    (a) Forehead > Back of hand > Palm

    (b) Forehead < Back of hand > Palm

    (c) Forehead < Back of hand < Palm

    (d) Forehead > Back of hand < Palm

10. Which of the following can influence permeation of the drug through the skin

    (a) Gender                      (b)    Race

    (c) pH of the body fluid        (d)    Buffer capacity of the body fluid

11. Which of the following can enhance the drug permeation through skin

    (a) Carbohydrate                (b)    Protein

    (c) Surfactant                  (d)    All of the above

12. In a membrane permeation-controlled TDDS
    (a) The drug is dispersed in an adhesive polymer
    (b) The drug remains in the form of dispersion within a polymer matrix
    (c) The drug remains in the form of reservoir
    (d) The drug remains as a combined form of dispersion and reservoir

13. Which of the following statements is correct?
    (a) Stratum corneum is structurally heterogeneous
    (b) Stratum corneum contains mainly carbohydrate
    (c) Stratum corneum is structurally homogeneous
    (d) Stratum corneum is a part of the dermis

14. Which of the following statements is correct?
    (a) Papillary and reticular regions are found in the epidermis.
    (b) Papillary and reticular regions are found in the dermis.
    (c) Papillary and reticular regions are found in the hypodermis.
    (d) None of the above.

15. Which of the following is a mechanical function of the skin?
    (a) Protection from radiation
    (b) Protection from the entry of some foreign substances
    (c) Protection from shock
    (d) None of the above

16. Which of the following excipients is not used as penetration enhancer?
    (a) DMSO                          (b)    Sorbitan trioleate
    (c) Isopropyl myristate           (d)    Carbon tetrachloride

17. Which of the following components of TDDS is responsible for fastening the device to the skin?
    (a) Backing membrane             (b)    PSA
    (c) Release Liner                (d)    Polymer matrix

18. A transdermal drug delivery system can be used for
    (a) Releasing the drug rapidly
    (b) Releasing the drug at a constant rate
    (c) Releasing the drug at a regular rate
    (d) All of the above

19. The adhesive layer of a TDDS should
    - (a)   Have a specific permeability
    - (b)   Have a uniform thickness throughout the layer
    - (c)   Provide adhesive diffusion-controlled delivery
    - (d)   All of the above

20. Microreservoir or micro sealed dissolution-controlled system
    - (a)   Contains micro-reservoir of drug
    - (b)   Is a combination of reservoir and matrix system
    - (c)   Is a matrix system
    - (d)   All of the above

## B. Short Questions

1. What are the advantages and disadvantages of TDDS?
2. What are skin appendages? Write down the functions of the skin appendages.
3. Explain briefly how can a drug penetrate through skin appendages.
4. What do you know about complex barriers and parallel barrier for diffusion through the skin?
5. What is permeation enhancer? What are different classes of the chemical penetration enhancer?
6. Describe the membrane permeation-controlled TDDS.

## C. Long Questions

1. Write down briefly the anatomy and physiology of the skin.
2. Discuss briefly the functions of the skin.
3. Describe briefly about transepidermal absorption.
4. Explain how the drug is diffused through the skin.
5. Discuss briefly the factors that affect the permeation of drug through the skin.
6. Discuss the components of TDDS briefly.

## CHAPTER 7

# Gastroretentive Drug Delivery Systems

*Introduction, advantages, disadvantages, approaches for GRDDS – Floating, high density systems, inflatable and gastro adhesive systems and their applications.*

## Introduction

Among all the routes, the oral route of administration is the preferred one. There are several well-established advantages. These formulations are also less expensive, easy to transport and store, flexible in terms of the constituents, and ready to administer. However, the products administered orally face various problems due to the heterogeneity of the gastrointestinal system. Moreover, several variables change throughout the gastrointestinal tract and greatly influence the absorption of drugs. Among these factors the most important are pH, the commensal flora, gastrointestinal transit time, enzymatic activity and surface area.

Traditional systems cannot overcome all these problems occur in the gastrointestinal tract. For example, these are unsuitable for drugs that are specially absorbed in the upper part of the gastrointestinal system. The conventional formulations do not possess the capacity to face gastric emptying; therefore, they cannot be released in the colon where they remain during the release time. Therefore, the incomplete release of drugs occurs and the effectiveness of the dose is reduced. These adversities are overcome by technological researchers through the development of pharmaceutical systems that can control drug release and the residence time, some of which are already available on the market.

The poor gastric retention time of the conventional systems resulted to the development of oral gastroretentive systems. Such delivery systems were designed to retain the dosage form in the upper gastrointestinal tract for a prolonged period of time, during which they release the drug on a controlled manner. The extended contact period of gastroretentive systems with the absorbing membrane allows an increase in drug bioavailability.

Several approaches have been tried to formulate successful controlled drug delivery systems to increase the gastric residence time such as bioadhesive or mucoadhesive systems, expandable systems, high-density systems, floating systems, microporous hydrogels, and magnetic systems.

## Anatomy and Physiology of Stomach

The gastrointestinal tract is primarily a tube about nine meters long that runs through the middle of the body from the mouth to the anus. It includes the throat (pharynx), oesophagus, stomach, small intestine (consisting of the duodenum, jejunum and ileum) and large intestine (consisting of the cecum, appendix, colon and rectum). The wall of the gastrointestinal tract has the same or similar general structure throughout most of its length from the oesophagus to the anus, with some local variations for each region (fig. 7.1). The stomach is an organ having a capacity for storage and mixing. The antrum region is responsible for mixing and grinding of gastric contents. The motility pattern of gastrointestinal tract is commonly called the 'migrating motor complex' (MMC) and is organized in cycles of activity and quiescence.

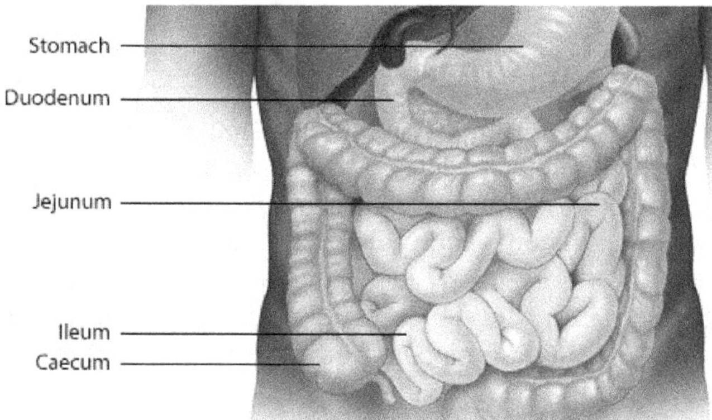


**Fig. 7.1:** Anatomy of gastro intestinal tract.

Each cycle persists for 90–120 minutes and consists of four phases. The concentration of the hormone motilin in the blood controls the duration of the phases. In the inter-digestive or fasted state, the MMC wave migrates from the stomach to lower part of the GI tract for every 90–120 minutes. A full cycle consists of four phases, beginning in the lower oesophageal sphincter/gastric pacemaker, propagating over the whole stomach, the duodenum and jejunum, and finishing at the ileum. Phase III is termed the 'housekeeper wave' as the powerful contractions in this phase tend to empty the stomach of its fasting contents and indigestible debris. The administration and subsequent ingestion of food quickly interrupts the MMC cycle, and the digestive phase is allowed to take place. The upper part of the stomach stores the ingested food initially, where it is compressed gradually by the phasic contractions.

The digestive or fed state is observed after ingestion of meal. It resembles the fasting Phase II and is not cyclical, but continuous, provided that the food remains in the stomach. Large objects are retained in the stomach during the fed pattern but are allowed to pass during Phase III of the inter-digestive MMC. It is thought that the sieving efficiency (i.e. the ability of the stomach to grind the food into smaller size) of the stomach is improved by the fed pattern or by the presence of food (fig. 7.2 and 7.3).

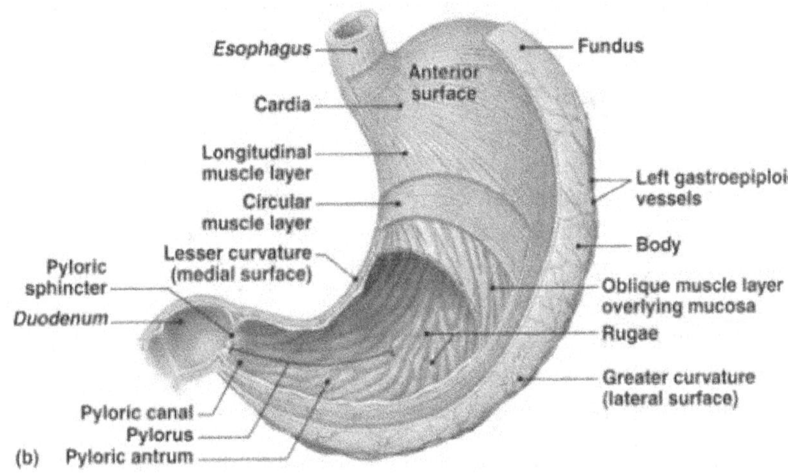


**Fig. 7.2:** Anatomy of stomach.

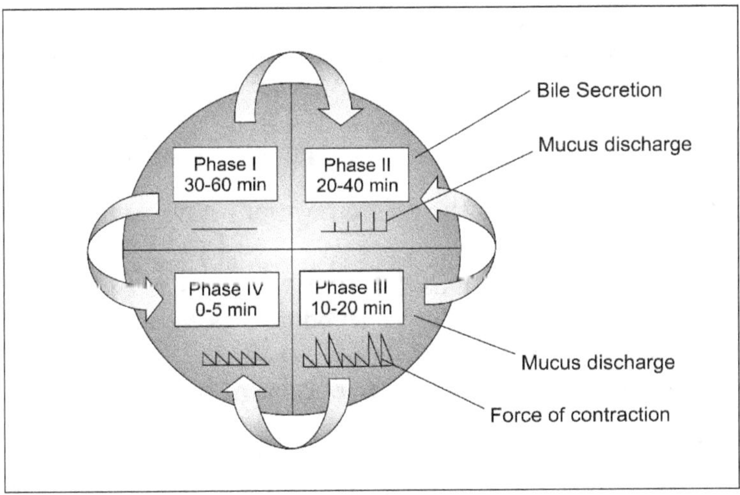


**Fig. 7.3:** Motility pattern of GIT.

## Need for GRDDS

- Conventional delivery system has many limitations and major limitation is non-site specificity.
- Some drugs are absorbed at specific site only. They require release at specific site or a release in such a way that maximum amount of drug can reach to the specific site.
- Gastro-retentive delivery is one of the site-specific delivery of drugs either at stomach or at intestine. It is possible by retaining dosage form into stomach and drug is released at controlled manner to specific site either in stomach, duodenum and intestine.

## Factors Affecting Gastro Retentive Drug Delivery

Many factors are there that affect the gastric emptying process which may seriously affect the release of a drug and its absorption. Hence, it is desirable to develop a drug delivery system that can exhibit an extended gastric residence and increases the drug release profile, independent of patient related variables. The factors that affect the gastric emptying and hence, the gastric retention of the drugs includes:

- During the fasting state an inter-digestive series of electrical events take place, which cycle both through stomach and intestine every 2 to 3 hours.
- In the fed state, this cycle is delayed and hence, the gastric emptying rate is slowed.
- Density, size and shape of the dosage form.
- The nature of the food, calorie content and its frequency of intake have considerable effect on the retention of drugs in stomach.
- Simultaneous administration of drugs such as anticholinergic agents such as, atropine, propantheline and opiates delay the gastric emptying while the prokinetic agents like metoclopramide and cisapride enhance the gastric emptying process.

## Advantages

The gastro retentive drug delivery system offers various advantages that are mentioned below:

- Enhanced bioavailability: The bioavailability of the drugs having absorption in the upper part of the GIT like riboflavin, levodopa has tremendously been increased than that of the conventional dosage forms.
- Sustained drug delivery and reduced frequency of dosing. This improves patient compliance.
- Targeted delivery of the drug at the upper part of the GIT making it suitable for the local treatment of the disease of the region such as antacids, anti-ulcer drugs, antibacterial for *H. pylori* infection.

➢ Suitable for the drugs which have pH dependent absorption from stomach such as Furosemide, Captopril, Diazepam, Verapamil, Cefpodoxime proxeti.

➢ Suitable for the drugs which degrade in the intestine or column such as Ranitidine hydrochloride.

➢ Drug level fluctuation is not observed and maintains the optimal therapeutic plasma and tissue concentrations over prolonged time period. This avoids sub-therapeutics as well as toxic concentration and minimizes the risk of failure of the medical treatment and undesirable side effects.

➢ Additional advantages of these systems include
   (i) An improvement in therapeutic effectiveness,
   (ii) A reduction in drug loss,
   (iii) An increase in drug solubility in cases with low solubility in a high pH environment, and
   (iv) Benefits due to the delivery of drugs that act locally in the stomach and duodenum.

## Disadvantages

Despite having various advantages, the GRDDS also have some limitations;

➢ Not suitable for drug substances having low aqueous solubility

➢ Not suitable for drugs susceptible for GI degradation

➢ Not suitable for drugs which undergoes first pass metabolism

➢ Not suitable for drug which are instable in GI environment or in acidic medium.

➢ Not suitable for drugs which are intended for lower GIT or absorbed in intestinal region

➢ Dose dumping is the major problem associated with GRDDS

➢ The pH of the GIT, gastric motility, amount and type of food significantly affect the gastric retention and drug absorption

➢ Poor *in vitro-in vivo* correlation

➢ Cost of formulation is high

➢ In case of drug poisoning, toxicity or hypersensitivity reaction, the drug retrieval is very difficult.

➢ GRDDS needs high level of fluid to float in the stomach.

## Approaches for GRDDS

Different approaches have been tried to increase the retention of oral dosage forms in the stomach. Some are formulated as single component whereas others are formulated as multicomponent dosage forms. GRDDS can be broadly categorized into floating and non-floating system (fig. 7.4).

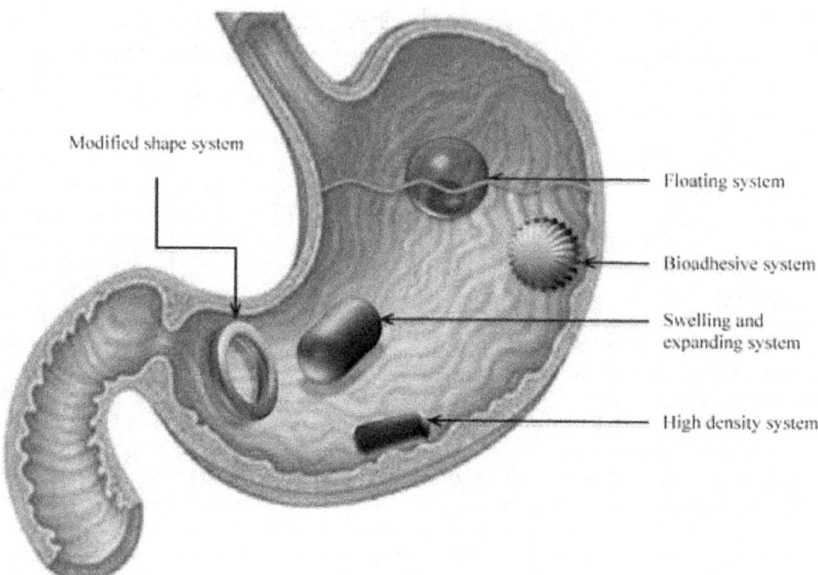



**Fig. 7.4:** Types of Gastro retentive system.

1. Non-floating system
   (a)  Bioadhesive/mucoadhesive system
   (b)  High density/sinking system
   (c)  Magnetic system
   (d)  Unfoldable system
2. Floating system
   (a)  Effervescent system
       (i)    Gas generation system
       (ii)   Volatile liquid
   (b)  Non-effervescent system
       (i)    Bilayer floating tablet
       (ii)   Single layer floating tablet /Hydrodynamically balanced system
       (iii)  Microballoons or hollow microspheres
       (iv)   Alginate beads
       (v)    Microporous compartment
       (vi)   Swelling system

1. **Non-floating system**
   (a)  ***Bioadhesive/mucoadhesive system***: Bioadhesive or mucoadhesive systems bind with the gastric epithelial cell surface, or mucin. The bound molecules extend the GRT by increasing the intimacy and duration of contact between the dosage form and the biological membrane. The concept is based on the self-protecting mechanism of the GIT. The specialized goblet cells present

throughout the GIT continuously secrete mucus and this mucus plays a cytoprotective role. Mucus is a viscoelastic, gel-like, stringy slime composed mainly of glycoproteins. The thickness of the mucus layer decreases from the membrane surface to the GI lumen. The primary function of mucus is to protect the surface mucosal cells from acid and peptidases. In addition, it acts as a lubricant for the passage of solids and as a barrier to antigens, bacteria, and viruses. The epithelial adhesive properties of mucin are well known and have been applied to the development of GRDDS through the use of bio/mucoadhesive polymers. The adherence between the delivery system and the gastric wall increases residence time at a particular site; hence, improves bioavailability. A bio/mucoadhesive substance is a natural or synthetic polymer capable of adhering to a biological membrane (bioadhesive polymer) or the mucus lining of the GIT (mucoadhesive polymer). The characteristics of these polymers are:

- Molecular flexibility,
- Hydrophilic functional groups, and
- Specific molecular weight,
- Chain length, and conformation.
- Nontoxicity and non absorbability,
- Capability of forming non covalent bonds with the mucin–epithelial surfaces,
- Ability of quick adherence to moist surfaces,
- Easy incorporation of the drug, and
- No hindrance to drug release,
- Having specific site of attachment and
- Economical.

The binding of polymers to the mucin epithelial surface can be subdivided into three broad categories: hydration-mediated adhesion, bonding mediated adhesion, and receptor-mediated adhesion. Materials commonly used for bioadhesion are poly (acrylic acid) (Carbopol, polycarbophil), Chitosan, Gantrez (Polymethyl vinyl ether/maleic anhydride copolymers), cholestyramine, tragacanth, sodium alginate, sucralfate, polyethylene glycol, dextran and polylactic acid.

***Hydration-mediated adhesion:*** Certain hydrophilic polymers absorb large amount of water and become sticky and acquire bioadhesive properties. The prolonged gastroretention of the bio/mucoadhesive drug delivery system is controlled by the dissolution rate of the polymer.

***Bonding-mediated adhesion:*** The adhesion of polymers to a mucus or epithelial cell surface involves various bonding mechanisms, including physical–mechanical bonding and chemical bonding. Physical–mechanical bonds can result from the insertion of the adhesive material into the crevices or folds of the mucosa. Chemical bonds may be either covalent (primary) or ionic (secondary) in nature. Secondary chemical bonds consist of dispersive interactions (i.e., van der Waals interactions) and stronger specific interactions such as hydrogen bonds. The hydrophilic functional groups such as hydroxyl and carboxylic groups are responsible for forming hydrogen bonds.

*Receptor-mediated adhesion*: Certain polymers can bind to specific receptor sites on the surface of cells; hence, can enhance the gastric retention of dosage forms. Certain plant lectins such as tomato lectins interact specifically with the sugar groups present in mucus or on the glycocalyx.

**(b)  High density/sinking system:** These systems have a density of about 3 $g/cm^3$ and can retain in the rugae of the stomach. These  are capable of withstanding its peristaltic movements. Above a threshold density of 2.4–2.8 $g/cm^3$, such systems can be retained in the lower part of the stomach. The major limitation with such systems is that it is technically difficult to manufacture these with a large amount of drug (>50 %) and to achieve the required density of 2.4–2.8 $g/cm^3$. Diluents such as barium sulphate (density = 4.9 $g/cm^3$), zinc oxide, titanium dioxide, and iron powder may be used to manufacture such high-density formulations.

**(c)  Magnetic system:** Magnetic systems signify an approach that is very different from those of all other gastroretentive delivery forms defined previously, as they are based on the attraction between two magnets. These systems are made of two components: the pharmaceutical dosage form itself, which comprises a small internal magnet, and an external magnet. The device is placed under the abdomen, near the stomach. The gastric residence time and bioavailability of acetaminophen can be increased when administered in the form of magnetic tablets. It is administered to beagle dogs with the simultaneous application of an external magnet.

The system is based on a simple idea that the dosage form containing a small internal magnet, and a magnet is to be placed on the abdomen over the position of the stomach. Ito et al. used this technique in rabbits with bioadhesive granules comprising ultrafine ferrite (g-Fe2O). They directed the granules to the oesophagus by use of an external magnet (~1700 G) for the initial 2 min and almost all the granules were reserved in the region after 2h. Similarly, Fujimori et al. prepared a magnetic tablet containing 50% w/w ultra-ferrite with hydroxy propyl cellulose and cinnarizine. In beagle dogs, the tablet stayed in the stomach for 8 h by the use of a magnetic field (1000 to 2600 G). Absorption of cinnarizine was extended and the area under the plasma concentration time-curve values (AUC $_{0-24\ h}$) were found to increase. Groning et al. developed a method for assessing the gastrointestinal transit of magnetic dosage forms under the control of an extracorporeal magnet, using a pH-telemetering capsule (Heidelberg capsule). Small magnets had been attached to the capsule and administered to human volunteers. With the extracorporeal magnet, gastric residence time of the dosage form could be increased to more than 6 h while the control delivery system showed only 2.5 h. After two years, the same group developed oral depot tablets of acyclovir with internal magnets. *In vivo* human studies exhibited that, in the presence of an extracorporeal magnet, the plasma concentrations of acyclovir had been significantly increased after 7, 8, 10 and 12 h. Furthermore, the mean AUC was found to be about 2800 ng h/mL using an external magnet and around 1600 ng h/mL without any magnet. However, these systems can work properly, if the external magnet is positioned with a degree of accuracy with cooperation of the patient.

2.  **Floating system:** Floating systems are low-density devices that possess sufficient buoyancy to float over the gastric contents and stay in the stomach for a prolonged period of time. When the device floats over the gastric contents, the drug release takes place slowly at the desired rate. As a result, the gastric retention time (GRT) is increased and the fluctuation in plasma drug concentration is reduced. For gastroretention the floating drug delivery system and bioadhesive drug delivery are extensively used technique and floating systems in particular has been widely investigated. Because, the floating systems do not adversely alter the motility of GI tract (fig. 7.5 and 7.6).

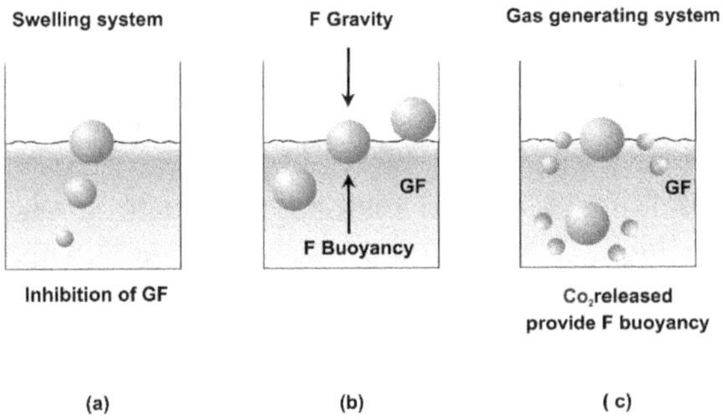


**Fig. 7.5:** Mechanism of Floating System; (a) floating due to swelling, (b) buoyancy and (c) gas generating system.

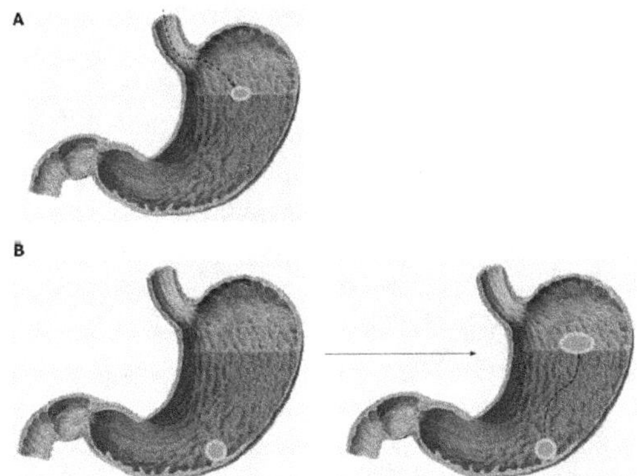


**Fig. 7.6:** Floating system; initially floats, then sink due to high density and further lowering the density of tablet after administration.

**(a) Effervescent system:** By incorporating a floating chamber filled with vacuum, air, or an inert gas floatation of a drug delivery system in the stomach can be attained. Gas can be incorporated into the floating chamber by the volatilizing an organic volatile solvent such as ether or cyclopentane, or by the $CO/CO_2$ formed as a result of an effervescent reaction between organic acids and carbonate–bicarbonate salts. These systems contain a hollow deformable unit that changes from a collapsed to an expanded position and can return to the collapsed position after a predetermined amount of time and after a spontaneous discharge of the inflatable system from the stomach.

     **(i) Gas generative system:** These buoyant systems contain matrices prepared by using

>    swellable polymers like methocel, polysaccharides such as chitosan,

>    effervescent components such as sodium bicarbonate, citric acid and tartaric acid,

>    chambers containing a liquid that gasifies at body temperature.

The ideal stoichiometric ratio of citric acid and sodium bicarbonate for generation of gas is reported to be 0.76:1. The commonly these systems are prepared by using resin beads loaded with bicarbonate and then, coated with ethylcellulose. The coating is insoluble in water but, allows permeation of water. Thus, carbon dioxide is released and the beads start to float in the stomach. Other methods and materials have been reported that highly swellable hydrocolloids and light mineral oils, a mixture of sodium alginate and sodium bicarbonate, multiple unit floating pills can produce carbon dioxide after ingestion. Floating minicapsules having a core of sodium bicarbonate, lactose and polyvinyl pyrrolidone are coated with hydroxypropyl methylcellulose (HPMC) and floating systems based on ion exchange resin technology, etc. (fig. 7.7 and 7.8).

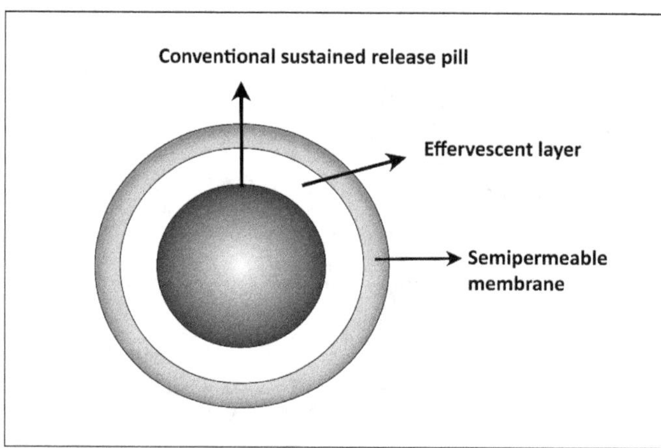


**Fig. 7.7:** Effervescent gas generating system.

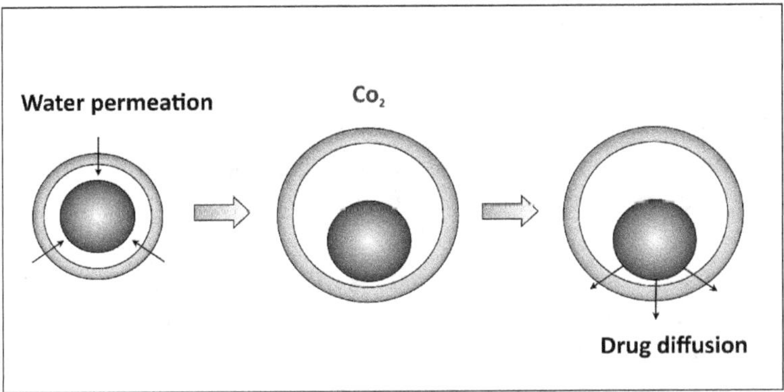



**Fig. 7.8:** Mechanism of drug release from gas generating effervescent system.

In single unit system, such as capsule or tablet, effervescent substances are mixed with the hydrophilic polymer, and CO bubbles are trapped in the swollen matrix. *In vitro*, the lag time before the unit floats is less than 1 min and the buoyancy are extended up to 8 - 10 h. *In vivo* experiments in fasted dogs exhibited a mean gastric residence time enhanced to 4 h. Bilayer or multilayer systems have also been developed. Drug and excipients are prepared individually and the gas-producing unit is incorporated into any of the layers. Further improvements can be made by coating the matrix with a polymer which is permeable to water; but not to $CO_2$. The chief difficulty of such formulation is to achieve a good compromise between elasticity, plasticity and permeability of the polymer (fig. 7.9).

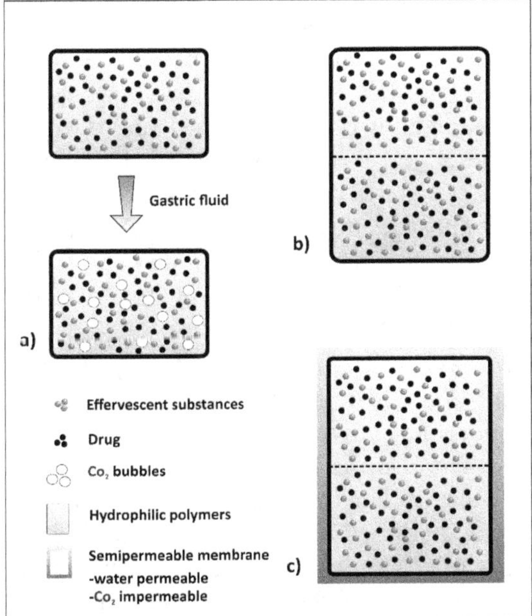



**Fig. 7.9:** Schematic representation of gas generating effervescent system (a) Bilayer system, (b) without semipermeable membrane, and (c) with semipermeable membrane.

**(ii)   Volatile liquid:** These have an inflatable chamber in which a liquid e.g. ether, cyclopentane is contained. The liquid can gasify at about 37°C (body temperature) and results the inflation of the chamber in the stomach. These floating systems are osmotically controlled systems comprising a hollow unit which can be deformed. There are two chambers in the system, one chamber contains the drug and the other contains the volatile system.

These are classified as:

(a) *Intra gastric floating gastro intestinal drug delivery system:* This system comprises a floatation chamber that contains no air (vacuum) or an inert, harmless gas, and a microporous compartment enclosing drug reservoir.

(b) *Inflatable gastro intestinal drug delivery system:* This system contains inflatable chamber containing liquid ether which gasifies at body temperature to inflate the stomach. Inflatable chamber is made of bioerodable polymer filament such as copolymer of poly vinyl alcohol and poly ethylene. The polymer gradually dissolves in gastric fluid and finally produces inflatable chamber to release gas and collapses.

(c) *Intra-gastric osmotically controlled drug delivery system:* It is an osmotic pressure-controlled drug delivery device and an inflatable floating capsule. In the stomach, inflatable capsule disintegrates and releases the drug at osmotically controlled rate. Such drug delivery system contains two components – drug reservoir compartment and osmotically active compartment.

**(b)   Non-effervescent system:** Non-effervescent systems is composed of a high level (20–75 % w/w) of one or more gel-forming, highly swellable, cellulosic hydrocolloids such as hydroxyethyl cellulose, hydroxypropyl cellulose, hydroxypropyl methylcellulose (HPMC), and sodium carboxymethylcellulose, polysaccharides, or matrix forming polymers such as polycarbophil, polyacrylates, and polystyrene inside the tablets or capsules. When such system comes in contact with gastric fluid, these gel forming polysaccharides and polymers hydrate and forms a colloidal gel barrier that controls the rate of penetration of fluid into the device and subsequently drug release. Since the exterior surface of the dosage form dissolves, the gel layer is maintained by the hydration of the adjacent hydrocolloid layer. The air trapped by the swollen polymer lowers the density and confers buoyancy to the dosage form.

(i) *Hydrodynamically balanced system:* These are single unit dosage forms. These are prepared with one or more gel forming hydrophilic polymers. HPMC is the most commonly used polymer; however, HEC, HPC NaCMC, agar and alginic acid are also used. The drug is mixed with polymer and generally administered in a gelatine capsule. The capsules rapidly dissolve in the gastric fluid, and surface polymer hydrates and swells and produce a floating mass. Drug release is controlled by the formation of hydrated boundary at the surface. Continuous erosion of the surface permits water penetration to the inner layer and maintains surface hydration and buoyancy. Inclusion of fatty excipients produces low density formulations and reduces penetration of water; thus, the erosion is decreased. The main limitation is the inactiveness of operation. It depends on the air sealed in the dry mass centre following hydration of gelatinous surface layer and hence the characteristics and amount of polymer. Effective drug delivery depends on the balance of drug loading and effect of polymer on its release profile.

(ii) ***Low density system/ Microballoons or hollow microspheres:*** Gas-generating system generally have a lag time before floating on the stomach contents. During this period the dosage form may experience premature evacuation through the pyloric sphincter. Low density system ($<1$ g/cm$^3$) with instant buoyancy have therefore been developed. These are made of low-density materials that can entrap oil or air. Most are multiple- unit systems and are also called "microballoons" because their cores are of low-density.

Microballoons / hollow microspheres loaded with drugs in other polymer-shelves were developed by simple solvent evaporation or solvent diffusion / evaporation methods to extend the gastric retention time (GRT) of the dosage form. Generally, the polymers used to develop these systems are polycarbonate, cellulose acetate, calcium alginate, Eudragit S, agar and low methoxylated pectin etc. Buoyancy and drug release from the dosage form depend on –

➢ quantity of polymers,

➢ the plasticizer polymer ratio, and

➢ the solvent used for formulation.

The microballoons floated continuously over the surface of an acidic dissolution media containing surfactant for >12 hours. At present hollow microspheres are considered to be one of the most promising buoyant systems because they combine the advantages of multiple-unit system and good floating (fig. 7.10).

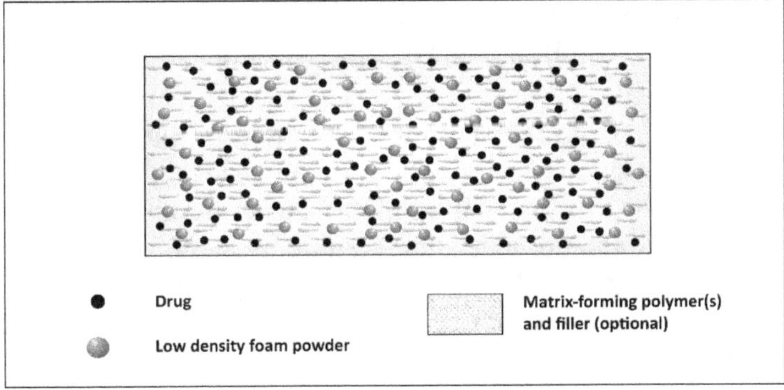


**Fig. 7.10:** Low density floating system.

**(iii)** *Alginate beads:* Talukdar and Fassihi currently developed a multiple-unit floating system based on cross-linked beads. They were prepared by using Ca and low methoxylated pectin (anionic polysaccharide) or $Ca^{2+}$ low methoxylated pectin and sodium alginate.   In this method, generally sodium alginate solution is dropped into aqueous solution of calcium chloride and causes the precipitation of calcium alginate. These beads are then separated and dried by air convection and freeze drying, leading to the formulation of a porous system, which can maintain a floating force for over 12 hrs. These beads improve gastric retention time (GRT) more than 5.5 hrs

**(iv)** *Microporous compartment:* This method is based on the principle of the encapsulation of a drug reservoir inside a microporous compartment with pores along its top and bottom walls. The peripheral walls of the device were completely sealed to present any direct contact of the gastric surface with the undissolved drug.  In the stomach the floatation chamber containing entrapped air causes the delivery system to float in the gastric fluid. Gastric fluid enters through the aperture, dissolves the drug and causes the dissolved drug for continuous transport across the intestine for drug absorption.

**(v)** *Swellable system:* After being swallowed, these dosage forms swell to a size that prevents their passage through the pylorus. As a result, the dosage form is retained in the stomach for a long period of time.  These systems are sometimes referred to as plug type systems because they tend to remain lodged at the pyloric sphincter. These polymeric matrices remain in the gastric cavity for several hours even in the fed state. Sustained and controlled drug release may be achieved by selecting a polymer with the proper molecular weight and swelling properties. Upon coming in contact with gastric fluid, the polymer imbibes water and swells. The extensive swelling of these polymers is a result of the presence of physical–chemical crosslinks in the hydrophilic polymer network. These crosslinks prevent the dissolution of the polymer and thus maintain the physical integrity of the dosage form. A balance between the extent and duration of swelling is maintained by the degree of cross linking between the polymeric chains. A high degree of cross-linking retards the swelling ability of the system and maintains its physical integrity for a prolonged period. On the other hand, a low degree of cross-linking results in extensive swelling followed by the rapid dissolution of the polymer (fig. 7.11).

An optimum amount of cross linking is required to maintain a balance between swelling and dissolution. The swollen system eventually will lose its integrity because of a loss of mechanical strength caused by abrasion or erosion or will burst into small fragments when the membrane ruptures because of continuous expansion. These systems also may erode in the presence of gastric juices so that after a predetermined time the device no longer can attain or retain the expanded configuration.

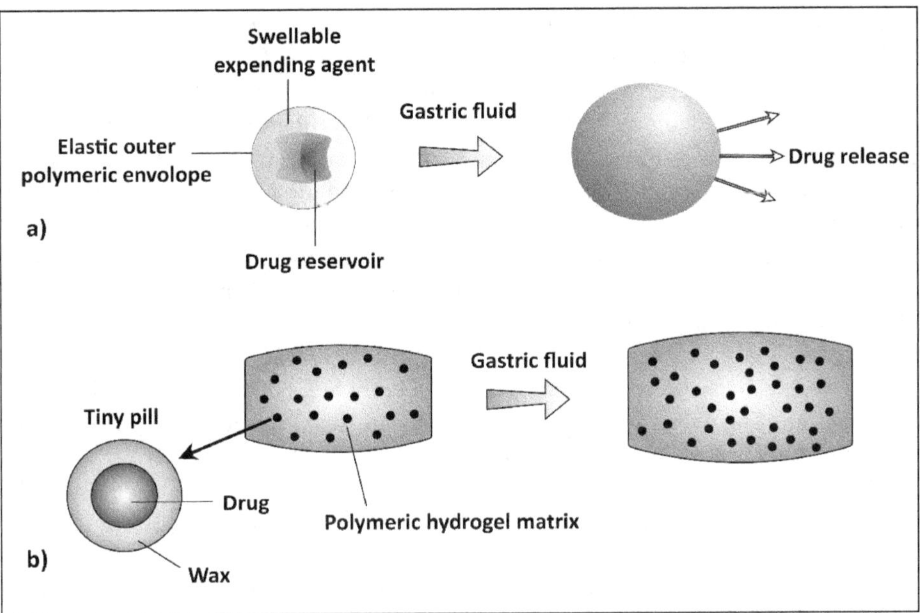


**Fig. 7.11:** Swellable system; (a) swellable system with expanding agent and (b) swellable pills with hydrogel matrix.

**Table 7.1** Application of GRDDS in Drug Delivery including various Marketed Formulations are as follows

| Active Ingredient | Brand Name |
| --- | --- |
| Ciprofloxacin | Cifran OD |
| L-Dopa and Benserazide | Madopar |
| Diazepam | Valrelease |
| Aluminium magnesium antacid | Topalkan |
| Aluminium magnesium antacid | Almagate Flat Coat |
| Aluminium hydroxide | Liquid Gavision |
| Ferrous sulphate | Conviron |
| Misoprostal | Cytotech |

# Bibliography


1. Alzaher, W., J. Shaw, and R. Al-Kassas, Gastroretentive Formulations for Improving Oral Bioavailability of Drugs-Focus on Microspheres and their Production. Curr Drug Deliv, 2016. 13(5): p. 646-61.
2. Bansal, D., et al., Development of liposomes entrapped in alginate beads for the treatment of colorectal cancer. Int J Biol Macromol, 2016. 82: p. 687-95.

3.    Bardonnet, P.L., et al., Gastroretentive dosage forms: overview and special case of Helicobacter pylori. J Control Release, 2006. 111(1-2): p. 1-18.

4.    Chavanpatil, M.D., et al., Novel sustained release, swellable and bioadhesive gastroretentive drug delivery system for ofloxacin. Int J Pharm, 2006. 316(1-2): p. 86-92.

5.    Chen, Y.-C., et al., Physical characterizations and sustained release profiling of gastroretentive drug delivery systems with improved floating and swelling capabilities. International Journal of Pharmaceutics, 2013. 441(1): p. 162-169.

6.    Chuong, M.C., J.M. Christensen, and J.W. Ayres, Sustained delivery of intact drug to the colon: mesalamine formulation and temporal gastrointestinal transit analysis. Pharm Dev Technol, 2009. 14(1): p. 116-25.

7.    Cora, L.A., et al., Gastrointestinal transit and disintegration of enteric coated magnetic tablets assessed by ac biosusceptometry. Eur J Pharm Sci, 2006. 27(1): p. 1-8.

8.    Du, H., et al., The design of pH-sensitive chitosan-based formulations for gastrointestinal delivery. Drug Discov Today, 2015. 20(8): p. 1004-11.

9.    Du, J., I.M. El-Sherbiny, and H.D. Smyth, Swellable ciprofloxacin-loaded nano-in-micro hydrogel particles for local lung drug delivery. AAPS PharmSciTech, 2014. 15(6): p. 1535-44.

10.    Liu, L., pH-Responsive carriers for oral drug delivery: challenges and opportunities of current platforms. Drug Deliv, 2017. 24(1): p. 569-581.

11.    Liu, P., Stabilization of layer-by-layer engineered multilayered hollow microspheres. Adv Colloid Interface Sci, 2014. 207: p. 178-88.

12.    Lopes, C.M., et al., Overview on gastroretentive drug delivery systems for improving drug bioavailability. Int J Pharm, 2016. 510(1): p. 144-58.

13.    Mandal, U.K., B. Chatterjee, and F.G. Senjoti, Gastro-retentive drug delivery systems and their in vivo success: A recent update. Asian Journal of Pharmaceutical Sciences, 2016. 11(5): p. 575-584.

14.    Moes, A.J., Gastroretentive dosage forms. Crit Rev Ther Drug Carrier Syst, 1993. 10(2): p. 143-95.

15.    Nupur, N., E.Y. Ashish, and M. Debnath, Preparation and Biochemical Property of Penicillin G Amidase-Loaded Alginate and Alginate/Chitosan Hydrogel Beads. Recent Pat Biotechnol, 2016. 10(1): p. 121-132.

16.    Patil, H., R.V. Tiwari, and M.A. Repka, Recent advancements in mucoadhesive floating drug delivery systems: A mini-review. Journal of Drug Delivery Science and Technology, 2016. 31: p. 65-71.

17.    Phillips, L.K., et al., Gastric emptying and glycaemia in health and diabetes mellitus. Nat Rev Endocrinol, 2015. 11(2): p. 112-28.

18.    Pinto, J.F., Site-specific drug delivery systems within the gastro-intestinal tract: from the mouth to the colon. Int J Pharm, 2010. 395(1-2): p. 44-52.

19.    Reddy, L.H. and R.S. Murthy, Floating dosage systems in drug delivery. Crit Rev Ther Drug Carrier Syst, 2002. 19(6): p. 553-85.

20.    Streubel, A., J. Siepmann, and R. Bodmeier, Drug delivery to the upper small intestine window using gastroretentive technologies. Curr Opin Pharmacol, 2006. 6(5): p. 501-8.

21.    Streubel, A., J. Siepmann, and R. Bodmeier, Gastroretentive drug delivery systems. Expert Opin Drug Deliv, 2006. 3(2): p. 217-33.

## Exercise

## A. Multiple Choice Questions

1. Gastroretentive drug delivery systems are
    (a) Less expensive
    (b) Administered parenterally
    (c) Administered orally
    (d) pH dependant

2. Gastroretentive drug delivery systems are developed
    (a) To extend the gastric retention time
    (b) To increase the rate of absorption of drug
    (c) To increase the extent of drug absorption
    (d) All of the above

3. Gastroretentive drug delivery systems are used to
    (a) Improve therapeutic effectiveness of drug
    (b) Increase the loss of drug in GIT
    (c) Administer the drugs only locally effective
    (d) Administer the drugs which are not affected in GIT.

4. Gastric emptying depends on
    (a) Density of the gastric fluid
    (b) Calorie content of the food
    (c) Nature of the drug administered
    (d) All of the above

5. Gastroretentive drug delivery systems are suitable
    (a) For drugs having low aqueous solubility
    (b) For drugs susceptible to GI degradation
    (c) For drugs which are pH dependent
    (d) When *in vitro-in vivo* correlation is high

6. The polymer used to prepare GRDDS should have
    (a) Molecular flexibility
    (b) Non-specific molecular weight
    (c) Hydrophobic functional groups
    (d) Ability to retard the release of drug

7. High density gastro-retentive drug delivery system
    (a) Have density less than $2.4 \text{g/cm}^3$
    (b) Have density more than $2.8 \text{g/cm}^3$
    (c) Have density within $2.4 - 2.5 \text{g/cm}^3$
    (d) Have density within $2.4 - 2.6 \text{g/cm}^3$

8. Drug content of a high-density gastro-retentive drug delivery system should be
   - (a) More than 50%
   - (b) More than 60%
   - (c) Less than 50%
   - (d) More than 70%

9. Magnetic gastro-retentive drug delivery system contains
   - (a) Two magnets, One internal and one external manet
   - (b) Numbers of internal magnets only
   - (c) Internal magnets and external magnets
   - (d) No magnets

10. Bioadhesive or mucoadhesive gastro-retentive drug delivery systems are based on
    - (a) Receptor-mediated adhesion
    - (b) Hydration-mediated adhesion
    - (c) Bonding-mediated adhesion
    - (d) All of the above

11. Gastro-retentive floating system are
    - (a) High-density devices
    - (b) Low-density devices
    - (c) All of the above
    - (d) None of the above

12. When gastro-retentive system floats over the gastric contents
    - (a) The drug-release rate would be reduced
    - (b) The drug-release rate would be increased
    - (c) The drug-release rate would not be changed
    - (d) None of the above

13. Effervescing gastro-retentive floating system is prepared with
    - (a) Swellable polymer
    - (b) Effervescent components
    - (c) Chambers containing a liquid that gasifies at body temperature
    - (d) All of the above

14. Non-effervescent gastro-retentive drug delivery systems may be
    - (a) Hydrodynamically balanced
    - (b) Hollow microspheres
    - (c) Swellable system
    - (d) All of the above

15. Which of the following statements is correct?
    - (a) Alginate beads belong to multiple-unit floating system
    - (b) Alginate beads are prepared by using Calcium alginate and low methoxylated pectin
    - (c) Alginate beads are prepared by using Calcium sulphate and high methoxylated pectin
    - (d) Alginate beads are prepared by using Calcium chloride and high methoxylated pectin

16. Microporous gastro-retentive drug delivery systems contains
    (a) Microporous compartment inside the drug reservoir
    (b) Drug reservoir inside the microporous compartment
    (c) Micropores inside the drug particles
    (d) All of the above

17. Swellable gastro-retentive drug delivery systems provide sustained release of drug due to
    (a) Extensive swelling of the polymer present in the device
    (b) High degree of cross-linking of the polymer
    (c) Optimum cross-linking of the polymer only
    (d) Low degree of cross-linking of the polymer

18. Which of the following statements is correct?
    (a) Buoyant systems contain matrices prepared by using polymers
    (b) Buoyant systems contain matrices prepared by using swellable polymers and effervescing agent
    (c) Buoyant systems are prepared by using effervescing polymers
    (d) Buoyant systems contain matrices prepared by using effervescing agent

19. Buoyancy and drug release from low density gastro-retentive drug delivery system depends on
    (a) Quantity of polymers present in the device
    (b) Polymer-drug ratio
    (c) Plasticizer-drug ratio
    (d) None of the above

20. Characteristics of bioadhesive polymer is
    (a) Capability of forming noncovalent bonds with the mucin-epithelial surfaces
    (b) Hydrophilic functional groups
    (c) There should be no hindrance to drug release
    (d) All of the above

## B. Short Questions

1. What is GRDDS? Why it is developed?
2. What are the factors that affect the functions of GRDDS?
3. What are the benefits and limitations of GRDDS?
4. Explain the gastro-retentive drug delivery system that works on the principle of magnetism.
5. Can evolution of a gas make a device floating in the gastrointestinal tract? If so, how?

6. Explain how a swelling can be related to floating of a device in the gastrointestinal tract to deliver a drug.

7. Explain how the volatile liquids can be utilized to formulate the gastroretentive drug delivery system.

## C. Long Questions

1. Explain why gastroretentive drug delivery systems are designed. Conventional oral solid dosage forms do not remain in the gastrointestinal tract for longer period of time; then how non-floating systems can stay in the GIT for longer period?

2. Write down briefly the methods employed to make the dosage form floating in the gastrointestinal tract.

3. Under normal conditions no matter can retain in the gastrointestinal tract beyond gastric retention time; then how the gastric retention time of a non-floating drug delivery system can be retained in the gastrointestinal tract beyond the gastric retention time?

4. Explain how the density of a drug delivery system can be utilized for development of a gastroretentive drug delivery system.

5. What are the various approaches used to develop a gastroretentive drug delivery system based on polymer properties?

## CHAPTER 8

# Nasopulmonary Drug Delivery System

*Introduction to Nasal and Pulmonary routes of drug delivery, Formulation of Inhalers (dry powder and metered dose), nasal sprays, nebulizers.*

## Introduction

### Nasal Drug Delivery

Now a day, the administration of drug through nasal route has gained a great popularity. It is a convenient and reliable method not only for local but also for systemic administration of drugs, particularly for those drugs that are orally ineffective and need to be administered by injection.

Investigations have revealed that the drugs with a wide variety of chemical structures are well absorbed through the nasal membranes of animals as well as man. On the basis of above observations, it has been recognized that the nasal route could be a promising route of administration of drugs having low dose, persistently used and are ineffective orally, but need to be rapidly present in the general circulation. The rate of absorption of drug through a physiological membrane can be greatly influenced by physicochemical properties of the drug molecule such as the extent of ionisation, lipophilicity of the compound, the molecular size as well as the ability of the compound to form hydrogen bond with the components of the membrane.

Several drugs such as, peptides, narcotic antagonists, male and female hormones are ineffective when administered orally, because these are metabolised in the gastrointestinal tract or due to the first-pass effects in the liver. These drugs may be absorbed through nasal mucosa and some of them are already in the market as prescription products. The penetration of bioactive molecules through the nasal mucosa has shown good bioavailability and nasal formulations also demonstrated better patients' compliance. The dosage forms suitable for nasal delivery are composed of: (1) the formulation and (2) the device that can deliver the desired amount of the formulation.

## Technological Aspects

To know the required absorption drug profile after intranasal administration the most suitable dosage form and delivery system should be identified. The selection of dosage form generally depends on the drug, clinical indication, number of patients and market requirements.

Various nasal dosage forms have been developed till this date such as drops, solution and suspension, sprays, powders, gels, emulsions and ointments; even some specialised systems such as liposomes and microspheres. Among all these forms, liquid forms are widely used. These are largely aqueous formulations. These are administered to the patients with help of suitable devices such as metered dose nasal actuator systems. Although liquid preparations are considered as the most common and convenient formulation for administration, this perception is simplistic; not realistic. Because, there are several factors such as the physicochemical stability of drug in solution, microbiological stability of the dosage form and the effect of the formulation on the physiological clearance mechanisms from the nasal mucosa have to be carefully considered.

Moreover, when a systemic pharmacological effect is expected, these formulations could show limited worth; because, simple solutions are readily cleared from the site of administration through the combined action of mucus secretion and the beating movements of cilia. Thus, even if the absorption of the drug is rapid, the extent of absorption becomes inadequate due to the short residence time in situ.

This problem has two feasible solutions: (1) increasing the contact time of the drug with the nasal mucosa by the use of appropriate excipients, (2) modification of the formulation by adding a suitable penetration enhancer. Thus, both rate and extent of drug absorption through the mucosa can be increased. As regards the increase in contact time, bioadhesive or microsphere-based formulations have become the subject of related scientific research. Excipients with bioadhesive property function as per their ability to adhere to a biological tissue for a prolonged period of time, thus limited to the clearance of the formulation. Microsphere-based formulations transport the drug by physical entrapment. These formulations when come in contact with nasal mucosa absorb water and form gels that adhere tightly for a prolonged time to the surface. The gels so prepared allow drug release *in situ* of the active from the formulation for a longer period. On the other hand, as far as penetration enhancers are concerned, most of these systems are based on surfactants and often the improvements in absorption are attached with tissue damages. Hence, providing high bioavailability is the important aim of formulation development for nasal products with minimum or no tissue side effects. This can be accomplished by using certain phospholipid compounds, and more particularly cationic polymers such as chitosan.

## Pulmonary Drug Delivery

The inhalation route of drug delivery offers an effective way of delivering drug therapies to the lung in the treatment of respiratory diseases. Recently delivering drug therapies through the lung for the treatment of a wide range of other disorders is of concern. Lung anatomy and lung physiology provides a number of advantages which makes the pulmonary route a good target for these drug delivery therapies. Among those advantages, the following are the most significant:

> - a large surface area of about 150 $m^2$
> - an extremely well vascularised and thin epithelial lining surface

These advantages lead to the following benefits for pulmonary drug delivery:

> - a non-invasive method of drug delivery providing the patient with an alternative to injection therapies
> - a direct entree to systemic circulation providing for a more rapid onset of action where such a response is important especially for acute treatments
> - an avoidance of first-pass metabolism and of gastrointestinal degradation resulting in lower doses of medication and concomitantly producing fewer unwanted side effects
> - a more convenient means of drug administration, i.e., a non-clinical setting

In order to use this route for drug administration, a number of technologies have been developed during the last half-century. The current pulmonary drug delivery systems include:

> - pressurised metered dose inhalers (pMDIs)
> - dry powder inhalers (DPIs)
> - classical nebulizers and, more recently, aqueous mist inhalers (AMIs)

Effective drug delivery to the lung includes an understanding of the drug formulation, the inhaler device and the patient. This review will briefly explore the above-mentioned aspects of their effects upon the various technology platforms before proceeding onto an examination of the therapeutic patents in the pulmonary drug delivery area.

## Formulation of Inhalers (Dry Powder and Metered Dose)

### Pressurised Metered Dose Inhalers

Pressurized metered dose inhalers (pMDIs) signify the most extensively used inhalation devices in the respiratory care in drug delivery area. This system is almost completely related to the treatment of asthma. These devices commonly contain β-agonists or corticosteroids. Riker Laboratories (a subsidiary of 3M Pharmaceuticals) first introduced this product in 1956. These devices utilise a number of chlorofluorocarbon propellants (CFCs), commonly called freons, to aerosolise and deliver micronized drug particles in suspension formulations. When actuated, these pMDIs deliver the aerosolised drug particles at very high speeds near about 30 m/sec. Unless actuation of the device is co-ordinated with the breathing process, a large amount of the drug accumulates at the back of the throat and is swallowed. Therefore, the major factor influencing the delivery of drugs by this route is inhaler technique (fig. 8.1).

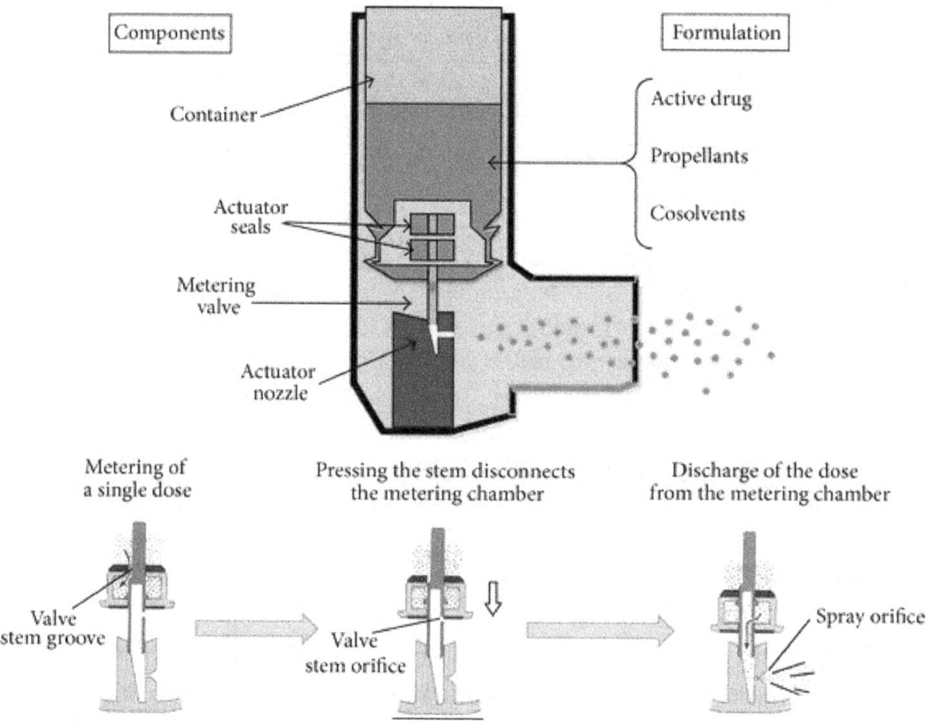


**Fig. 8.1:** Schematic representation of metered dose inhaler.

To moderate the effects of the disadvantages of conventional pMDIs, a number of device enhancements have been developed. Breath actuated devices (for example, the Autohaler® and Easi-Breathe) have established to be effective in improving the co-ordination problems often related with these devices. Similarly, integrated (Azmacort®) and add-on (Spacehaler®) spacers have established to be beneficial in reducing oropharyngeal deposition.

## Dry Powder Inhalers

In order to further report some of the disadvantages of the pMDI, the DPI was developed in the late 1960s and in the early 1970s to provide the patient with an alternative to the pMDI. However, the 'Montreal Protocol' of 1987 named for a phase-out of CFCs and other environmentally injurious chemicals, and the desire to deliver biotherapeutics via the inhalation route, has spurred a rapid development of devices in this area. Using this device the patient inhales micronized drug particles with or without a drug carrier (usually lactose). Whereas early DPIs were single dose capsule-based devices (Fisons' Spinhaler® and GlaxoWellcome's Rotohaler), improved multiple dose devices (GlaxoWellcome's Diskhaler® and Diskus® as well as Astra Draco's Turbuhaler®) are now available. As these devices dispense only during inhalation, they require less co-ordination than pMDIs. Improved powder processing and the use of impellers (Dura Pharmaceuticals' Spiros®) to help the patient with aerosolization represent attempts to address some of the disadvantages of DPIs.

## Nebulizers and Aqueous Mist Inhalers

The metered dose and powder inhalers are not suitable for geriatric patients and infants. The aqueous mist inhalers or compressed air nebulizer or ultrasonic nebulizers offers an alternative approach for such condition. It composed of a device that nebulizes the ethanolic or aqueous solution of drug into the smaller size droplets (generally 2-5 µ) suitable for inhalation. The nebulizer therapy takes usually longer time than the aforementioned therapies which lasts for 15 to 20 mins and can occurs with normal tidal breathing. The nebulizer is able to deliver all the drugs and biotherapeutics at any virtual dosage. On the other hand the size of conventional nebulizer is too large to carry and also not portable. Thus, to resolve the limitations of the conventional nebulizer AMIs have been evolved. It is a compact device which can deliver approximately 50µ*l* of the liquid aerosol in a metered fashion.

## Nasal Sprays

Nasal spray drug products contain therapeutically active ingredients (drug substances) dissolved or suspended in solutions or mixtures of excipients (e.g., preservatives, viscosity modifiers, emulsifiers, buffering agents) in non-pressurized dispensers that deliver a spray containing a metered dose of the active ingredient. The dose can be metered by the spray pump or could have been pre-metered during manufacture. A nasal spray unit can be intended for unit dosing or can discharge up to several hundred metered sprays of formulation containing the drug substance. Nasal sprays are applied to the nasal cavity for local and/or systemic effects (fig. 8.2).

Although similar in many aspects to other drug products, some aspects of nasal sprays may be unique (e.g., formulation, container closure system, manufacturing, stability, controls of critical steps, intermediates, and drug product). These features should be considered carefully during the development program because changes can influence the ability of the product to deliver reproducible doses to patients during the product's shelf life. Some of the unique features of nasal sprays are listed below:

1. Metering and spray producing (e.g., orifice, nozzle, jet) pump mechanisms and components are used for reproducible delivery of drug formulation, and these can be constructed of many parts of different design that are exactly controlled in terms of dimensions and composition.

2. Energy is required for dispersion of the formulation as a spray. This is typically accomplished by forcing the formulation through the nasal actuator and its orifice.

3. The formulation and the container closure system (container, closure, pump, and any protective packaging) collectively create the drug product. The design of the container closure system influences the dosing performance of the drug product

4. The concept of classical bioequivalence and bioavailability may not be applicable for all nasal sprays, depending on the intended site of action. The doses administered are typically so small that blood or serum concentrations are generally undetectable by routine analytical procedures.

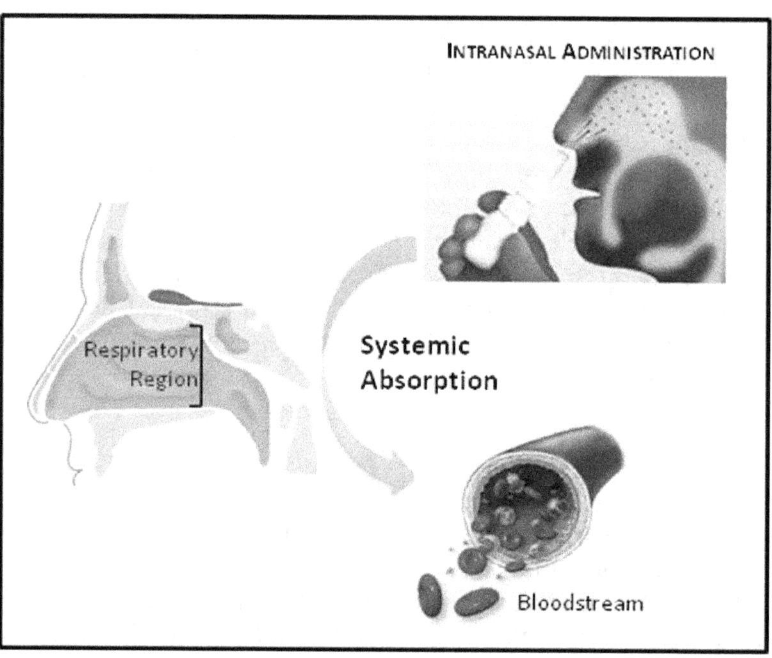


**Fig. 8.2:** Systemic drug delivery through nasal spray.

## Nebulizers

Nebulizers are used regularly as a part of the management of a wide variety of respiratory problems, most commonly to administer anti-cholinergic and $\beta_2$-agonist drugs. More recently, they have been used for aerosol administration of deoxyribonuclease in the treatment of cystic fibrosis, and more viscous drugs such as pentamidine for prophylaxis against Pneumocystis pneumonia in patients infected with the HIV virus. Nebulizer systems are now in common use, but we still do not fully understand the functional operation of these systems. The effects of evaporation of the diluent and drug, and whether the speed of delivery of the drug to the patient plays an important role on the efficacy of drug therapy by this mode, are not fully-evaluated. While these pose interesting problems, there remain a number of everyday practical problems which can easily be addressed. Effective delivery of any aerosol is important to provide maximum possible benefit to the patient. Instrumentation of a commercial nebulizer was shown in figure 8.3.

## Fill Volume and Residual Volume

Each nebulizer chamber has a residual volume in which a small amount of drug and diluent remain when the nebulizer is run 'dry'. The consequence of this is that the amount of drug nebulized is less than the amount initially placed in the chamber. Thus, if a 2.5 m*l* ampoule of drug is placed in a nebulizer chamber with a residual volume of 1.75 m*l*, only 0.75 m*l* of the solution is actually available to the patient, whereas, if a chamber with a 0.5 m*l* residual volume is used, 2 m*l* of solution is available. Simply increasing the fill volume, to say 4 ml, would increase the volume of respirable solution available to the patient, but has the limitations of increased cost and inefficiency, and will prolong the total time of nebulization.

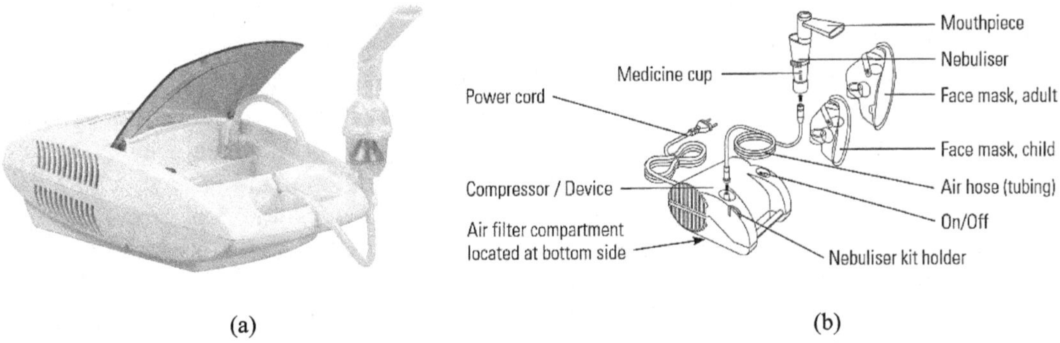


**Fig. 8.3:** (a) a commercial nebulizer system and (b) schematic representation of nebulizer instrumentation.

In 1983, when Clay et al. recommended for a 4 mL fill volume for bronchodilator drugs, no nebulizer chambers existed with a residual volume of less than 1 mL. A similar recommendation has been made for antibiotic drugs. Consequently, many protocols require a fill volume of 4 mL in the nebulizer. These recommendations are based on nebulizer chambers which have a residual volume of 1 mL or more. Since then, a number of new nebulizer chambers have become available that have a residual volume of less than 1 mL, and therefore do not require to have fill volumes of 4 mL. Where there is a large residual volume, the percentage of drug delivered to the patient will increase with increased fill volume if nebulization continues to dryness. However, for most nebulizers with a small residual volume, the percentage increase is less than 25% for either bronchodilator drugs or antibiotics. While this increased drug delivery may benefit the patient; less compliance may possibly occur because of the inherently longer nebulization times required.

The fill volume does not appear to influence the particle size distribution. Particle size should ideally be 3~$\mu$m – 5~$\mu$m to achieve effective lung deposition. The flow-rate and pressure of gas from the compressor are correlated; so, higher is the pressure, higher is the flow-rate at the nebulizer. The higher the flow-rate at the nebulizer, the smaller the particle size of the aerosol will be. To compare different systems, the mass median aerodynamic diameter (MMAD) is calculated. This is the particle diameter above which 50% of the mass of the aerosol particles is distributed. Comparing the MMAD at a fill volume of 2.5 m*l* and at 5 m*l*, the relationship of MMAD to flow-rate is not significantly different. Therefore, choosing a higher fill volume will not significantly increase the effective deposition of aerosol particles.

Drug companies now supply bronchodilator drugs in ampoule sizes of 2 m*l* or 2.5 m*l*. To our knowledge, there is no evidence to show that increasing the fill volume to 4 m*l*, either subjectively or objectively, improves the quality of life of the patient. The practice of adding diluent to the nebulizer solution from these ampoules, may well further decrease the compliance with therapy. Furthermore, adding saline increases the overall costs of drug therapy with the additional need for saline, needles and syringes. This leads to more potential needle-stick injuries for both patients and healthcare workers, and increased staff costs when this practice is used in health centres or hospital units.

In conclusion, the view that the fill volume of nebulizers should be 4 m*l* is not supported by current evidence regarding nebulizer performance, for either bronchodilator drugs or antibiotics. This is particularly true when using the newer nebulizer chambers that have a residual volume of less than 1 m*l*. The increased nebulization time, additional staff and consumable costs simply do not justify using a 4 ml volume as a routine. We therefore recommend that the nebulizers in routine use should have as small a residual volume as possible, that users should know what this volume is, and that a fill volume of no less than 2 m*l* should be used. This does not preclude the use of chambers with larger residual volumes, but these should be reserved for cases where larger volumes of drugs need to be nebulized.

## Characterization of Nasopulmonary Drug Delivery System

For nasal spray and inhalation solution, suspension, and spray drug products, certain studies should be performed to characterize the performance properties of the drug product and to provide support in defining the optimal labelling statements regarding use (e.g., storage, cleaning, shaking). Delivery systems for nasal and inhalation spray drug products can vary in both design and mode of operation, and these characteristics may be unique to a particular drug product. Studies to define these characteristics will help facilitate correct use and maintenance of the drug product and contribute to patient compliance. For the most part, these should be one-time studies, preferably performed on multiple batches (e.g., two or three) of drug product representative of the product intended for distribution. Additionally, this information will provide a baseline for comparison if, at a later time, the performance characteristics of a drug product are in question. For ANDAs, the applicability of each of the characterization studies outlined below for a given drug product can be discussed with the responsible review division.

1. **Priming and Repriming in Various Orientations:** For multiple-dose nasal and inhalation spray drug products, studies should be performed to characterize the priming and repriming required for the product after storage in multiple orientations (upright and inverted or upright and horizontal) and after different periods of non-use. SCU and other pertinent parameters should be evaluated. The following information should be established:
   - The approximate interval that can pass before the drug product should be reprimed to deliver the labelled amount of medication.
   - The number of sprays recommended to prime or reprime the unit
   - Multiple orientation studies should be performed with initial sprays and with sprays near the label claim number. Priming and repriming information will be used to support the proposed labelling statements.

2. **Effect of Resting Time:** For multiple-dose inhalation spray drug products, a study is recommended to determine the effect of increasing resting time on the first spray of unprimed units, followed immediately by the second and the third sprays. Units should be primed only before initiation of the study. After resting for increasing periods of time (e.g., 6, 12, 24, 48 hours), uniformity of the medication delivered in the first, second, and third sprays (no priming) should be determined. Testing should be performed on units that have been stored in different orientations (i.e., upright and inverted or upright and horizontal). To shorten the length of the study, testing can be performed concurrently on separate samples with progressively longer resting periods.

3. **Temperature Cycling :** For nasal spray, inhalation suspension, and inhalation spray drug products, a stress temperature cyclic study should be performed to evaluate the effects of high and low temperature variations that may be encountered during shipping and handling on the quality and performance of the drug product. Such a study can consist of 12-hour cycles, with temperatures ranging between freezer temperature (-10 to -20°C) and 40°C for a period of at least 4 weeks. Alternative conditions and duration can be used with appropriate justification. Periodically throughout the study, at the end of a predetermined number of cycles, the samples should be analysed for appropriate parameters and compared with the control drug product.

Test parameters for cycling studies should include, where applicable, droplet size distribution, particle size distribution, microscopic evaluation, appearance, color, clarity, assay, SCU, sterility, and functionality of pump components. A validated container closure integrity test, instead of sterility testing, can be used to assess sterility and demonstrate maintenance of the integrity of the microbial barrier provided by the container closure system. With regard to appearance of the nasal spray and inhalation drug products, one should consider, as applicable, the discoloration of the formulation, distortion of pump components, pump clogging, and adherence of the drug to the walls of the container, closure, and/or pump components.

4. ***In Vitro* Dose Proportionality:** For nasal and inhalation spray drug products with multiple strength suspension formulations, studies should address *in vitro* dose proportionality between strengths by determining SCU and particle/droplet size distribution.

5. **Cleaning Instructions:** For nasal and inhalation spray drug products, in-use studies should be performed to determine the frequency of cleaning and related instructions to be included in the labelling.

6. **Device Robustness:** Device robustness should be studied for nasal and inhalation spray drug products and should address the following:
   - For devices that can be reused repeatedly with replaceable reservoirs, a study should be conducted to establish the product performance characteristics in terms of SCU and particle/droplet size distribution throughout the nominal number of sprays of the device.
   - Limits of use related to failure of critical device mechanisms should be studied to determine the appropriate replacement intervals for the device.
   - The performance characteristics of the device should be studied after different handling situations (e.g., dropping, shaking, vibrating).

7. **Effect of Dosing Orientation:** For nasal and inhalation spray drug products, studies should be undertaken to determine the comparative performance of the devices in terms of SCU and particle/droplet size distribution at various dosing orientations.

8. **Effect of Varying Flow Rates:** The effect of varying flow rate should be studied for inhalation spray drug products and should address the following:
   - For breath-activated drug products or those that are intended to be marketed with an expansion or holding chamber, spacer, or similar component, a study should be undertaken to determine the SCU and the particle/droplet size distribution as a function of different testing flow rates at a constant volume. The total volume should be limited to 2 litres.

> This study assesses the sensitivity of the device to widely changing flow rates generated by patients of different age and gender and with diverse severity of disease.

> Another study for breath-activated products should assess the triggering ranges of flow rates that generate the amount of delivered dose and the corresponding particle/droplet size distribution.

For drug products with an expansion or holding chamber, spacer, or similar component, a separate study is encouraged to assess the effect of increasing waiting periods (e.g., 0, 5, 10 seconds) between actuation and initiation of inflow, at a specified flow rate, on the SCU and particle/droplet size distribution.

9. **Profiling of Sprays Near Container Exhaustion (Tail Off Characteristics):** For nasal and inhalation spray drug products, a study should be conducted to determine the profiles of SCU and droplet (solution) or particle/droplet (suspension) size distribution of each individual spray after the point at which the labelled number of sprays have been dispensed until no more sprays are possible (i.e., the container is empty). SCU testing can be replaced by pump delivery testing for solution formulations. These studies help determine if the target fill and any proposed overfill of the containers are justified, since the tail off characteristics can vary as a function of pump design, container geometry, and formulation. A graphical representation of the findings is also recommended.

10. **Effect of Storage on the Particle Size Distribution:** For suspension spray drug products, the stability studies on the primary stability batches should determine the effect of storage time and conditions on particle size distribution through unit life (beginning to end for device-metered products). If stability studies demonstrate an effect on the particle size distribution within unit life, then the routine stability protocol should include particle size distribution testing through unit life.

11. **Plume Geometry:** For nasal spray drug products, plume geometry of the spray should be characterized. Plume geometry does not distinguish between drug substance particles and formulation droplets in the spray or indicate any density gradient for the drug substance but determines the shape of the entire plume. Therefore, this test is complementary to the spray pattern test. The plume geometry characteristics can be used as a baseline to compare similar nasal spray drug products by different manufacturers or when certain changes are introduced to an already approved drug product.

12. **Preservative Effectiveness and Sterility Maintenance:** If preservatives are used in the formulation, the minimum content limit should be demonstrated as microbiologically effective by performing a microbial challenge assay of the drug formulated with an amount of preservative equal to or less than the minimum amount specified. For details for this characterization, see the stability guidance.

For device-metered, aqueous-based inhalation spray drug products, studies should be performed to demonstrate the appropriate microbiological quality through the life of the reservoir and during the period of reservoir use. Such testing could assess the ability of the container closure system to prevent microbial ingress into the formulation and/or the growth inhibiting properties of the formulation.

13.  **Characterization of Nebulizer Specified in the Labelling:** For inhalation solution and suspension drug products, a study should be undertaken to determine the delivered dose and the particle/droplet size distribution as per the specified operating parameters and ranges for a given nebulizer.

14.  **Photostability:** Photostability studies should be performed using appropriate test conditions, if warranted by the immediate container, i.e., the formulation in the primary container can receive light exposure. These studies should be conducted in the absence of any additional packaging (e.g., foil overwrap).

15.  **Stability of Primary (Unprotected) Package:** For a drug product labelled for storage at room temperature, if additional packaging (e.g., foil overwrap for LDPE-contained product) is used to protect the drug product from degradation and/or evaporative effects, adequate stability data conducted at a minimum of 25°C and a maximum of 40 percent RH should be generated for these units without the protective packaging for pertinent parameters. This data can support the establishment of the maximum length of time for product use after the protective packaging is removed. Drug products both newly manufactured and near the end of the proposed expiration dating period should be evaluated.

## Labelling Considerations

To achieve consistency and uniformity in the content, the product title, and the format of the labelling of nasal spray and inhalation solution, suspension, and spray drug products, the following pertinent information is recommended in the labelling. These comments are not all inclusive, and they are directed mainly at labelling issues unique to NDAs for prescription nasal spray and inhalation solution, suspension, and spray drug products.

1.  **Nasal and Inhalation Spray Drug Products**

    (a)  *Product Title*: To standardize the nomenclature for oral inhalation sprays, the established name of all such drug products should include the designation *(Drug Substance) Inhalation Spray*. For nasal sprays, the drug product would include the name *(Drug Substance) Nasal Spray*. The established name should be followed by a phrase such as *For Oral Inhalation Only*, or *For Nasal Use Only*, as appropriate.

    (b)  *Label*

    The label should bear the following information:

    ➢ Established name of the drug product

- ➢ Amounts of the drug substance delivered from the pump nasal actuator or mouthpiece
- ➢ Number of medication sprays per container
- ➢ Net content (fill) weight
- ➢ Usual dosage
- ➢ Excipients (established names)
- ➢ Route of administration
- ➢ Recommended storage conditions including any warning statements regarding temperature or light exposure
- ➢ Manufacturer's and/or distributor's name and address
- ➢ "Rx Only" or "L Only" statement
- ➢ Lot number
- ➢ Expiration date
- ➢ Use period once drug product is removed from protective packaging (if applicable)
- ➢ Instructions regarding shaking of suspension drug products
- ➢ NDC number

For nasal and inhalation spray drug product devices that can be reused repeatedly with multiple reservoirs, each reservoir should be labelled adequately.

In the case of small labels, only some of the information listed above must be included in the label (21 CFR 201.10(i)). However, all labelling information required by the Federal Food, Drug, and Cosmetic Act (the Act) and the regulations in Title 21 of the Code of Federal Regulations must be included on the carton, outer container, wrapper, and leaflet as appropriate.

2. **Inhalation Solutions and Suspensions**

   (a) ***Product Title***: To standardize the nomenclature for inhalation solutions, the established name of all such drug products should include the designation *(Drug Substance) Inhalation Solution*. For inhalation suspensions, the drug product would include the name *(Drug Substance) Inhalation Suspension*. The established name should be followed by a phrase such as *For oral inhalation only*.

   (b) ***Label***

The label should bear the following information:

- ➢ Established name of the drug product
- ➢ Amount of the drug substance per container and concentration of drug substance in the formulation
- ➢ Net content (fill) weight
- ➢ Usual dosage

> Excipients (established names)

> Route of administration

> Recommended storage conditions including any warning statements regarding temperature and light exposure

> Manufacturer's and/or distributor's name and address

> "Rx Only" or "L Only" statement

> Lot number

> Expiration date

> Use period once drug product is removed from protective packaging (if applicable)

> Instructions regarding shaking of suspension drug products

> NDC number (recommended)

In the case of small labels, only some of the information listed above must be included in the label (21 CFR 201.10(i)). However, all labelling information required by the Act and the regulations in Title 21 must be included on the carton, outer container, wrapper, and leaflet as appropriate.

# Bibliography


1. Ali, M., CHAPTER 9 - Pulmonary Drug Delivery, in Handbook of Non-Invasive Drug Delivery Systems, V.S. Kulkarni, Editor. 2010, William Andrew Publishing: Boston. p. 209-246.

2. Brocklebank, D., et al., Comparison of the effectiveness of inhaler devices in asthma and chronic obstructive airways disease: a systematic review of the literature. Health Technol Assess, 2001. 5(26): p. 1-149.

3. Denyer, J., K. Nikander, and N.J. Smith, Adaptive Aerosol Delivery (AAD) technology. Expert Opin Drug Deliv, 2004. 1(1): p. 165-76.

4. DiBlasi, R.M., Clinical Controversies in Aerosol Therapy for Infants and Children. Respir Care, 2015. 60(6): p. 894-914; discussion 914-6.

5. Elphick, M., et al., Factors to consider when selecting a nebulizer for a new inhaled drug product development program. Expert Opin Drug Deliv, 2015. 12(8): p. 1375-87.

6. Frijlink, H.W. and A.H. De Boer, Dry powder inhalers for pulmonary drug delivery. Expert Opin Drug Deliv, 2004. 1(1): p. 67-86.

7. Geller, D.E., Comparing clinical features of the nebulizer, metered-dose inhaler, and dry powder inhaler. Respir Care, 2005. 50(10): p. 1313-21; discussion 1321-2.

8. Geller, D.E., New liquid aerosol generation devices: systems that force pressurized liquids through nozzles. Respir Care, 2002. 47(12): p. 1392-404; discussion 1404-5.

9. Groneberg, D.A., et al., Fundamentals of pulmonary drug delivery. Respir Med, 2003. 97(4): p. 382-7.

10. Jia, Y., L. Krishnan, and A. Omri, Nasal and pulmonary vaccine delivery using particulate carriers. Expert Opin Drug Deliv, 2015. 12(6): p. 993-1008.

11. Kendrick, A.H., E.C. Smith, and J. Denyer, Nebulizers--fill volume, residual volume and matching of nebulizer to compressor. Respir Med, 1995. 89(3): p. 157-9.

12. Laube, B.L., The expanding role of aerosols in systemic drug delivery, gene therapy, and vaccination. Respir Care, 2005. 50(9): p. 1161-76.

13. Martin, A.R. and W.H. Finlay, Nebulizers for drug delivery to the lungs. Expert Opin Drug Deliv, 2015. 12(6): p. 889-900.

14. Martini, A., L. Muggetti, and M.P. Warchol, Nasal and pulmonary drug delivery systems. Expert Opinion on Therapeutic Patents, 2000. 10(3): p. 315-323.

15. Miller, C.J., Chapter 172 - Inhaled Medications, in Small Animal Critical Care Medicine (Second Edition), D.C. Silverstein and K. Hopper, Editors. 2015, W.B. Saunders: St. Louis. p. 903-906.

16. Mortensen, N.P. and A.J. Hickey, Targeting inhaled therapy beyond the lungs. Respiration, 2014. 88(5): p. 353-4.

17. Nanjwade, B.K., et al., Pulmonary drug delivery: novel pharmaceutical technologies breathe new life into the lungs. PDA J Pharm Sci Technol, 2011. 65(5): p. 513-34.

18. Patil, J.S. and S. Sarasija, Pulmonary drug delivery strategies: A concise, systematic review. Lung India, 2012. 29(1): p. 44-9.

19. Pleasants, R.A. and D.R. Hess, Aerosol Delivery Devices for Obstructive Lung Diseases. Respir Care, 2018. 63(6): p. 708-733.

20. Ram, F.S., et al., Pressurised metered-dose inhalers versus all other hand-held inhalers devices to deliver bronchodilators for chronic obstructive pulmonary disease. Cochrane Database Syst Rev, 2002(1): p. Cd002170.

21. Rogueda, P.G. and D. Traini, The nanoscale in pulmonary delivery. Part 2: formulation platforms. Expert Opin Drug Deliv, 2007. 4(6): p. 607-20.

22. Tashkin, D.P., et al., Comparing COPD treatment: nebulizer, metered dose inhaler, and concomitant therapy. Am J Med, 2007. 120(5): p. 435-41.

23. Watts, A.B., J.T. McConville, and R.O. Williams, 3rd, Current therapies and technological advances in aqueous aerosol drug delivery. Drug Dev Ind Pharm, 2008. 34(9): p. 913-22.

## Exercise

## A. Multiple Choice Questions

1. The extent of drug absorption from nasal preparation is not adequate due to

    (a)  Poor rate of administration
    (b)  Short residence time
    (c)  Increased biological half-life
    (d)  Biological half-life

2. The extent of drug absorption from nasal preparation can be improved by

    (a)  Increasing the contact time of the drug with nasal mucosa
    (b)  Modification of the formulation by adding penetration enhancer
    (c)  Incorporating the penetration enhancer
    (d)  All of the above

3. The dosage form used for pulmonary action of drug is by
   - (a) Inhalation
   - (b) Nasal drop
   - (c) Ointment
   - (d) All of the above

4. When pulmonary drug delivery system is used
   - (a) Onset of action is equivalent to that obtained after oral administration
   - (b) Onset of action is slow
   - (c) Onset of action is rapid
   - (d) None of the above

5. Dry powder inhaler contains
   - (a) Drug powders
   - (b) Micronized drug powders
   - (c) Coarse drug powders
   - (d) None of the above

6. Nebulizers contain
   - (a) Solution of drug in hydro alcohol
   - (b) Solution of drug in carbon tetrachloride
   - (c) Solution of drug in benzene
   - (d) Solution of drug in chloroform

7. Excipients present in nasal spray do not include
   - (a) Preservative
   - (b) Viscosity modifier
   - (c) Buffering agent
   - (d) Flavour

8. Nasal spray drug product constitutes
   - (a) Drug and container
   - (b) Drug, container and closure
   - (c) Drug, container, closure and pump
   - (d) None of the above

9. When a nebulizer is run 'dry'
   - (a) The container does not contain any drug
   - (b) The container contains a small amount of drug and diluent
   - (c) The container does not contain any diluent
   - (d) The container does not contain any amount of drug and diluent

10. Ideal size of particle sprayed by a nebulizer is
    - (a) Within $3 - 5\mu m$
    - (b) Within $5 - 10\mu m$
    - (c) Within $10 - 15\mu m$
    - (d) Within $20 - 25\mu m$

11. Stress temperature cycling test on nasal spray or inhalation spray is done to evaluate
    - (a) The effect of only high temperature on the product's performance
    - (b) The effect of only low temperature on the product's performance
    - (c) The effect of high and low temperatures on the product's performance
    - (d) Particle size in the product.

12. The performance characteristics of nasal spray or inhalation spray devices should be studied
    (a) After dropping  (b)  After shaking
    (c) After vibrating  (d)  All of these

13. Nasal preparation containing preservative should be tested for
    (a) Microbial challenge assay of the drug
    (b) The amount of preservative equal to the minimum amount specified
    (c) The amount of preservative less than the minimum amount specified
    (d) All of the above

14. Inhalation spray is prepared to administer the drug
    (a) Through oral and nasal routes
    (b) Through oral route only
    (c) Through nasal route only
    (d) All of the above

15. The effect of resting time should be conducted on multiple-dose inhalation spray product for
    (a) First spray  (b)  Second spray
    (c) Third spray  (d)  First, second and third sprays

16. For dispersion of the formulation as a spray
    (a) No energy is required
    (b) Energy is required
    (c) Orifice of proper aperture is only required
    (d) Particles of adequate size range is only required

17. For reproducible delivery of drug formulation from a metered and spray producing device
    (a) Only suitable pump is required
    (b) Pump with suitable orifice would be required
    (c) Pump with suitable orifice, nozzle, jet would be required
    (d) Pump with suitable jet would be required

18. Pressurized metered dose inhalers uses
    (a) Liquified freon as propellent
    (b) Liquified argon gas as propellent
    (c) Liquified carbon dioxide gas as propellent
    (d) Liquified nitrogen gas as propellent

19. On actuation, the pressurized metered dose inhaler delivers the formulation at a speed of
    (a) 20m/sec  (b)  30m/sec
    (c) 10m/sec  (d)  5m/sec

20. The nasopulmonary drug delivery system is suitable for
    (a) Drugs of low molecular weight only
    (b) Drugs of high molecular weight only
    (c) All drugs
    (d) Drugs which are susceptible metabolic first pass effect.

## B. Short Questions

1. Why the nasopulmonary route has gained importance?
2. Explain the advantages of nasopulmonary drug delivery system.
3. What is an inhaler? What is metered dose inhaler?
4. What are nebulizers and nasal spray?
5. What are fill volume and residual volume?
6. What do you understand by 'temperature cycling'?

## C. Long Questions

1. How the nasopulmonary drug delivery system can be characterized?
2. Write down the information to be provided through the label of a Nasal and Inhalation spray product.
3. Write down the information to be provided through the label of an Inhalation product containing solution or suspension.
4. 'Recently the administration of drug through nasal route has a great popularity'– explain the statement. Write down the technological aspects of this type of formulation.
5. Explain the construction and function of a system used to administer a specific amount of drug.
6. Explain in detail the importance of 'fill volume' and 'residual volume' with reference to administration of drug through nasopulmonary route.

## CHAPTER 9

# Nanotechnology and its Concepts

*Concepts and approaches for targeted drug delivery systems, advantages and disadvantages, introduction to liposomes, niosomes, nanoparticles, monoclonal antibodies and their applications.*

## Introduction

## Concepts

The term nanotechnology originates from the combination of two words: the Greek numerical prefix nano referring to a billionth and the word technology. As an outcome, Nanotechnology or Nanoscaled Technology is generally considered to be at a size below 0.1 μm or 100 nm (a nanometer is one billionth of a meter, $10^{-9}$ m). Nanoscale science or nanoscience studies the phenomena, properties, and responses of materials at atomic, molecular, and macromolecular scales, and in general at sizes between 1 and 100 nm. In this scale, and especially below 5 nm, the properties of matter differ significantly (i.e., quantum-scale effects play an important role) from that at a larger particulate scale. Nanotechnology is then the design, the manipulation, the building, the production and application, by controlling the shape and size, the properties-responses and functionality of structures, and devices and systems of the order or less than 100 nm.

Nanotechnology is considered an emerging technology. There is greater possibility of advancement well-established products and to make new products with totally new characteristics and functions with huge potential in a wide range of applications. Moreover, the possibility of various industrial uses, great innovations are expected in information and communication technology, in biology and biotechnology, in medicine and medical technology, in metrology, etc. Significant applications of nanosciences and nanoengineering are there in the fields of pharmaceutics, cosmetics, processed food, chemical engineering, high-performance materials, electronics, precision mechanics, optics, energy production, and environmental sciences. Nanotechnology is a dynamic field where over 50,000 nanotechnology articles have been published annually worldwide in recent years, and more than 2,500 patents have been filed at major patent offices such as the European Patent Office.

Targeted drug delivery is one of the smart drug delivery systems which is remarkable in delivering the drug to a patient. The conventional drug delivery system is done by the absorption of the drug across a biological membrane, whereas the targeted release system is that the drug is released from a dosage form at predetermined specific target area of the body.

Targeted drug delivery, sometimes called smart drug delivery, is a method of delivering medication to a patient in a manner that increases the concentration of the drug in some parts of the body relative to others. This means of delivery is largely founded on nanomedicine, which plans to use nanoparticle-mediated drug delivery to combat the downfalls of conventional drug delivery. These nanoparticles would be loaded with drugs and targeted to specific parts of the body where there is solely diseased tissue, thereby avoiding interaction with healthy tissue (fig. 9.1). The goal of a targeted drug delivery system is to prolong, localize, target and have a protected drug interaction with the diseased tissue. The conventional drug delivery system is the absorption of the drug across a biological membrane, whereas the targeted release system releases the drug from a dosage form at the diseased site. The advantages to the targeted release system are;

➢ the reduction in the frequency of the dosages taken by the patient,
➢ delivering a more uniform effect of the drug,
➢ reduction of drug side-effects, and
➢ reduced fluctuation in circulating drug levels.

The disadvantages of the system are

➢ high cost, which makes productivity more difficult and
➢ the reduced ability to adjust the dosages.

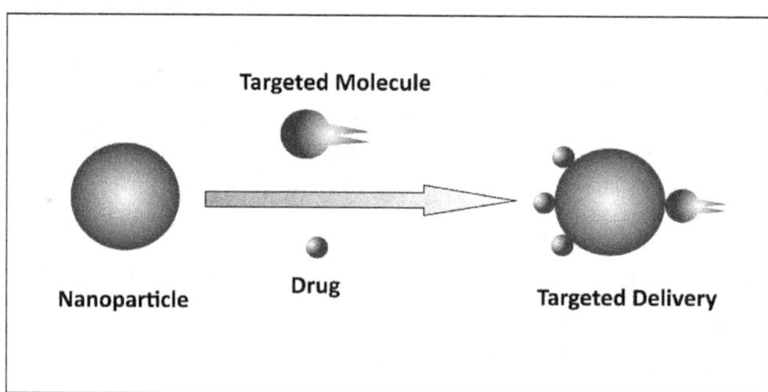


**Fig. 9.1:** Schematic representation of drug targeting.

Targeted drug delivery system is based on a method that delivers a certain amount of a therapeutic agent for a prolonged period of time to a targeted diseased area within the body. This helps to maintain the required plasma and tissue drug levels in the body;

therefore, avoiding any damage to the healthy tissue via the drug. The drug delivery system is highly integrated and requires various disciplines, such as chemists, biologist and engineers, to join forces to optimize this system. When, implementing a targeted release system, the following design criteria for the system need to take into account: the drug properties, side effects of the drugs, the route taken for the delivery of the drug, the targeted site, and the disease.

## Ideal Properties of Targeted Drug Delivery System

Products based on such a delivery system are being prepared by considering the specific properties of target cells, nature of markers or transport carriers or vehicles which convey the drug to specific receptors and ligands and physically modulated components. Ideal properties of targeted drug delivery systems are as follows:

- It should be biochemically inert (non-toxic)
- It should be non-immunogenic
- The targeted drug delivery system should be physically and chemically stable *in vivo* and *in vitro* conditions
- It should have controlled drug distribution to target cells or tissues or organs
- It should have uniform capillary distribution
- It should have controllable and predictable rate of drug release and also drug release should not affect the drug action.
- It should have therapeutic amount of drug release
- should have minimal drug leakage during transition
- The carriers used should be bio-degradable or readily eliminated from the body without any problem.
- The preparation of the delivery system should be easy or reasonably simple, reproducible and cost effective.

## Approaches of Targeted Drug Delivery

As discussed, targeting a drug to a specific area does not only increase the therapeutic efficacy of a drug, it can decrease the toxicity associated with the drug to allow lower doses of the drug to be used in therapy. For the fulfilment of such conditions, various approaches used extensively are discussed below (fig. 9.2):

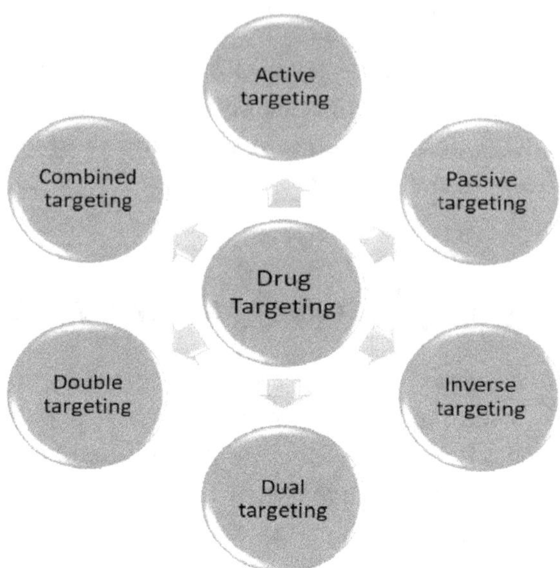


**Fig. 9.2:** Approaches of drug targeting

## Passive Targeting

It refers to the accumulation of drug or drug-carrier system at a specific site such as anti-cancerous drug whose explanation may be credited to physicochemical or pharmacological factors of the disease. Hence, in case of cancer treatment the size and surface properties of drug delivery nano-particles must be controlled specifically to avoid uptake by the reticuloendothelial system (RES) to increase circulation times and targeting ability. The bottom line is called passive targeting as misnomer which is simple drug delivery system via blood circulation. Drug release or drug actions are limited to selective sites within the body such as a tumour but not the liver. Other examples include targeting of antimalarial drugs for treatment of leishmiansis, brucellosis, candidacies.

## Active Targeting

Active targeting means a specific ligand receptor type interaction for intracellular localization which happens only after blood circulation and extravasations. This active targeting method can be further classified into three different levels of targeting which are:

1.  First order targeting refers to restricted distribution of the drug carrier systems to the capillary bed of a predetermined target site, organ or tissue e.g. compartmental targeting in lymphatics, peritoneal cavity, plural cavity, cerebral ventricles and eyes, joints.

2.  Second order targeting denotes to selective delivery of drugs to specific cell types such as tumour cells and not to the normal cells e.g. selective drug delivery to Kupffer cells in the liver.

3. Third order targeting refers to drug delivery specifically to the intracellular site of targeted cells e.g. receptor-based ligand mediated entry of a drug complex into a cell by endocytosis.

## Inverse Targeting

This approach leads to saturation of RES and suppression of defence mechanism. This type of targeting is an effective method to target drug(s) to non-RES organs.

## Dual Targeting

In this targeting method the carrier molecule itself have therapeutic activity and thus increase the therapeutic effect of drug. For example, a carrier molecule having its own antiviral activity can be loaded with antiviral drug and the net synergistic effect of drug conjugate was observed.

## Double Targeting

When temporal and spatial methodologies are combined to target a carrier system, then targeting may be called double targeting. Spatial placement relates to targeting drugs to specific organs tissues, cells or even subcellular compartment. Whereas temporal delivery refers to controlling the rate of drug delivery to target site.

## Combination Targeting

These targeting systems are equipped with carriers, polymers and homing devices of molecular specificity that could provide a direct approach to target site.

# Carrier System for Drug Targeting

Drug delivery vehicles are at the most important entity required for successful transportation of the loaded drug at the specific site

## Liposomes

Liposomes are small artificially designed vesicles containing phospholipid bilayers around themselves with the size ranging from 20 to 10,000 nm. Many liposome formulations are rapidly taken up by macrophages and this can be used either for macrophage-specific delivery of drugs or for passive drug targeting which allow slow release of the drug over time from these cells into the general circulation. Cationic liposomes and lipoplexes have been extensively researched for their application in non-viral vector mediated gene therapy.

## Monoclonal Antibodies and Fragments

The most of approaches based on antigen recognition by antibodies have been developed more specifically for cancer therapy. These approaches are mostly aimed at tumor associated antigens being present or in more specific term expressed by tumor cells. Antibody-drug conjugates (ADC) is complex of a drug with a monoclonal antibody which delivers selective targeting for tumoral cell masses or lymphomas. The drug is released by enzymatic cleavage of the linker under physiological conditions. An example of Antibody-drug conjugates (ADC) is Mylotarg (emtuzamabozogamicin) which was approved by the U.S. Food and Drug Administration (FDA), but later voluntarily withdrawn from the US market. Another ADC has been submitted for approval and at least 15 antibody conjugates are currently being investigated in clinical trials.

### Modified (plasma) proteins

Modified plasma proteins can be used as an intelligent drug vehicle for drug transportation because they have solubility and are of relatively small molecular weight. They can easily be modified by the attachment of different molecules like peptides, sugars, and other ligands to transport the drugs of interest makes them a suitable mode of drug delivery. In the case of liver cell targeting, extensive modifications of protein backbones such as albumins have been carried out effective delivery of the drug. Soluble synthetic polymers have been extensively researched as multipurpose drug carrier systems. Polymer chemistry permits the development of tailor-made conjugates in which target moieties as well as drugs can be entrapped into the carrier molecule. For cancer therapy, the well-established N (-2-hydroxypropyl) methacrylamide (HMPA) polymers have been extensively studied. Also, it provides a solution for selective and targeted chemotherapy.

## Microspheres and Nanoparticles

Microspheres and nanoparticles consist of biocompatible polymers and belong either to the soluble or the particle type carriers. HPMA polymeric backbone carriers have also been prepared using dextrans, ficoll, sepharose or poly-L-lysine as the main carrier body for the drugs. Nanoparticles are smaller (0.2– 0.5 µm) than microspheres (30–200 µm) and may have a smaller drug loading capacity than the soluble polymers. Formulation of drugs into the nanoparticles can occur at the surface of the particles and in nucleus, depending on the physicochemical characteristics of the drug. The site of incorporation of drug significantly influences its release rate from the particle. After systemic administration or transportation, they quickly distribute to the target, sit and then become internalized by the cells of the phagocytic system. Besides, microspheres and nanoparticles which are mostly used for cell selective delivery of drugs, they have more recently been studied for their application in oral delivery of peptides and peptidomimetics.

## Lipoproteins

Lipid particles such as LDL and HDL and an apoprotein moiety is termed as natural targeted liposomes and its core can be used to incorporate lipophilic drugs or lipophilic pro-drugs. It does not require covalent bonding with the drug. Modifications at the level of glycolipid incorporation can be used to introduce new targeting moieties. The majority of the research on the use of LDL and HDL particles has been done and improved at the level of targeting the drugs to the liver.

## Quantum Dots

A quantum dot is a semiconductor nanostructure that confines the motion of conduction band electrons, valence band holes or bound pairs of conduction band electrons and valence band holes in all three spatial directions. The ability to tune the size of quantum dots is advantageous for many applications and it is one of the most promising candidates as vehicle for drug transportation with its in solid-state quantum computation used for diagnosis, drug delivery, Tissue engineering, catalysis, filtration and textiles technologies too.

## Folate Targeting

Folate targeting is a method utilized in biotechnology for development of drug delivery. It involves the attachment of the vitamin, folate (folic acid) to drug to form folate conjugate. Based on the natural high affinity of folate for the folate receptor protein (FR) which is commonly expressed on the surface of cancer cells and folate-drug conjugates also bind tightly to the folate receptor protein (FR) which in turn, trigger cellular uptake via endocytosis. The folate receptor protein (FR) is also a recognized tumor-antigen/biomarker. Because of this inherent property of folate receptor protein (FR), exploits its use in diagnostic and therapeutic methods especially for the treatment of cancer.

## Advantages

The drug targeting provides various advantages in drug delivery system and promises to improves the drug efficiency. Common advantages of targeted drug delivery system over conventional system are mentioned below:
- Directly delivers the drug to particular site of action
- Improves the potency and efficacy of drug
- Reduces the side effect of drug
- Reduces the dosing frequency and improves the patient convenience
- Minimises the dose of drug

## Disadvantages

Along with this, it also has some disadvantages which are as follows:

- Rapid clearance of targeted system
- Sometimes it initiates the immunological responses
- Insufficient localization of targeted system in tumor cells
- Diffusion and redistribution of released drug
- High cost of the formulation

## Introduction to Liposomes

Liposomes are small artificial vesicles of spherical shape that can be prepared from cholesterol and natural nontoxic phospholipids. Due to their size and hydrophobic and hydrophilic character (besides biocompatibility), liposomes are promising systems for drug delivery. Liposome properties differ considerably with lipid composition, surface charge, size, and the method of preparation. Moreover, the selection of bilayer components determines the 'rigidity' or 'fluidity' and the charge of the bilayer. For example, unsaturated phosphatidyl choline species obtained from natural sources (egg or soybean phosphatidyl choline) give much more permeable and less stable bilayers, whereas the saturated phospholipids with long acyl chains (for example, dipalmitoylphos phatidyl choline) form a rigid, rather impermeable bilayer structure.

It has been displayed that phospholipids impulsively form closed structures when they are hydrated in aqueous solutions. Such vesicles which have one or more phospholipid bilayer membranes can transport aqueous or lipid drugs, depending on the nature of those drugs. Because lipids are amphipathic (both hydrophobic and hydrophilic) in aqueous media, their thermodynamic phase properties and self-assembling characteristics influence entropically focused confiscation of their hydrophobic sections into spherical bilayers. Those layers are referred to as lamellae. Generally, liposomes are definite as spherical vesicles with particle sizes ranging from 30 nm to several micrometers. They consist of one or more lipid bilayers surrounding aqueous units, where the polar head groups are oriented in the pathway of the interior and exterior aqueous phases (fig. 9.3). On the other hand, self-aggregation of polar lipids is not limited to conventional bilayer structures which rely on molecular shape, temperature, and environmental and preparation conditions but may self-assemble into various types of colloidal particles.

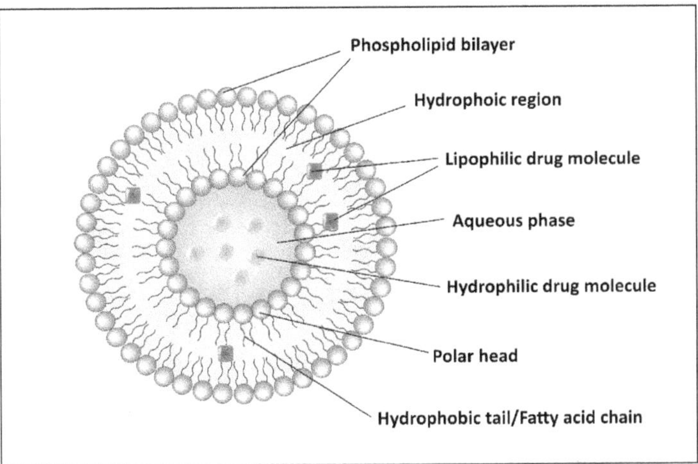


**Fig. 9.3:** Structure of liposome, illustrating the outer phospholipid bilayer enclosing the aqueous core inside. The lipophilic drug substances are intercalated in the phospholipid bilayer while the hydrophilic drugs are encapsulated in the aqueous core.

Liposomes are extensively used as carriers for numerous molecules in cosmetic and pharmaceutical industries. Additionally, food and farming industries have extensively studied the use of liposome encapsulation to grow delivery systems that can entrap unstable compounds (for example, antimicrobials, antioxidants, flavours and bioactive elements) and shield their functionality. Liposomes can trap both hydrophobic and hydrophilic compounds, avoid decomposition of the entrapped combinations, and release the entrapped at designated targets.

## Classification of Liposomes

The liposome size can vary from very small (0.025 µm) to large (2.5 µm) vesicles. Moreover, liposomes may have one or bilayer membranes. The vesicle size is an acute parameter in determining the circulation half-life of liposomes, and both size and number of bilayers affect the amount of drug encapsulation in the liposomes. On the basis of their size and number of bilayers, liposomes can be classified into one of two categories: (1) multilamellar vesicles (MLV) (2) unilamellar vesicles. Unilamellar vesicles can also be classified into two categories: (1) large unilamellar vesicles (LUV) and (2) small unilamellar vesicles (SUV). In unilamellar liposomes, the vesicle has a single phospholipid bilayer sphere enclosing the aqueous solution. In multilamellar liposomes, vesicles have an onion structure. Classically, several unilamellar vesicles will form on the inside of the other with smaller size, making a multilamellar structure of concentric phospholipid spheres separated by layers of water (fig. 9.4).

Liposomes can be classified in terms of composition and mechanism of intracellular delivery into five types

    (i)   Conventional liposomes

(ii)   pH-sensitive liposomes
(iii)  Cationic liposomes
(iv)   Immunoliposomes
(v)    Long-circulating liposomes

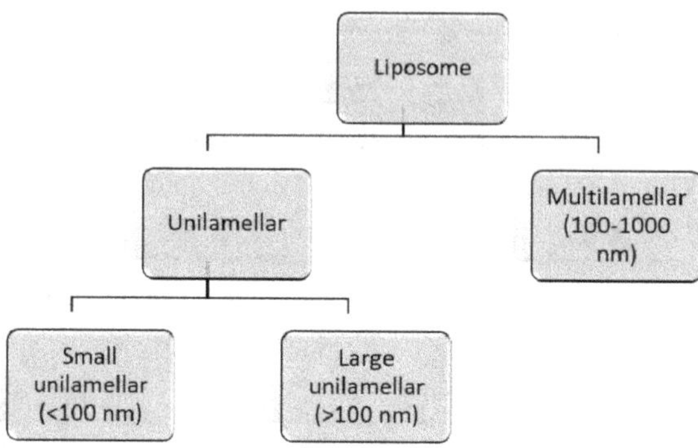


**Fig. 9.4:** Classification of Liposome on the basis of size and layers.

Liposomes have been used in a broad range of pharmaceutical applications. Liposomes are showing particular promise as intracellular delivery systems for anti-sense molecules, ribosomes, proteins/peptides, and DNA. Liposomes with enhanced drug delivery to disease locations, by ability of long circulation residence times, are now achieving clinical acceptance. Also, liposomes promote targeting of particular diseased cells within the disease site.

## Niosomes

Niosomes are a novel drug delivery system, in which the medication is encapsulated in a vesicle. The vesicle is composed of a bilayer of non-ionic surface-active agents and hence the name niosomes. The niosomes are very small, and microscopic in size. Their size lies in the nanometric scale. Although structurally similar to liposomes, they offer several advantages over them. Niosomes have recently been shown to greatly increase transdermal drug delivery and also can be used in targeted drug delivery, and thus increased study in these structures can provide new methods for drug delivery.

## Structure of Niosomes

Niosomes are microscopic lamellar structures, which are formed on the admixture of non-ionic surfactant of the alkyl or dialkyl polyglycerol ether class and cholesterol with subsequent hydration in aqueous media. Structurally, niosomes are similar to liposomes, in that they are also made up of a bilayer. However, the bilayer in the case of niosomes is made up of non-ionic surface-active agents rather than phospholipids as seen in the case of liposomes. Most surface-active agents when immersed in water yield micellar structures, however some surfactants can yield bilayer vesicles which are niosomes (fig. 9.5).

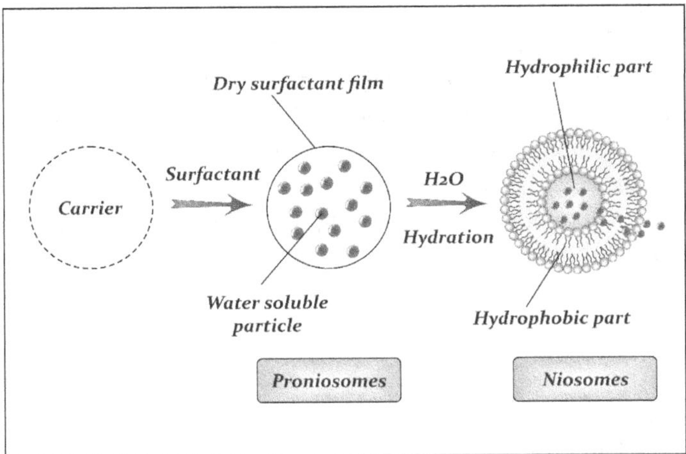


**Fig. 9.5:** Structure of niosome, prepared from the combination of a carrier system and surfactant.

Niosomes may be unilamellar or multilamellar depending on the method used to prepare them. The niosome is made of a surfactant bilayer with its hydrophilic ends are exposed on the outside and inside of the vesicle, while the hydrophobic chains face each other within the bilayer. Hence, the vesicle holds hydrophilic drugs within the space enclosed in the vesicle, while hydrophobic drugs are embedded within the bilayer itself. The figure below will give a better idea of what a niosomes looks like and where the drug is located within the vesicle.

## Advantages of Niosomes

Use of niosomes in cosmetics was first done by L'Oreal as they offered the following advantages:

1. The vesicle suspension being water based offers greater patient compliance over oil-based systems
2. Since the structure of the niosome offers place to accommodate hydrophilic, lipophilic as well as amphiphilic drug moieties, they can be used for a variety of drugs.
3. The characteristics such as size, lamellarity etc. of the vesicle can be varied depending on the requirement.
4. The vesicles can act as a depot to release the drug slowly and offer a controlled release.

Other advantages of niosomes are:
1. They are osmotically active and stable.

2. They increase the stability of the entrapped drug
3. Handling and storage of surfactants do not require any special conditions
4. Can increase the oral bioavailability of drugs
5. Can enhance the skin penetration of drugs
6. They can be used for oral, parenteral as well topical use
7. The surfactants are biodegradable, biocompatible, and non-immunogenic
8. Improve the therapeutic performance of the drug by protecting it from the biological environment and restricting effects to target cells, thereby reducing the clearance of the drug.
9. The niosomal dispersions in an aqueous phase can be emulsified in a non-aqueous phase to control the release rate of the drug and administer normal vesicles in external non-aqueous phase.

# Nanoparticles

Nanoparticles have been in use in pottery and medicine since ancient times. There are different ideal methods for nanoparticle to get synthesized. The following aspects involved for synthesizing nanoparticle are neutral pH, low cost and environmentally friendly condition. Nanoparticles get produced by plants are more stable and the rate of synthesis is faster than that in other case of organism. Mainly these methods for synthesizing nanoparticle have been developed in different methods in upcoming days because of the cost efficient and require little or no maintenance.

Nanoparticles get classified mainly into two groups they are organic nanoparticles and inorganic nanoparticles. Organic nanoparticles are carbon nanoparticle and inorganic nanoparticles are magnetic nanoparticle, semiconductor nanoparticle.

## Types of Nanoparticles

Depending upon the nature and composition of the material different types of nanoparticles are discussed below (fig. 9.6):

1. **Inorganic nanoparticles:** In the field of modern material science inorganic nanoparticles have been developed on the role based upon their unique physical properties and particularly in biotechnology. Based upon these two factors of inorganic nanoparticles they have certain physical properties that mainly include size dependent optical, magnetic, electronic, and catalytic properties. Bio related application are involved for the preparation of these interesting nanoparticles like iron oxides, gold, silver, silica, quantum dots etc. Novel physical properties mainly related because of their size approaches nanometer scale dimension.

2. **Polymeric nanoparticles:** Polymeric nanoparticle is also a type of nanoparticle. In recent years polymeric nanoparticle has a tremendous development in the field of research. The dispersion of preformed polymers and the polymerization of

monomers are two strong strategies mainly involved for preparation. 10-1000 it is the range of size involved with solid particles.

3.  **Solid lipid nanoparticles:** For controlling the drug delivery in 1990s Solid lipid nanoparticles played a dominant role. There are certain alternate carrier systems to emulsions, liposomes and polymeric nanoparticles as a colloidal Carrier system.

4.  **Liposomes:** Liposomes are one of the methods based upon the different types of nanoparticles. Structure of liposomes consists of one or more phospholipid bilayers and they are sphere-shaped vesicles to carry compound of interest. Today liposomes have been useful in the field of reagent and is a tool in various scientific disciplines. The numerous features of liposomes, evolved them to stand unique in the market. Liposomes acts as carries to many molecules used in cosmetic & pharmaceutical industry and in the field of Food and farming industries, liposomes are involved in encapsulation to enhance delivery system that can entrap unstable compounds.

5.  **Nanocrystal:** A nanocrystal is a type of based upon nanoparticle particle having at least one dimension smaller than 100 nanometres and is mainly composed of atoms in either a single or polycrystalline arrangement. Nanocrystals are aggregates of around hundreds and thousands of molecules that combine in a crystalline form, composed of pure drug with only a thin coating comprised of surfactant or combination of surfactants.

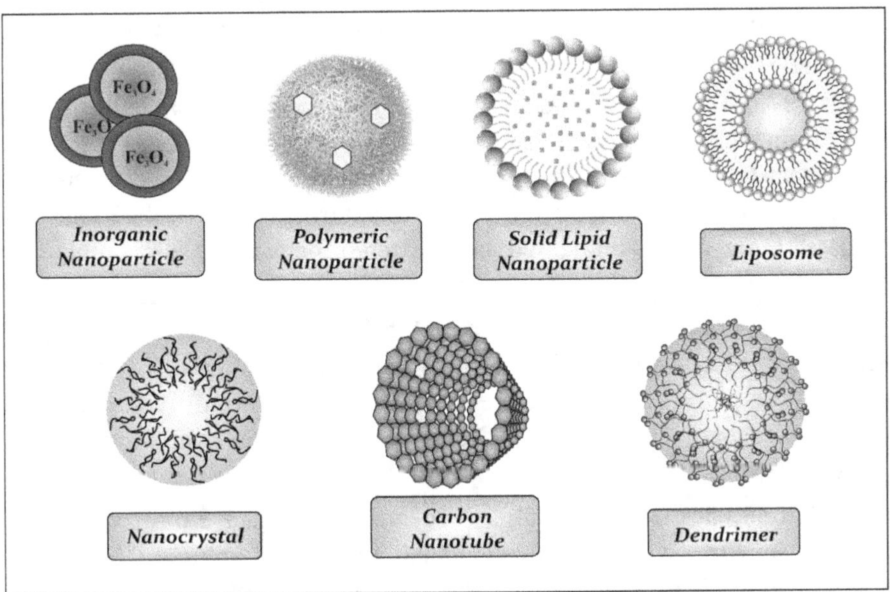


**Fig. 9.6:** Different types of nanoparticles.

6.  **Nanotube:** A nanotube is a nanometer scale tube like structure. Nanotubes are members of the fullerene structural family. Their name is derived from their long, hollow structure with the walls formed by one-atom-thick sheets of carbon called

graphene. These sheets are rolled at specific and discrete ("chiral") angles and the combination of the rolling angle and radius decides the nanotube properties; for example, whether the individual nanotube shell is a metal or semiconductor. Nanotubes are categorized as single-walled nanotubes (SWNTs) and multi-walled nanotubes.

7.  **Dendrimers:** Dendrimers arise from two Greek words: 'Dendron' meaning tree and 'Meros' meaning part.

    Structure of dendrimers has a well-defined size, shape and defined molecular weight and also Dendrimers are hyper-branched, globular, monodisperse, three dimensional nanoscales synthetic Polymers. Molecular chemistry and polymer chemistry both exhibit well-defined characteristics features of Dendrites.

## Monoclonal Antibodies

Monoclonal antibodies (mAb or moAb) are antibodies that are made by identical immune cells that are all clones of a unique parent cell. Monoclonal antibodies can have monovalent affinity, in that they bind to the same epitope (the part of an antigen that is recognized by the antibody). In contrast, polyclonal antibodies bind to multiple epitopes and are usually made by several different plasma cell (antibody secreting immune cell) lineages. Bispecific monoclonal antibodies can also be engineered, by increasing the therapeutic targets of one single monoclonal antibody to two epitopes (fig. 9.7).

In the year 1975, Kohler and Milsten provided the proof of clonal selection theory by the fusion of normal cells and the constantly dividing myeloma cells. This discovery was so spectacular that they were awarded with the prestigious Nobel Prize in the year 1984. There were few immunological reactions due to the murine nature of the older antibodies. In the year 1988 Greg Winter pioneered and mastered the technique of humanizing these antibodies.

The first FDA-approved therapeutic monoclonal antibody was a murine IgG2a CD3 specific transplant rejection drug, OKT3 (also called muromonab), in 1986. This drug found use in solid organ transplant recipients who became steroid resistant. Hundreds of therapies are undergoing clinical trials. Most are concerned with immunological and oncological targets.

Monoclonal antibodies were typically produced by fusing myeloma cells with splenic cells from a mouse which was immunized against a particular antigen. Mouse antibodies, being slightly different from human antibodies, produced an inflammatory reaction when injected into humans, resulting in infusion reactions and the production of neutralizing antibodies which would render the MAbs useless in a small percentage of patients. In order to overcome these difficulties various different kinds of approaches have been used, leading to the production off chimeric (partly mouse and partly human) and fully humanized antibodies.

## Types of Monoclonal Antibodies

Murine source MAbs: rodent MAbs with excellent affinities and specificities generated using conventional hybridoma technology.

1. Murine source MAbs: rodent MAbs with excellent affinities and specificities generated using conventional hybridoma technology.
2. Chimeric MAbs: chimers combine the human constant regions with the intact rodent variable regions. Affinity and specificity unchanged (fig. 9.7).
3. Humanized MAbs: contained only the CDRs of the rodent variable region grafted onto human variable region framework (fig. 9.7).
4. Recombinant DNA engineered MAbs.

Monoclonal antibodies (MAbs) are an integral part of targeted therapy approach for various diseases which result in decrease in adverse effects and increase in efficacy. MAbs are antibodies that are identical because they are produced by one type of immune cell; all are clones of a single parent cell. Treatment with monoclonal antibodies does not usually result in a "cure". Unlike antibiotics, which have the ability to eliminate pathogens, and thus result in a cure, MAbs are designed to target and modulate specific immune pathways. Discontinuation of treatment with an MAbs may result in re-occurrence of disease activity.

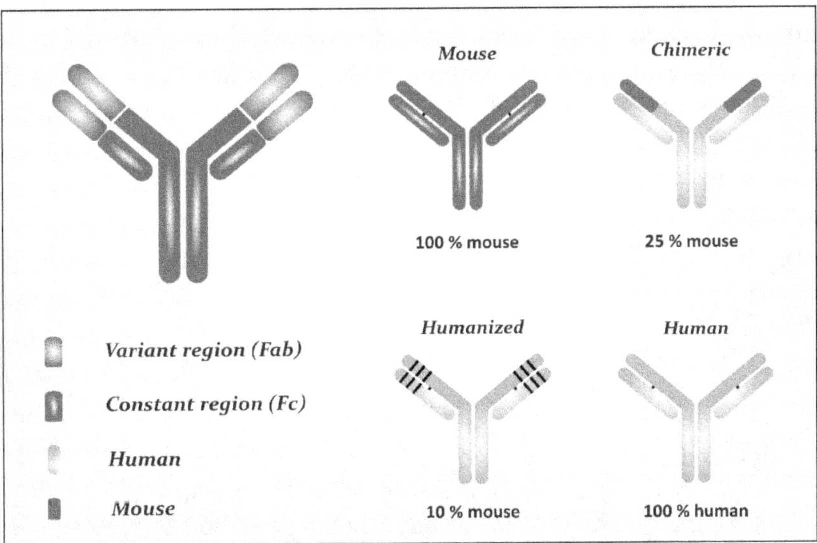


**Fig. 9.7:** Structure of monoclonal antibody; showing mouse, chimeric, humanized and human monoclonal antibodies.

## Structure and Function of Monoclonal Antibody

Immunoglobulins or antibodies are a group of glycoproteins that constitute one of the most important specific defence mechanisms in vertebrate animals. All of them have a very similar structure in a Y form (fig. 9.7) of bifunctional molecules with two identical domains for antigen recognition (Fab fragment), and two identical domains with effector functions (Fc fragment). The antigen-binding region is highly specific, and varies among the antibodies. Thousands of millions of different antibodies can be generated, each one with a distinct specificity.

Antibodies have two identical light chains of 24-25 kD and two heavy chains, also identical, of 55–70kD ($\gamma$, $\varepsilon$, $\delta$, $\alpha$, or $\mu$) bound by disulphur bridges. The type of immunoglobulin produced depends on the type of heavy chain and, therefore, in vertebrate animals five classes or isotypes of immunoglobulins (IgG, IgE, IgD, IgA, and IgM) can be distinguished, each one with a distinct functionality. In addition to the disulphur bridges between the chains, there are intracatenary disulphur bridges which provide stability to the molecule. The light chain (L) is formed by two domains of around 100 residues, known as the variable domain ($V_L$), at its aminoterminal end, and the constant domain (CL). The heavy chain (H) contains a variable domain ($V_H$) and three or four constant domains ($C_H1$, $C_H2$, $C_H3$, $C_H4$), depending on the isotype. The variable regions are the zones of the molecule involved in antigen binding, where the most divergent hypervariable regions, or complementary determining regions (CDR), are three in the VL domain and three in the VH domain. These regions are separated by structural regions called framework (FRW), which have highly conserved sequences.

Immunoglobulins (Igs) are found as membrane receptors in B lymphocytes, which are a subpopulation of leukocytes. After activation mediated by antigen (virus, bacteria, parasite), and in collaboration with other immune cells (such as T lymphocytes), the B lymphocytes become plasma cells secreting antibodies. The antibodies can then be released from the cell and have different effector functions.

Among their most important functions are the following:
1. Neutralization and blocking of pathogens and toxins;
2. Activation of complement: The IgM and IgG activate a proteolytic cascade, which leads eventually to the opening of pores in the membrane of the pathogens or target cells;
3. Phagocytosis: The IgG are the main type of antibodies capable of facilitating phagocytosis of pathogens, by binding to receptors of macrophages and dendritic cells;
4. Antibody-dependent cellular cytotoxicity (ADCC), natural Killer (NK) cells, and macrophages lyse cells in the presence of antibodies directed at target cells, to achieve this, the Fc portion of the antibody binds to the target cells, which secrete granular proteins that mediate in cytolytic functions;
5. Responses to parasites and allergic responses: The IgE is involved in allergic responses through the activation of mastocytes, which release their charged granules (of histamine, prostaglandins, etc.). It also participates in the elimination of parasites, with the help of eosinophils;
6. Mucosal protection: The IgA undertakes mucosal protection (respiratory, digestive) and is present in secretions, such as breast milk.

# Applications

1. **Nanoparticles are used in drug delivery:** The nanoparticles entrap the drugs either enhance delivery to, or uptake by, target cells and/or a reduction in the toxicity of the free drug to non-target organs.

2. **Applications of nanoparticles in food:** Nanofood is a term used to describe foods that use nanotechnology techniques, tools or manufactured nanomaterials that have been added during cultivation, production, processing or packaging. There are several purposes for the development of nanofood. These include improvement of food safety, enhancement of nutrition and flavour, and cutting production and consumer costs. In addition, nanofood provides various benefits by which include health promoting additives, longer shelf lives and new flavour varieties. The application of nanotechnology in food is rapidly emerging and is involving all areas of the food chain from agricultural applications to food processing and enhancing bioavailability of nutrients.

3. **Application of nanoparticle in gene delivery:** Gene delivery is a technique which plays a vital role, where it can efficiently introduce a gene of interest in order to express its encoded protein in a suitable host or host cell. Now a days, there are different types of primary gene delivery systems that mainly employ viral vectors like retroviruses and adenoviruses, nucleic acid electroporation, and nucleic acid transfection.

4. **Application of nanoparticle in cancer treatment:** There are a variety of nanoparticle systems currently investigated and explored for biomedical applications with some particular emphasis for cancer therapeutics; hence some precious metals (mainly gold and silver systems, Au, and Ag) and some magnetic oxides (in particular magnetite $Fe_3O_4$) received much interest including quantum dots and some of what is called natural nanoparticles. The unique conversion process of UCNPs may be utilized to activate photosensitive therapeutic agents for applications in cancer treatment.

5. **Other applications of nanoparticles:** In recent years nanoparticles are involved with new applications in areas like information & communication technology, power engineering, industrial engineering, environmental engineering, chemical industry, medicine, in pharmaceuticals and cosmetics etc. For decades some nanoscale materials have been involved (for e.g. they are used in window glass, sunglasses, car bumpers, paints), whereas others are newly discovered are used as sunscreens and cosmetics, textiles, coatings, sports goods, explosives, propellants and pyrotechnics or their applications are currently under development (e.g. in batteries, solar cells, fuel cells, light sources, electronic storage media, display technologies, bioanalysis and bio detectors, drug delivery systems, medical implants and new organs). All in all, the number of nano products and methods of their use increase continually.

# Bibliography


1.  Abrahamse, H., et al., Nanoparticles for Advanced Photodynamic Therapy of Cancer. Photomed Laser Surg, 2017. 35(11): p. 581-588.

2.  Alexander, A., et al., Recent expansion of pharmaceutical nanotechnologies and targeting strategies in the field of phytopharmaceuticals for the delivery of herbal extracts and bioactives. J Control Release, 2016. 241: p. 110-124.

3.  Agrawal, M., et al., Recent advancements in the field of nanotechnology for the delivery of anti-Alzheimer drug in the brain region. Expert Opin Drug Deliv, 2018. 15(6): p. 589-617.

4.  Akbarzadeh, A., et al., Liposome: classification, preparation, and applications. Nanoscale Res Lett, 2013. 8(1): p. 102.

5.  Arora, P., et al., Nano-regenerative medicine towards clinical outcome of stem cell and tissue engineering in humans. J Cell Mol Med, 2012. 16(9): p. 1991-2000.

6.  Arora, R., et al., Solid lipid nanoparticles and nanostructured lipid carrier-based nanotherapeutics in treatment of psoriasis: a comparative study. Expert Opin Drug Deliv, 2017. 14(2): p. 165-177.

7.  Bamrungsap, S., et al., Nanotechnology in therapeutics: a focus on nanoparticles as a drug delivery system. Nanomedicine (Lond), 2012. 7(8): p. 1253-71.

8.  Banerjee, T., et al., Preparation, characterization and biodistribution of ultrafine chitosan nanoparticles. Int J Pharm, 2002. 243(1-2): p. 93-105.

9.  Beber, T.C., et al., Cationic Polymeric Nanocapsules as a Strategy to Target Dexamethasone to Viable Epidermis: Skin Penetration and Permeation Studies. J Nanosci Nanotechnol, 2016. 16(2): p. 1331-8.

10. Beloqui, A., et al., Nanostructured lipid carriers: Promising drug delivery systems for future clinics. Nanomedicine, 2016. 12(1): p. 143-61.

11. Bernal, G.M., et al., Convection-enhanced delivery and in vivo imaging of polymeric nanoparticles for the treatment of malignant glioma. Nanomedicine, 2014. 10(1): p. 149-57.

12. Bonifacio, B.V., et al., Nanotechnology-based drug delivery systems and herbal medicines: a review. Int J Nanomedicine, 2014. 9: p. 1-15.

13. Ferreira, L., et al., New opportunities: the use of nanotechnologies to manipulate and track stem cells. Cell Stem Cell, 2008. 3(2): p. 136-46.

14. Goyal, R., et al., Nanoparticles and nanofibers for topical drug delivery. J Control Release, 2016. 240: p. 77-92.

15. Hao, J., et al., Fabrication of an ionic-sensitive in situ gel loaded with resveratrol nanosuspensions intended for direct nose-to-brain delivery. Colloids Surf B Biointerfaces, 2016. 147: p. 376-386.

16. Hussain, A., et al., Nanoemulsion gel-based topical delivery of an antifungal drug: in vitro activity and in vivo evaluation. Drug Deliv, 2016. 23(2): p. 642-47.

17.  Canovi, M., et al., The binding affinity of anti-Abeta1-42 MAb-decorated nanoliposomes to Abeta1-42 peptides in vitro and to amyloid deposits in post-mortem tissue. Biomaterials, 2011. 32(23): p. 5489-97.

18.  Geskin, L.J., Monoclonal Antibodies. Dermatol Clin, 2015. 33(4): p. 777-86.

19.  Hanack, K., K. Messerschmidt, and M. Listek, Antibodies and Selection of Monoclonal Antibodies. Adv Exp Med Biol, 2016. 917: p. 11-22.

20.  da Silva Santos, S., E. Igne Ferreira, and J. Giarolla, Dendrimer Prodrugs. Molecules, 2016. 21(6).

21.  Shcharbin, D., et al., Dendrimer-protein interactions versus dendrimer-based nanomedicine. Colloids Surf B Biointerfaces, 2017. 152: p. 414-422.

22.  Hsu, H.J., et al., Dendrimer-based nanocarriers: a versatile platform for drug delivery. Wiley Interdiscip Rev Nanomed Nanobiotechnol, 2017. 9(1).

## Exercise

## A. Multiple Choice Questions

1.  The size range of nano particles is
    (a)  Below 100 nm                     (b)   $1 - 100$ μm
    (c)  $1 - 100$ mm                     (d)   $10 - 100$ μm

2.  The targeted drug delivery system is developed for
    (a)  Producing a higher extent of therapeutic action of a drug
    (b)  Producing a relatively uniform effect of the drug
    (c)  Producing localized effect of the drug
    (d)  Reducing the frequency of dosing.

3.  Which of the following statements is correct?
    (a)  Targeted drug delivery system may be biochemically inert
    (b)  Targeted drug delivery system should be biochemically inert
    (c)  Targeted drug delivery system may be immunogenic
    (d)  Targeted drug delivery system may be therapeutically inert

4.  Which of the following statements is correct?
    (a)  Targeted drug delivery system should have less therapeutic amount of drug release
    (b)  Targeted drug delivery system should have slightly less therapeutic amount of drug release
    (c)  Targeted drug delivery system should have therapeutic amount of drug release
    (d)  Targeted drug delivery system should have more therapeutic amount of drug release

5. Which of the following statements is correct?
   (a) The carriers used in targeted drug delivery system should be eliminated from the body without any problem.
   (b) The carriers used in targeted drug delivery system should be bio-degradable
   (c) The carriers used in targeted drug delivery system should be readily eliminated from the body without any problem.
   (d) The carriers used in targeted drug delivery system should be bio-degradable or readily eliminated from the body without any problem.

6. Which of the following statements is correct?
   (a) The preparation of the targeted drug delivery system should be reasonably simple, reproducible and cost effective.
   (b) The preparation of the targeted drug delivery system should be easy
   (c) The preparation of the targeted drug delivery system should be reasonably simple, reproducible and cost effective.
   (d) The preparation of the targeted drug delivery system should be cost effective.

7. Which of the following statements is correct?
   (a) First order targeting denotes to selective delivery of drugs to specific cell types such as tumour cells and not to the normal cells e.g. selective drug delivery to kupffer cells in the liver.
   (b) Third order targeting denotes to selective delivery of drugs to specific cell types such as tumour cells and not to the normal cells e.g. selective drug delivery to kupffer cells in the liver.
   (c) Second order targeting denotes to selective delivery of drugs to specific cell types such as tumour cells and not to the normal cells e.g. selective drug delivery to kupffer cells in the liver.
   (d) Second order targeting denotes to non-selective delivery of drugs to specific cell types such as tumour cells and not to the normal cells e.g. selective drug delivery to kupffer cells in the liver.

8. Which of the following statements is correct?
   (a) Third order targeting refers to drug delivery to the receptors for entry of a drug complex into a cell by endocytosis.
   (b) Third order targeting refers to drug delivery specifically to the intracellular site of targeted cells such as receptor-based ligand mediated entry of a drug complex into a cell by endocytosis.
   (c) First order targeting refers to drug delivery specifically to the intracellular site of targeted cells such as receptor-based ligand mediated entry of a drug complex into a cell by endocytosis.
   (d) Second order targeting refers to drug delivery specifically to the intracellular site of targeted cells such as receptor-based ligand mediated entry of a drug complex into a cell by endocytosis.

9. Which of the following statements is correct?
   (a) Drug release from a targeted drug delivery system takes place within the body.
   (b) Drug release from a targeted drug delivery system are not limited to selective sites within the body.
   (c) Drug release from a targeted drug delivery system takes place within the body such as a tumour.
   (d) Drug release from a targeted drug delivery system are limited to selective sites within the body such as a tumour but not the liver.

10. Which of the following statements is correct?
    (a) In dual targeting method the carrier molecule itself have therapeutic activity and thus, increase the therapeutic effect of drug.
    (b) In dual targeting method a molecule other than the drug have therapeutic activity and the carrier molecule does not have any therapeutic effect.
    (c) In dual targeting method two drug molecules are used having therapeutic activity and thus, increase the therapeutic effect of drug.
    (d) In dual targeting method two carrier molecules are present and thus increase the therapeutic effect of drug.

11. Which of the following statements is correct?
    (a) Microspheres and nanoparticles consist of compatible, soluble polymers.
    (b) Microspheres and nanoparticles consist of compatible polymers which function as carriers.
    (c) Microspheres and nanoparticles consist of biocompatible polymers and belong either to the soluble or the particle type carriers.
    (d) Microspheres and nanoparticles consist of biocompatible, insoluble polymers which work as carriers.

12. Lipoproteins are
    (a) Lipid particles or a protein moiety naturally available for targeting liposomes and its core can be used to incorporate lipophilic drugs or lipophilic pro-drugs.
    (b) Lipid particles such as LDL and HDL and an apoprotein moiety is termed as natural targeted liposomes and its core can be used to incorporate lipophilic drugs or lipophilic pro-drugs.
    (c) A protein molecule which is used to incorporate lipophilic drugs.
    (d) Lipid particles such as LDL and HDL and an apoprotein moiety is termed as natural targeted liposomes and its core can be used to incorporate hydrophilic or lipophilic drugs.

13. Which of the following statements is correct?

    (a) Folate targeting involves the attachment of the vitamin, folate (folic acid) to drug to form folate conjugate.

    (b) Folate targeting involves the use of a drug containing folic acid.

    (c) Folate targeting involves the attachment of the folic acid-enzyme to drug to form folate conjugate.

    (d) Folate targeting involves the use of a vitamin to drug to form folate conjugate.

14. Which of the following statements is correct?

    (a) The structure of niosomes are not similar to liposomes, they are also made up of a bilayer.

    (b) The structure of niosomes are similar to liposomes, they are of monolayer.

    (c) The structure of niosomes are similar to liposomes, they are composed of drug molecule.

    (d) The structure of niosomes are similar to liposomes, in that they are also made up of a bilayer.

15. Which of the following statements is correct?

    (a) The niosomes are made of a surfactant with its hydrophobic ends exposed on the outside and inside of the vesicle, while the hydrophilic chains face each other within the bilayer.

    (b) The niosomes are made of a surfactant bilayer with its hydrophobic ends exposed on the outside and inside of the vesicle, while the hydrophilic chains face each other within the bilayer.

    (c) The niosomes are made of a surfactant bilayer with its hydrophilic ends exposed on the outside and inside of the vesicle, while the hydrophobic chains face each other within the bilayer.

    (d) The niosomes are made of a surfactant unilayer with its hydrophilic ends exposed on the outside and inside of the vesicle, while the hydrophobic chains face each other within the bilayer.

16. Which of the following statements is correct?

    (a) The structure of the niosome can accommodate hydrophilic, lipophilic as well as amphiphilic drug moieties.

    (b) The structure of the niosome can accommodate hydrophilic drugs.

    (c) The structure of the niosome can accommodate only lipophilic drugs.

    (d) The structure of the niosome can accommodate only amphiphilic drugs.

17. Which of the following statements is correct?
    (a) The aspect involved for synthesizing nanoparticle is only neutral pH.
    (b) The aspects involved for synthesizing nanoparticle are neutral pH, low cost and environmentally friendly condition.
    (c) The aspect involved for synthesizing nanoparticle is only environmentally friendly condition.
    (d) The aspect involved for synthesizing nanoparticle is the low cost.

18. Which of the following statements is correct?
    (a) Monoclonal antibodies are antibodies that are made by immune cells some of which are not clones of a unique parent cell.
    (b) Monoclonal antibodies are antibodies made by immune cells some of those are clones of a unique parent cell.
    (c) Monoclonal antibodies are antibodies made by identical immune cells that are all clones of a unique parent cell.
    (d) Monoclonal antibodies are antibodies made by immune cells.

19. Which of the following statements is correct?
    (a) The IgM and IgG lead to the opening of pores in the membrane of the pathogens or target cells
    (b) The IgM and IgG activate a proteolytic enzyme, which leads to the opening of pores in the membrane.
    (c) The IgM and IgG activate a proteolytic enzyme, which leads to the closing of pores in the membrane of the pathogens or target cells
    (d) The IgM and IgG activate a proteolytic cascade, which leads eventually to the opening of pores in the membrane of the pathogens or target cells

20. Which of the following statements is correct?
    (a) The IgE is involved in allergic responses through the activation of mastocytes, which release their charged granules of histamine, prostaglandins, etc.
    (b) The IgE is involved in non-allergic responses through the activation of mastocytes.
    (c) The IgE does not involve in allergic responses through the activation of mastocytes, which release their charged granules.
    (d) The IgE releases the charged granules of histamine, prostaglandins, etc.

## B. Short Questions

1. Write down the concept of nanotechnology.
2. What are the approaches of drug formulation utilizing nanotechnology?

3.  What should be ideal properties of targeted drug delivery system?
4.  Write down the advantages and disadvantages of targeted drug delivery system.
5.  What do you know about liposome?
6.  What do you know about the structure of niosomes.
7.  Write a note about monoclonal antibodies.

## C. Long Questions

1.  Explain the carrier systems used for drug targeting.
2.  Explain the concept of targeted drug delivery system.
3.  Discuss briefly the methods applied for developing targeted drug delivery system.
4.  Explain the various carrier systems used for developing targeted drug delivery system
5.  Write a note about different types of nanoparticles.
6.  Discuss the structure and function of monoclonal antibody.
7.  Write a note on applications of nanoparticles.

## CHAPTER 10

# Ocular Drug Delivery Systems

*Introduction, intra ocular barriers and methods to overcome –Preliminary study, ocular formulations and Occuserts.*

## Introduction

Ophthalmic drug delivery is one of the most interesting and challenging endeavours facing the pharmaceutical scientist. The anatomy, physiology, and biochemistry of the eye render this organ highly impervious to foreign substances. Drug delivery to the eye can be broadly classified into anterior and posterior segments (fig. 10.1).

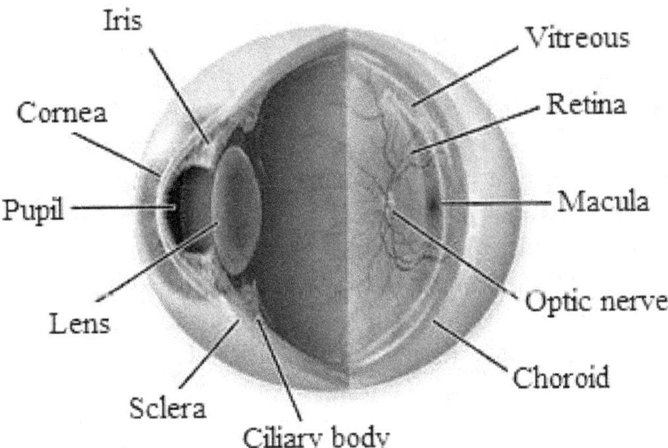


**Fig. 10.1:** Structure of human eye.

Conventional systems like eye drops, suspensions, and ointments cannot be considered optimal in the treatment of vision-threatening ocular diseases. However, more than 90%

of the marketed ophthalmic formulations are in the form of eye drops. These formulations mainly target the diseases in the anterior segment of eye. Topical ocular medications do not reach the posterior segment of the eye. Posterior segment (retina, vitreous, choroid) can be treated by high drug dosage regimen given intravenously or by intravitreal administration or implants or by periocular injections. Currently, the posterior segment drug delivery is a rapidly growing interest area in ophthalmic drug delivery.

The goal of pharmacotherapeutics is to treat a disease in a consistent and predictable fashion. A significant challenge to the formulator is to circumvent the protective barriers of the eye without causing permanent tissue damage. Development of newer, more sensitive diagnostic techniques and novel therapeutic agents continue to provide ocular delivery systems with high therapeutic efficacy. An assumption is made that a correlation exists between the concentration of a drug at its intended site of action and the resulting pharmacological effect. The specific aim of designing a therapeutic system is to achieve an optimal concentration of a drug at the active site for the appropriate duration. Ocular disposition and elimination of a therapeutic agent is dependent upon its physicochemical properties as well as the relevant ocular anatomy and physiology. A successful design of a drug delivery system, therefore, requires an integrated knowledge of the drug molecule and the constraints offered by the ocular route of administration.

The active sites for the antibiotics, antiviral, and steroids are the infected or inflamed areas within the anterior as well as the posterior segments of the eye. A host of different tissues are involved, each of which may pose its own challenge to the formulator of ophthalmic delivery systems. Hence, the drug entities need to be targeted to many sites within the globe.

The eye consists of transparent cornea, lens, and vitreous body without blood vessels. The oxygen and nutrients are transported to this non-vascular tissue by aqueous humour which is having high oxygen and same osmotic pressure as blood. The aqueous humour in human is having volume of 300 $\mu l$ that fills the anterior chamber of the eye which is in front of lens. The cornea is covered by a thin epithelial layer continuous with the conjunctiva at the cornea-sclerotic junction. The main bulk of cornea is formed of criss-crossing layers of collagen and is bounded by elastic lamina on both front and back. Its posterior surface is covered by a layer of endothelium. The cornea is richly supplied with free nerve endings. The transparent cornea is continued posteriorly into the opaque white sclera which consists of tough fibrous tissue. Both cornea and sclera withstand the intra ocular tension constantly maintained in the eye. The eye is constantly cleansed and lubricated by the lacrimal apparatus which consists of four structures. lacrimal glands, lacrimal canals, lacrimal sac, nasolacrimal duct. The lacrimal fluid secreted by lacrimal glands is emptied on the surface of the conjunctiva of the upper eye lid at a turnover rate of 16% per min. It washes over the eye ball and is swept up by the blinking action of eye lids. Muscles associated with the blinking reflux compress the lacrimal sac, when these muscles relax; the sac expands, pulling the lacrimal fluid from the edges of the eye lids along the lacrimal canals, into the lacrimal sacs. The lacrimal fluid volume in humans is 7 $\mu L$ and is an isotonic aqueous solution of bicarbonate and sodium chloride of pH 7.4. It serves to dilute irritants or to wash the foreign bodies out of the conjunctival sac. It contains lysozyme, whose bactericidal activity reduces the bacterial count in the conjunctival sac.

The physiological barriers to diffusion and productive absorption of topically applied drug exist in the precorneal and corneal spaces. The precorneal constraints that are responsible for poor bioavailability of conventional ophthalmic dosage forms are solution drainage, lacrimation, tear dilution, tear turn over and conjunctival absorption.

## Advantages of Ocular Drug Delivery Systems

1. Increased accurate dosing.
2. To overcome the side effects of pulsed dosing produced by conventional systems.
3. To provide sustained and controlled drug delivery.
4. To increase the ocular bioavailability of drug by increasing the corneal contact time. This can be achieved by effective adherence to corneal surface.
5. To provide targeting within the ocular globe so as to prevent the loss to other ocular tissues.
6. To avoid the protective barriers like drainage, lacrimation and conjunctival absorption.
7. To provide comfort, better compliance to the patient and to improve therapeutic performance of drug.
8. To provide better housing of delivery system.

## Disadvantages

Various disadvantages of ocular drug delivery system are given below:

1. The physiological restriction is the limited permeability of cornea resulting into low absorption of ophthalmic drugs.
2. A major portion of the administered dose drains into the lacrimal duct and thus can cause unwanted systemic side effects.
3. The rapid elimination of the drug through the eye blinking and tear flow results in a short duration of the therapeutic effect resulting in a frequent dosing regimen.

## Physiological Considerations

The extent of absorption of an ophthalmic drug is extremely limited by physiological constraints. Among the factors that limit ocular absorption is the relatively impermeable corneal barrier. The cornea consists of three membranes: the epithelium, the endothelium, and inner stroma which are the main absorptive barriers. The epithelium facing the tears with lipophilic cellular layers acts as a barrier to ion transport. The tight junctions of the corneal epithelium serve as a selective barrier for small molecules and prevent the diffusion of macromolecules through the paracellular route. The stroma beneath the epithelium is a highly hydrophilic layer making up 90% of the cornea. The corneal endothelium is responsible for maintaining normal corneal hydration. Clearly then, the more lipophilic the drugs are, the more resistance they will find crossing the stroma.

The more hydrophilic is the drug, the more resistant the epithelium; though the stroma and endothelium are limited in their resistance. Physicochemical drug properties, such as lipophilicity, solubility, molecular size and shape, charge and degree of ionization affect the route and rate of permeation through the corneal membrane in the cul-de-sac.

## Pharmacokinetic Considerations

Various pharmacokinetic consideration of ocular formulations are as follows:

- Transcorneal permeation from the lachrymal fluid into the anterior chamber,
- Noncorneal drug permeation across the conjunctiva and sclera into the anterior uvea,
- Drug distribution from the blood stream through blood-aqueous barrier into the anterior chamber,
- Elimination of drug from the anterior chamber by the aqueous humour turnover to the trabecular meshwork and Sclemm's canal,
- Drug elimination from the aqueous humour into the systemic circulation across the blood-aqueous barrier,
- Drug distribution from the blood into the posterior eye across Intravitreal drug administration,
- Drug elimination from the vitreous via posterior route across the blood-retina barrier, and
- Drug elimination from the vitreous via anterior route to the posterior chamber.

## Intra Ocular Barriers and Methods to Overcome

Ocular drug delivery systems are developed to treat eye locally, whereas past formulations are targeted to reach systemic circulation and these are designed to overcome all the disadvantages of conventional dosage forms such as ophthalmic solutions. The main problem with conventional dosage forms is eye irritation (due to drug particle size and shape) which induces lacrimation i.e. overflow on to lids, tear turn over, and due to pharmacokinetic responses like metabolism, non-specific binding and different mechanisms like diffusion, dissolution and erosion the conventional dosage forms are less advantageous.

The eye drop dosage form is easy to instil but suffers from the inherent draw back that the majority of the medication it contains is immediately diluted in the tear film as soon as the eye drop solution is instilled into the cul-de-sac and is rapidly drained away from the precorneal cavity by constant tear flow, a process that proceeds more intensively in inflamed than in the normal eyes, and lacrimal-nasal drainage. Therefore, only a very small fraction of the instilled dose is absorbed into the target tissues i.e. about 1.2% is available to the aqueous humor and relatively concentrated solution is required for instillation to achieve an adequate level of therapeutic effect. The frequent periodic instillation of eye drops becomes necessary to maintain a continuous sustained level of medication. If there is high drug concentration in eye drop solution it may give, the eye massive and unpredictable dose of medication as well as it creates greater loss of lacrimal-nasal drainage system. Subsequently this may lead to systemic side effects. The major barriers which limits the intraocular drug absorption are as follows:

1. **Tear:** One of the precorneal barriers is tear film which reduces the effective concentration of the administrated drugs due to dilution by the tear turnover (approximately 1 µL/min), accelerated clearance, and binding of the drug molecule to the tear proteins. In addition, the dosing volume of instillation is usually 20–50 µL whereas the size of cul-de-sac is only 7–10 µL. The excess volume may spill out on the cheek or exit through the nasolacrimal duct. For details of structure and function of tear film.

2. **Cornea:** The cornea consists of three layers; epithelium, stroma and endothelium, and a mechanical barrier to inhibit transport of exogenous substances into the eye (fig. 10.2). Each layer possesses a different polarity and a rate-limiting structure for drug permeation. The corneal epithelium is of a lipophilic nature, and tight junctions among cells are formed to restrict paracellular drug permeation from the tear film. The stroma is composed of an extracellular matrix of a lamellar arrangement of collagen fibrils. The highly hydrated structure of the stroma acts as a barrier to permeation of lipophilic drug molecules. Corneal endothelium is the innermost monolayer of hexagonal-shaped cells, and acts as a separating barrier between the stroma and aqueous humor. The endothelial junctions are leaky and facilitate the passage of macromolecules between the aqueous humor and stroma.

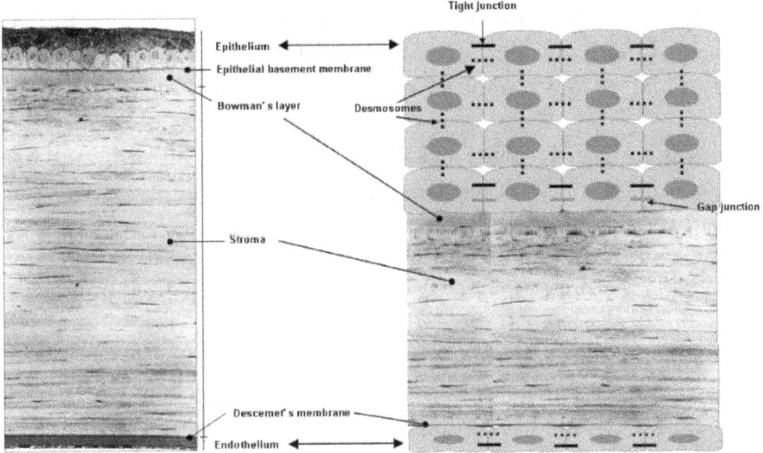


**Fig. 10.2:** Cellular structure of cornea as transport limiting barrier.

3. **Conjunctiva:** Conjunctiva of the eyelids and globe is a thin and transparent membrane, which is involved in the formation and maintenance of the tear film. In addition, conjunctiva or episclera has a rich supply of capillaries and lymphatics (fig. 10.3); therefore, administrated drugs in the conjunctival or episcleral space may be cleared through blood and lymph. The conjunctival blood vessels do not form a tight junction barrier, which means drug molecules can enter into the blood circulation by pinocytosis and/or convective transport through paracellular pores in the vascular endothelial layer. The conjunctival lymphatics act as an efflux system for the efficient elimination from the conjunctival space.

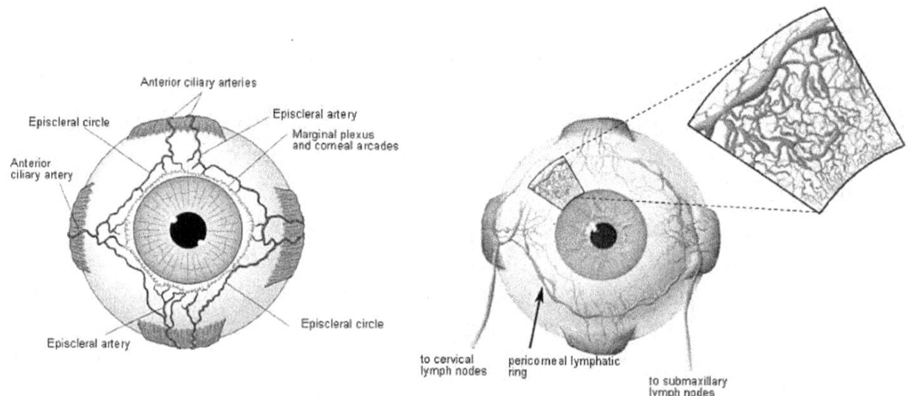


**Fig. 10.3:** Subconjunctival blood vessel and lymphatic network in the eye.

Recently, it has been reported that at least 10% of a small molecular weight hydrophilic model compound (sodium fluorescein), administered in the subconjunctival space, is eliminated via the lymphatics within the first hour in rat eyes. Therefore, drugs transported by lymphatics in conjunction with the elimination by blood circulation can contribute to systemic exposure, since the interstitial fluid is returned to the systemic circulation after filtration through lymph nodes.

4. **Sclera:** The sclera mainly consists of collagen fibres and proteoglycans embedded in an extracellular matrix. Scleral permeability has been shown to have a strong dependence on the molecular radius; scleral permeability decreases roughly exponentially with molecular radius. Additionally, the posterior sclera is composed of a looser weave of collagen fibres than the anterior sclera, and the human sclera is relatively thick near the limbus (0.53 ± 0.14 mm), thin at the equator (0.39 ± 0.17 mm), and much thicker near the optic nerve (0.9–1.0 mm). Thus, the ideal location for transscleral drug delivery is near the equator at 12–17 mm posterior to the corneoscleral limbus. Hydrophobicity of drugs affects scleral permeability; increase of lipophilicity shows lower permeability; and hydrophilic drugs may diffuse through the aqueous medium of proteoglycans in the fibre matrix pores more easily than lipophilic drugs. Furthermore, the charge of the drug molecule

also affects its permeability across the sclera. Positively charged compounds may exhibit poor permeability due to their binding to the negatively charged proteoglycan matrix.

5. **Choroid/Bruch's Membrane:** Choroid is one of the most highly vascularized tissues of the body to supply the blood to the retina. Its blood flow per unit tissue weight is ten-fold higher than in the brain. In addition, the choroidal capillary endothelial cells are fenestrated and, in humans, are relatively large in diameter (20–40 μm) (fig. 10.4). An Optical Coherence Tomography (OCT) can noninvasively measure the thickness of retina and choroid. Using an OCT, it has been shown, choroidal thickness becomes thinner with age. Histological studies have shown choroidal thickness changes from 200 μm at birth decreasing to about 80 μm by age 90. In addition, chorioretinal diseases including AMD with pigment epithelial detachment, central serous chorioretinopathy, age-related choroidal atrophy, and high myopia, affect choroidal thickness.

   In contrast, Bruch's membrane (BM) causes thickening with age. These changes cause increased calcification of elastic fibres, increased cross-linkage of collagen fibres and increased turnover of glycosaminoglycans. In addition, advanced glycation end products and lipofuscin accumulate in BM. Thickness changes of choroid and BM might affect drug permeability from subconjunctiva or episcleral space into the retina and the vitreous.

6. **Retina:** The drugs in the vitreous are eliminated by two main routes from anterior and posterior segments. All drugs are able to eliminate via the anterior route. This means drugs can diffuse across the vitreous to the posterior chamber and, thereafter, eliminate via aqueous turnover and uveal blood flow. Elimination via the posterior route takes place by permeation across the retina. One of the barriers restricting drug penetration from the vitreous to the retina is the internal limiting membrane (ILM) (fig. 10.4). The ILM separates the retina and the vitreous and is composed of 10 distinct extracellular matrix proteins. Although a previous study using primates has suggested that molecules exceeding 100 kDa cannot cross the retinal layers into the subretinal space, it has been confirmed by immunohistochemical analysis, a full-length, humanized, anti-vascular endothelial growth factor (VEGF) monoclonal antibody (Bevacizumab, Avastin®, Genentech Inc.), composed of 214 amino acids with a molecular weight of 149 kDa, injected into the vitreous cavity, can penetrate through the sensory retina into retinal pigment epitheliums (RPE), subretinal and choroidal space, in monkey and rabbit. In addition, nanometer-sized particles whose mean diameter is below 200 nm can penetrate across the sensory retina into RPE after intravitreal injection in rabbit. In intact retina, theoretically, the drugs in the subretinal fluid could either be absorbed by the sensory retinal blood vessels or transported across the RPE, where it may be absorbed into the choroidal vessels or pass through the sclera. Drug transport across the RPE takes place both by transcellular and paracellular routes. The driving forces of outward transport of molecules from the subretinal spaces are hydrostatic and osmotic, and small molecules might transport through the

paracellular inter-RPE cellular clefts and by active transport through the transcellular route.

7. **Blood-Retinal Barrier:** Blood-retinal barrier (BRB) restricts drug transport from blood into the retina. BRB is composed of tight junctions of retinal capillary endothelial cells and RPE, called iBRB for the inner and oBRB for the outer BRB, respectively (fig. 10.4). The function of iBRB is supported by Müller cells and astrocytes. The retinal capillary endothelial cells are not fenestrated and have a paucity of vesicles (fig. 10.4). The function of these endothelial vesicles has been described as endocytosis or transcytosis that may be receptor mediated or fluid phase requiring adenosine triphosphate. A close spatial relationship exists between Müller cells and retinal capillary vessels to maintain the iBRB in the uptake of nutrients and in the disposal of metabolites under normal conditions.

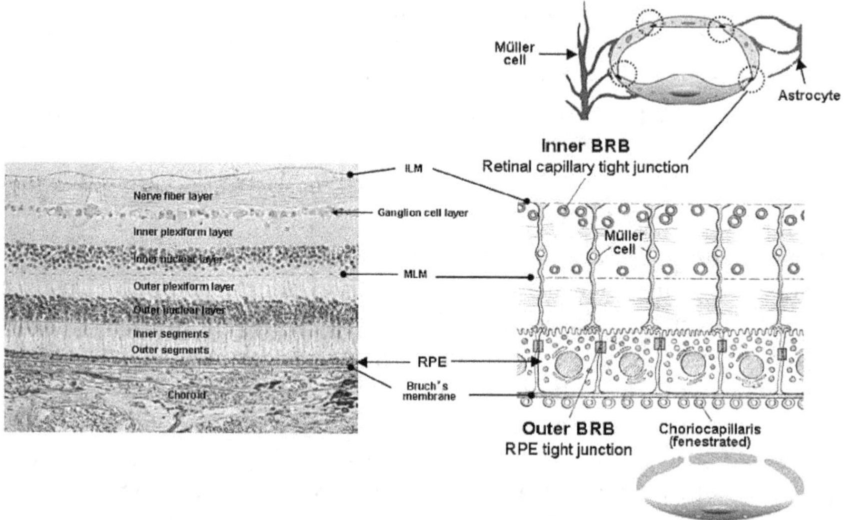



**Fig. 10.4:** Structure of blood retinal barrier showing capillary wall of the retina and choroid.

Müller cells are known to support neuronal activity and maintain the proper functioning of the iBRB under conditions. They are involved in the control and homeostasis of K+ and other ions signalling molecules, and in the control of extracellular pH. Dysfunction of Müller cells may contribute to a breakdown of the iBRB in many pathological conditions, such as diabetes. Müller cells enhance the secretion of VEGF under hypoxic and inflammatory conditions. *In vitro* study has shown that VEGF-induced occluding phosphorylation and ubiquitination causes trafficking of tight junction and leads to increased retinal vascular permeability. The astrocytes originate from the optic nerve and migrate to the nerve fibre layer during development. They are closely associated with the retinal capillary vessels and help to maintain the capillary integrity. Astrocytes are known to increase the barrier properties of the retinal vascular endothelium by enhancing the expression of the tight junction protein ZO-1 and modifying endothelial morphology.

Following systemic drug administration, drugs can easily enter into the choroid since choroid is highly vascularized tissue compared to retina. The choriocapillaris are fenestrated resulting in rapid equilibration of drug molecules present in the bloodstream with the extravascular space of the choroid. Therefore, oBRB (RPE) restricts further entry of drugs from the choroid into the retina. RPE is a monolayer of highly specialized hexagonal-shaped cells, located between the sensory retina and the choroid. The tight junctions of the RPE efficiently restrict intercellular permeation into the sensory retina.

## Preliminary Study

Formulation of ophthalmic drug delivery system is associated with several critical parameters to maintain the intact nature of the eye. Hence, preliminary investigations involve the following parameters:

1. **Clarity:** Ophthalmic solution by definition contains no undissolved ingredients and is essentially free from foreign particles. Clarity may be enhanced in some cases by filtration. It is essential that the filtration equipment be clean and well rinsed so that particulate matter is not contributed to the solution by equipment designed to remove it. Operations performed in clean surroundings, the use of laminar-flow hoods, and proper non-shedding garments will contribute collectively to the preparation of clear solutions essentially free from foreign particles. In many instances clarity and sterility may be achieved in the same filtration step. If viscosity-imparting polymers are used, a polish-filtering step may be required prior to the final filtration. Both container and closure must be thoroughly clean, sterile, and non-shedding, neither contributing particulate matter to the solution during prolonged contact for the duration of the shelf life. Normally this is established by thorough stability testing, which also will indicate if insoluble particles are generated by drug degradation (by-products with lower solubility). Solution formulations also may contain viscosity imparting polymers that can diminish clarity. In these situations, it may be important both to define the visual clarity of the product and monitor its stability. The European pharmacopoeia describes visual clarity and recommends that can be used for clarity specifications.

2. **Stability:** The stability of a drug in an ophthalmic product depends on a number of factors including the chemical nature of the drug substance, whether it is in solution or suspension, product pH, method of preparation (particularly temperature exposure), solution additives, and type of packaging. A pharmaceutical manufacturer strives for a shelf-life measured in years at controlled room temperature conditions whereas the compounding pharmacist often is not certain about the shelf life of his preparation and thus provides relatively small quantities at one time and assigns a shelf life in terms of days or weeks and may specify

refrigerated storage as a further precaution. The attainment of optimum stability often imposes some compromises in the formulation, packaging and preparation of the final product. The product's pH is often the stability-controlling factor for many drugs. Drugs such as pilocarpine and physostigmine are both active and comfortable in the eye at a pH of 6.8; however, at this pH chemical stability (or instability) can be measured in days or months. With either drug, a substantial loss in chemical stability will occur in less than 1 year. On the other hand, at pH 5 both drugs are stable for a period of several years. In addition to optimal pH, if oxygen sensitivity is a factory, adequate stability may require inclusion of an antioxidant or special packaging. Plastic packaging, i.e., the low-density polyethylene containers such as the Drrop-Tainer (Alcon) that represents a patient convenience, may prove detrimental to stability by permitting oxygen permeation resulting in oxidative decomposition of the drug substance. To develop an epinephrine solution with 2 to 3 years stability in a plastic package requires the use as a pH of about 3 for protection from oxidation whereas an epinephrine borate solution formulated at a pH of about 7, which is more comfortable to the patient, requires an antioxidant system and the use of glass packaging. The prodrug of epinephrine, dipivefrin, significantly increases ocular bioavailability and is effective at one-tenth the concentration of epinephrine. The structure of the chemical derivative protects the active epinephrine portion from oxidation enabling it to be packaged in plastic. However, the prodrug introduces a labile ester linkage and as a result must be formulated at a pH of about 3 to minimize hydrolysis and still can only achieve a room temperature shelf life of less than 18 months.

Some of the newer classes of ophthalmic drugs, like prostaglandins are very hydrophobic and have very low concentrations. For example, in the product Xalatan latanoprost is present at 0.005% and in the product Travatan travoprost is present at 0.004% Actives at such low concentration present a challenge for formulators since the loss of even small amounts of drug, e.g., from adsorption losses to packaging, may become significant. Pharmacia's Xalatan requires refrigerated storage, and as indicated earlier, temperature cycling also can reduce the concentration of active ingredients. It is important for the pharmacist to know the properties of the drug substance so that product to know the properties of the drug substances so that product quality is maintained is maintained throughout the shelf life of the product.

3. **Buffer and pH:** Ideally, ophthalmic preparations should be formulated at a pH equivalent to the tear fluid of 7.4. Practically this seldom is achieved. The large majority of active ingredients used in ophthalmology is salts of weak bases and are most stable at an acid pH. This generally can be extended to suspensions of insoluble corticosteroids. Such suspensions usually are most stable at acid pH. Optimum pH adjustment generally requires a compromise on the part of the formulator. The pH selected should have capacity adequate to maintain pH within the stability range for the duration of product shelf life. Buffer capacity is the key in this situation.

In general, it is accepted that a low (acid) pH necessarily will not cause stinging or discomfort on instillation. If the overall pH of tears, after instillation, reverts rapidly to pH 7.4, discomfort is minimal. On the other hand, if the buffer capacity is sufficient to resist adjustment by tear fluid and the overall eye pH remains acid for an appreciable period of time, then stinging and discomfort may result. Consequently, buffer capacity should be adequate for stability but minimized, so far as possible, to allow the overall pH of the tear fluid to be disrupted only momentarily. Special care in formulating intraocular products is required regarding their pH and buffer capacity. The corneal endothelium can tolerate much less deviation from physiological conditions compared to the external corneal epithelium.

4. **Tonicity:** Tonicity refers to the osmotic pressure exerted by salts in aqueous solution. An ophthalmic solution is isotonic when the magnitudes of the colligative properties of the solution are equal. An ophthalmic solution is considered isotonic when its tonicity is equal to that of a 0.9% sodium chloride solution (290 mOsm). However, the osmotic pressure of the aqueous intraocular fluid is slightly higher than tears measuring about 305 mOsm.

   In actuality the external eye is much more tolerate of tonicity variations that was at one time suggested and usually can tolerate solutions equivalent to a range of 0.5 to 1.8% sodium chloride. Given a choice, isotonicity is desirable and particularly is important in intraocular solutions. However, in certain cases a non-isotonic topical product is desirable. Tear fluid in some cases of dry eye is reported to be hypertonic and a hypotonic artificial tear product is used to counteract this condition. Hypertonic ophthalmic products are used to relieve corneal edema and solutions and ointments containing 2% or 5% sodium chloride are available for this use.

   The tonicity of ophthalmic solutions has been investigated intensively over the years. These studies have resulted in the accumulation and publication of a large number of sodium chloride equivalents that are useful in calculating tonicity values.

5. **Viscosity:** Ophthalmic solution and suspension eye drops may contain viscosity-imparting polymers to thicken the tear film and increase corneal contact time, i.e., reduce the rate of tear fluid drainage. For suspensions, the increased viscosity also serves to retard the settling of particles between uses and at the same time maintains their suspension for uniform dosing. However, added viscosity may make initial resuspension more difficult particularly in a suspension that has a tendency to cake during storage. The hydrophilic polymers most often used for these purposes are methylcellulose, hydroxypropyl methylcellulose, hydroxyethyl cellulose and polyvinyl alcohol. They are used at concentrations that produce viscosities in the range of about 5 to 100cps. These polymers are also used themselves as the active ingredients in artificial tear solutions for their lubrication and moisturizing properties in dry eye therapy. Viscosity agents can have several disadvantages in that they sometimes produce blurring of vision and can leave a

residue on the eyelids. These effects are most often seen at the higher end of the viscosity range. The added viscosity can make filtration more difficult particularly for the small pore size filters used to sterilize solutions.

Newer ophthalmic dosage forms such as gel-forming solutions and semi-solid aqueous gels utilize increased viscosity and gel elasticity to improve significantly drug bioavailability and duration of effect. With these advances, the frequency of dosing can be reduced and patient compliance improved. These newer dosage forms utilize novel polymer systems with special rheological properties to enhance their effect. Their complex rheology and intricate dependence on environment, however, increase the complexity of the sterile manufacturing process.

6. **Additives:** Additives or pharmaceutical excipients are used as inactive ingredients in most ophthalmic dosage forms. Because of the need for tissue compatibility, the use of additives is perhaps more limited in ophthalmic, particularly in intraocular products.

The most common inactive ingredient is the product's vehicle. For topical dosage forms, Purified Water USP is used. Because of the requirement for non-pyrogenicity, Water for Injection USP is used for intraocular products. While a mineral oil and petrolatum combination is the vehicle used for ophthalmic ointments, nonaqueous liquids are rarely used in topical eye drops due to their potential for ocular irritation and poor patient tolerance. Some mineral and vegetable oils have been used for very moisture-sensitive or poorly water-soluble drugs. The purest grade of oil such as those used for parenteral products should be used.

Microbiological preservatives are commonly used in multiple dose topical ophthalmic products and will be discussed in a later section. Other commonly used additives in topical eye products are ingredients to adjust and buffer pH and adjust tonicity in addition to the viscosity agents previously discussed. Ingredients to adjust pH and tonicity and buffer pH are essentially the same as those used in parenteral products. Less commonly used additives are antioxidants such as sodium bisulfite, ascorbic acid and acetyl cysteine.

Surfactants are sometimes used in topical eye products for dispersing insoluble ingredients or to aid in solubilization. They are used in the smallest concentration possible to perform the desired function since they can be irritating to sensitive ocular tissues. Non-ionic surfactants are used most often since they are generally less irritating than ionic surfactants. Polysorbate 80 is used in the preparation of an ophthalmic emulsion. Polyoxyl 40 stearate and polyethylene glycol have been used to solubilize a drug in an anhydrous ointment so that it can be filter sterilized. Surfactants are often used to stabilize more hydrophobic drugs, for example preventing loss to adsorption on the container walls. For example, a nonionic surfactant like polyoxyl 40 hydrogenated castor oil (HCO-40) has been used to stabilize travoprost, a prostaglandin derivative. Similarly, Cremophore EL has been used to stabilize diclofenac in the Voltaren formulation marketed by Novartis.

## Ocular Formulations

A wide range of ocular formulation are available for drug delivery to eye, these are classified on the basis of their physical state. Different ophthalmic formulations are as follows:

(A) **Liquids:** Solutions, Suspensions, Sol to gel systems, Sprays

(B) **Solids:** Ocular inserts, Contact lenses, corneal shield, Artificial tear inserts, Filter paper strips

(C) **Semi-solids:** Ointments, Gels

(D) **Miscellaneous:** Ocular iontophoresis, Vesicular systems, Mucoadhesive dosage forms, Particulates, Ocular penetration.

(A) **Liquids Ophthalmic Dosage Forms:** Liquids are the most popular and desirable state of dosage forms for the eye. This is because the drug absorption is fastest from this state. The slow release of the drug from the suspended solids provides a sustained effect for a short duration of time.

1. **Solutions and Suspensions:** Solutions are the pharmaceutical forms most widely used to administer drugs that must be active on the eye surface or in the eye after passage through the cornea or the conjunctiva. The drug in the solution is in the solved state and may be immediately active. This form also have disadvantages; the very short time the solution stays at the eye surface, its poor bioavailability (a major portion i.e. 75% is lost via nasolacrimal drainage), the instability of the dissolved drug, and the necessity of using preservatives. A considerable disadvantage of using eye drops is the rapid elimination of the solution and their poor bioavailability. This rapid elimination is due to solution state of the preparation and may be influenced by the composition of the solution. The retention of a solution in the eye is influenced by viscosity, hydrogen ion concentration, the osmolality and the instilled volume. Extensive work has been done to prolong ocular retention of drugs in the solution state by enhancing the viscosity or altering the pH of the solution.

   *Eye-Drops:* To prolong the retention time of topically applied drugs, anterior DDSs for eye-drops utilizing interaction between drug carrier (excipients) and physiological environment of cornea and/or subconjunctiva are being developed. Durasite® DDS (InSite Vision Inc., Alameda, CA, U.S.) is based on a polycarbophil aqueous solution. Polycarbophil is polyacrylic acid cross-linked with divinyl glycol, and forms hydrogen-bonding with the mucus, and corneal and conjunctival epitheliums, which are all negatively charged, to extend the effects of drug to several hours.

   A broad-spectrum antibiotic, azithromycin ophthalmic solution, formulated with Durasite® (AzaSite®, Inspire Pharmaceuticals Inc., Durham, NC, U.S.) for the treatment of bacterial conjunctivitis was launched in the United States in 2007. This utilizes Durasite®, a combination of azithromycin and dexamethasone (DEX) (ISV-502; AzaSite Plus™, InSite Vision Inc.), for the treatment of conjunctivitis and is currently in Phase III. Bromfenac in DuraSite® (ISV-303, InSite Vision Inc.) is in Phase I/II to reduce inflammation and pain after ocular surgery.

Methylcellulose (MC) has a lower critical solution temperature (LCST) at approximately 50 °C, and sol-gel phase transition occurs. Since the temperature of ocular surface is 32-34 °C, LCST needs to be lower to gel MC solution at ocular surface quickly after instillation as eye-drops. In general, high concentration of electrolytes leads to salting-out and gelation of MC. Wakamoto Pharmaceutical Co., Ltd. (Tokyo, Japan) has developed temperature-responsive eye-drops formulated timolol maleate for glaucoma therapy (Rysmon® TG) available in Japan, using combinations of MC, sodium citrate and polyethylene glycol, which can act by lowering LCST of MC.

A strong cationic ion exchange resin, Amberlite® IRP-69 is polystyrene sulfonic acid resin cross-linked with divinyl benzene. Betoptic S® marketed from 1990 (Alcon Laboratories, Inc., Fort Worth, TX, U.S.), whose active ingredient is betaxolol for glaucoma therapy, is consisted of this resin. Positively charged betaxolol is bound to the negatively charged sulfonic acid groups in the resin. When betaxolol-bound resin is applied to the eye, the cationic ions such as $Na^+$ or $K^+$ in the tear fluid induce the release of betaxolol molecules from resin matrix into the tear film and lead to betaxolol penetration across the cornea.

Gellan gum is an anionic deacetylated polysaccharide with a tetrasaccharide repeating unit of one β-L-rhamnose, one β-D-glucuronic acid and two β-D-glucuronic acid residues. *In situ* gelation occurs in the presence of mono- and divalent cations including $Ca^{2+}$, $Mg^{2+}$, $K^+$ and $Na^+$. Timoptic-XE® (Merck & Co., Inc., Whitehouse Station, NJ, U.S.) formulated using gellan gum, is on the market, and shows administration once a day is equally effective in lowering intraocular pressure (IOP) as the equivalent concentration of simple eye-drops of aqueous solution of timolol maleate (Timoptic®, Merck & Co., Inc.) administered twice a day. Novasorb® (Novagali Pharma S.A., Evry, France) is a cationic emulsion, based on electrostatic attraction that occurs between the oily droplets of a positively-charged emulsion loaded with active ingredient, and negatively charged ocular surface. Therefore, Novasorb® improves solubility and absorption of lipophilic drugs, reduces the number of instillation times and side effects, leading to better efficacy and compliance. Cationorm®, which is composed of only cationic emulsion without any active ingredients, has been launched for mild dry eye. NOVA22007, a cationic emulsion incorporated cyclosporine, has completed Phase III studies for dry eye and Phase II/III studies for vernal keratoconjunctivitis.

2. ***Sol to gel Systems:*** The new concept of producing a gel *in situ*; for example, in the cul-de-sac of the eye was suggested for the first time in the early 1980s. It is widely accepted that increasing the viscosity of a drug formulation in the precorneal region will leads to an increased bioavailability, due to slower drainage from the cornea. Several concepts for the in-situ gelling systems have been investigated. These systems can be triggered by pH, temperature or by ion activation. An anionic polymeric dispersion shows a low viscosity up to pH 5.0, and will coacervate in contact with tear fluid due to presence of a carbonic buffer system which regulates the pH of tears. *In situ* gelling by a temperature change is produced when the temperature of polymeric dispersion is raised from 25 to 37°C. Ion activation of polymeric dispersion occurred due to the presence of cations in the tear fluid.

3. ***Sprays:*** Although not commonly used, some practitioners use mydriatics or cycloplegics alone or in combination in the form of eye spray. These sprays are used in the eye for dilating the pupil or for cycloplegic examination.

**(B)** **Solids:** The concept of using solids for the eye is based on providing sustained release characteristics.

1. ***Ocular inserts:*** Ocular inserts are solid dosage form and can overcome the disadvantage reported with traditional ophthalmic systems like aqueous solutions, suspensions and ointments. The typical pulse entry type drug release behaviour observed with ocular aqueous solutions (eye drops), suspensions and ointments are replaced by more controlled, sustained and continuous drug delivery using a controlled release ocular drug delivery system. The eye drops provided pulse entry pattern of drug administration in the eye which is characterized by transient overdose, relatively short period of acceptable dosing, followed by prolonged periods of under dosing. The ocular inserts maintain an effective drug concentration in the target tissues and yet minimize the number of applications consonants with the function of controlled release systems. Limited popularity of ocular inserts has been attributed to psychological factors, such as reluctance of patients to abandon the traditional liquid and semisolid medications, and to occasional therapeutic failures (e.g. unnoticed expulsion from the eye, membrane ruptures etc.). A number of ocular inserts were prepared utilizing different techniques to make soluble, erodible, non-erodible, and hydrogel inserts.

2. ***Contact Lens:*** Contact lenses can absorb water soluble drugs when soaked in drug solutions. These drug saturated contact lenses are placed in the eye for releasing the drug for long period of time. The hydrophilic contact lenses can be used to prolong the ocular residence time of the drugs. In humans, the Bionite lens which was made from hydrophilic polymer (2-hydroxy ethyl methacrylate) has been shown to produce a greater penetration of fluorescein.

3. ***Corneal shield:*** A non-cross-linked homogenized, porcine scleral collagen slice is developed by a company (Biocor (Bausch and Lomb pharmaceuticals). Topically applied antibiotics have been used in conjunction with the shield to promote healing of corneal ulcers. Collagen shields are fabricated with foetal calf skin tissue and originally developed as a corneal bandage. These devices, once softened by the tear fluid, form a thin pliable film that confirms exactly to the corneal surface, and undergoes dissolution up to 10, 24 or 72 hours. Collagen film proved as a promising carrier for ophthalmic drug delivery system because of its biological inertness, structural stability and good biocompatibility. Gussler et al investigated the delivery of trifluoro thymidine (TFT) in collagen shields and in topical drops in the cornea of normal rabbits and corneas with experimental epithelial defects. It was found that highest drug concentrations were found in the eyes treated with shields as compared to eye drops.

4. ***Artificial tear inserts:*** A rod-shaped pellet of hydroxypropyl cellulose without preservative is commercially available (Lacrisert). This device is designed as a sustained release artificial tear for the treatment of dry eye disorders. It was developed by Merck, Sharp and Dohme in 1981.

5. ***Filter paper strips:*** Sodium fluorescein and rose Bengal dyes are commercially available as drug impregnated filter paper strips. These dyes are used diagnostically to disclose corneal injuries and infections such as herpes simplex, and dry eye disorders.

**(C) Semi-solids:** A wide variety of semisolids vehicles are used for topical ocular delivery which falls into two general categories: simple and compound bases. Simple bases refer to a single continuous phase. These include white petrolatum, lanolin and viscous gels prepared from polymers such as PVA, carbopol etc. Compound bases are usually of a biphasic type forming either water in oil or oil in water emulsions. A drug in either a simple or compound base provide an increase in the duration of action due to reduction in dilution by tears, reduction in drainage by way of a sustained release effect, and prolonged corneal contact time. The most commonly used semisolid preparation is ointments consisting of dispersion of a solid drug in an appropriate vehicle base. Semi-solids dosage forms are applied once or twice daily and provide sustained effects. The primary purpose of the ophthalmic ointment vehicle is to prolong drug contact time with the external ocular surface. But they present a disadvantage of causing blurring of vision and matting of eyelids. Ophthalmic gels are similar in viscosity and clinical usage to ophthalmic ointments. Pilopine HS is one of the ophthalmic preparations available in gel form and is intended to provide sustained action of pilocarpine over a period of 24 hours. Semi-solids vehicles were found to prolong the ocular contact time of many drugs, which ultimately leads to an enhanced bioavailability.

1. ***Ointments and Gels***: Prolongation of drug contact time with the external ocular surface can be achieved using ophthalmic ointment vehicle but, the major drawback of this dosage form like, blurring of vision and matting of eyelids can limits its use. Pilopine HS gel containing pilocarpine was used to provide sustain action over a period of 24 hours. A number of workers reported that ointments and gels vehicles can prolong the corneal contact time of many drugs administered by topical ocular route, thus prolonging duration of action and enhancing ocular bioavailability of drugs.

**(D) Novel formulations to overcome intraocular barriers**

1. ***Microemulsion***: Due to their intrinsic properties and specific structures, microemulsions are a promising dosage form for the natural defence of the eye. Indeed, because they are prepared by inexpensive processes through auto emulsification or supply of energy and can be easily sterilized, they are stable and have a high capacity of dissolving the drugs.

2. ***Collagen Shield***: Collagen is regarded as one of the most useful biomaterials. The excellent biocompatibility and safety due to its biological characteristics, such as biodegradability and weak antigenicity, made collagen the primary resource in medical applications. Collasomes show promise among drug delivery systems to the human eye. They are first fabricated from porcine scleral tissue, which bears a collagen composition similar to that of the human cornea. The shields are hydrated before they are placed on the eye.

3. ***Ocular Iontophoresis***: Iontophoresis is the process in which direct current drives ions into cells or tissues. Ocular iontophoresis offers a drug delivery system that is fast, painless and safe; and in most cases; it results in the delivery of a high concentration of the drug to a specific site. But the role of iontophoresis in clinical ophthalmology remains to be identified.

4. ***Liposomes***: Liposomes are phospholipid-lipid vesicles for targeting drugs to the specific sites in the body; provide the controlled and selective drug delivery and improved bioavailability. Liposomes offer the advantages of being completely biodegradable and relatively non-toxic but are less stable than particulate polymeric drug delivery systems.

5. ***Niosomes***: In order to circumvent the limitations of liposomes, such as chemical instability, oxidative degradation of phospholipids, cost and purity of natural phospholipids, Niosomes have been developed as they are chemically stable compared to liposomes and can entrap both hydrophilic and hydrophobic drugs. They are non-toxic and do not require special handling techniques.

6. ***Mucoadhesive Dosage Forms***: The successful development of fewer mucoadhesive dosage forms for ocular delivery still poses numerable challenges. This approach relies on vehicles containing polymers, which will attach, via noncovalent bonds to conjunctival mucin.

7. ***Nanoparticles & Microparticles:*** Particulate polymeric drug delivery systems include Micro and Nanoparticles. The upper size limit for microparticles for ocular delivery is about 5-10 mm. above this size; a scratching feeling in the eye can result after ocular application. After optimal drug binding to microspheres or Nanoparticles, the drug absorption in the eye enhanced significantly in comparison to eye drops.

8. ***Prodrugs:*** Prodrugs are simple, chemically or enzymatically liable derivatives of drugs, which are converted to their active parent drug typically as a result of hydrolysis within the eye. Prodrug technology is generally considered as a useful technique in improving corneal permeability of drugs. It is also useful in solving pharmaceutical formulation problems such as poor solubility and stability.

9. ***Hydrogels:*** Hydrogels are three-dimensional, hydrophilic, polymeric networks capable of imbibing large amount of water or biological fluids. The environmental conditions to which a hydrogel can be made responsive by pH, temperature, electric field, ionic strength, salt type, solvent, external stress, light, or a combination of these. Due to their elastic properties, hydrogels can also represent an ocular drainage-resistance device. In addition, they may offer better feeling, with less of a gritty sensation to patients. In particular, *in-situ* forming hydrogels are attractive as an ocular drug delivery system because of their facility in dosing as a liquid, and their long-term retention property as a gel after dosing.

10. ***Sol to Gel Systems:*** Several new preparations have been developed for ophthalmic use not only to prolong the contact time of the vehicle at ocular surface, but at the same time slow down the elimination of the drug.

## Ocuserts

Ophthalmic inserts/Occusert are sterile preparations with a solid or a semisolid consistency, and whose size and shape are especially designed for ophthalmic application. The inserts are placed in the lower fornix and less frequently, in the upper fornix or on the cornea. Ocular inserts can overcome the disadvantages reported with traditional.

Ophthalmic systems like eye drops, suspensions and ointments. The typical pulse entry type drug release behaviour observed with eye drops, suspensions and ointments is replaced by more controlled, sustained and continuous drug delivery using a controlled release ocular drug delivery system. In the recent years, there has been explosion of interest in the polymer-based delivery devices, adding further dimension to topical drug delivery thereby promoting the use of polymers such as collagen and fibrin fabricated into erodible inserts for placement in cul-de-sac. Utilization of the principles of controlled release as embodied by ocular inserts offers an attractive approach to the problem of prolonging precorneal drug residence times. Ocular inserts also offer the potential advantage of improving patient compliance by reducing the dosing frequency. The main objective of the ophthalmic inserts is to increase the contact time between the preparation and the conjunctival tissue to ensure a sustained release suited to topical or systemic treatment. They are composed of polymeric support with or without drugs, the latter being incorporated as dispersion or a solution in the polymeric support (fig. 10.5).

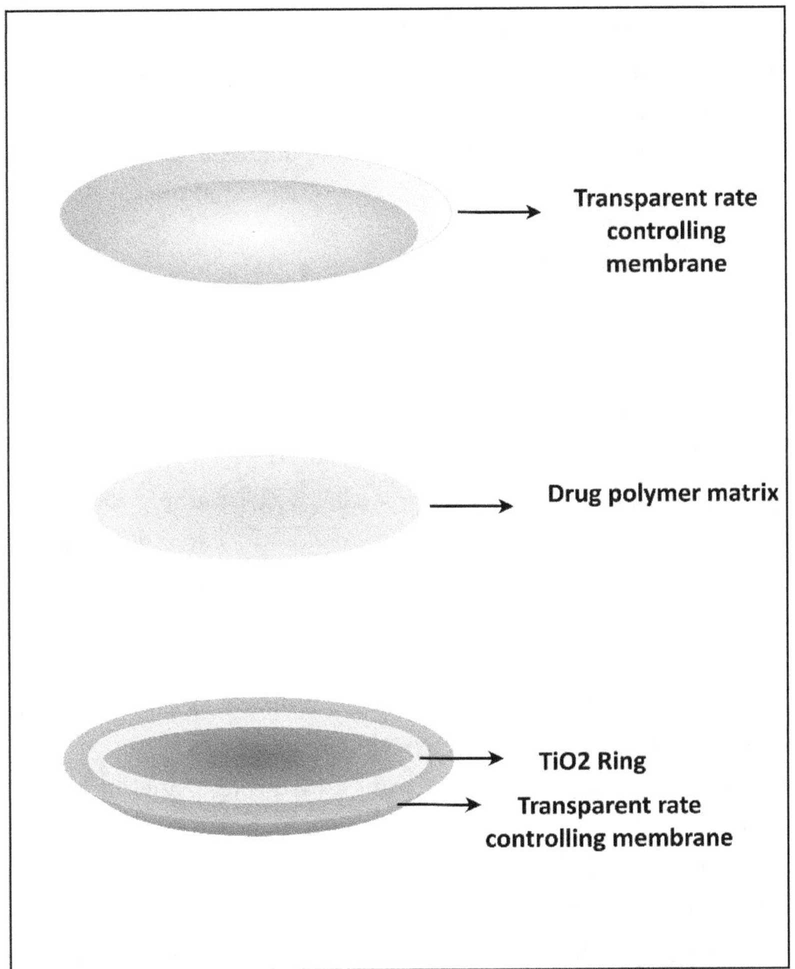


**Fig. 10.5:** Structure of a typical ocusert.

Ocusert® provides uniform controlled release (20 or 40 µg/hour for 7 days) of pilocarpine as an ocular hypotensive drug and has been commercialized in 1974. Ocusert® consists of two outer layers of ethylene-vinyl acetate copolymer (EVA), and an inner layer of pilocarpine in alginate gel within di-(ethylhexyl) phthalate for a release enhancer, sandwiched between EVA layers. However, Ocusert® has not become widely used because of unsatisfactory IOP control due to various causes, including difficulty of inserting the device, ejection of the device from eye, and irritation during insertion.

Lacrisert® (Aton Pharma, Inc., Lawrenceville, NJ, U.S.) is a rod-shaped, water-soluble cul-de-sac insert composed of hydroxypropyl cellulose without preservatives and other ingredients (1.27 mm diameter, 3.5 mm long), and is indicated in moderate to severe dry eye syndrome. Lacrisert® has not been applied as a drug delivery carrier as yet. Although previously many inserts including collagen shield, Ocufit SR®, New Ophthalmic Delivery System, and Minidisc ocular therapeutic system have been developed, there are no further activities at present. The commercial failure of inserts might be attributed to psychological factors including the reluctance to abandon the traditional droppable formulations, and occasional ejection from the eye observed in the case of Ocusert®.

## Advantages of Ocular Inserts

The advantages of ocular inserts over other ocular dosage forms are as follows:

- Increased ocular residence, hence a prolonged drug activity and a higher bioavailability with respect to standard vehicles.
- Possibility of releasing drugs at a slow, constant rate;
- Accurate dosing (contrary to eye drops that can be improperly instilled by the patient and are partially lost after administration, each insert can be made to contain a precise dose which is fully retained at the administration site).
- Reduction of systemic absorption (which occurs freely with eye drops via the nasolacrimal duct and nasal mucosa)
- Better patient compliance, resulting from a reduced frequency of administration and a lower incidence of visual and systemic side-effects
- Possibility of targeting internal ocular tissues through non-corneal (conjunctival scleral) routes
- Increased shelf life with respect to aqueous solutions
- Exclusion of preservatives, thus reducing the risk of sensitivity reactions;
- Possibility of incorporating various novel chemical/technological approaches.

## Disadvantages of Ocular Inserts

- A capital disadvantage of ocular inserts resides in their 'solidity', i.e., in the fact that they are felt by the (often oversensitive) patients as an extraneous body in the eye.
- The occasional inadvertent loss during sleep or while rubbing the eyes.
- Their interference with vision.
- Difficult placement of the ocular inserts (and removal, for insoluble types).

## Formulation Methods of Ocusert

### Solvent Casting Method

In this method using different ratios of drug and polymer a no. of batches are prepared. The polymer is dissolved in distilled water. A plasticizer is added to this solution under stirring conditions. The weighed amount of drug was added to above solution and stirred to get a uniform dispersion. After proper mixing the casting solution was poured in clean glass petridish and covered with an inverted funnel to allow slow and uniform evaporation at room temperature for 48 h. The dried films thus obtained were cut by cork borer into circular pieces of definite size containing drug. The ocular inserts were then stored in an airtight container (desiccator) under ambient condition.

### Drug Reservoir Film

1% w/w polymer for example chitosan was soaked in 1% v/v Acetic acid solution for 24hrs, to get a clear solution of chitosan in acetic acid solution. The solution was filtered through a muslin cloth to remove undissolved portion of the polymer (chitin). Required quantity of drug-$\beta$ CD complex was added and vortexed for 15 minutes to dissolve the complex in chitosan solution. 1% w/v propylene glycol (plasticizer) was added to it and mixed well with stirrer. The viscous solution was kept aside for 30 minutes for complete expulsion of air bubbles. The rate controlling films were prepared. The films were casted by pouring solution into the centre of levelled glass mould and allowing it to dry at room temperature for 24hrs. After drying, films were cut into occuserts of desired size so that each contains equal quantity of the drug. Then, the matrix was sandwiched between the rate controlling membranes using non-toxic, nonirritating, water insoluble gum. They were wrapped in aluminium foil separately and stored in a desiccator.

### Melt Extrusion Technique

Drug for example, acyclovir and the polymer were sieved through 60#, weighed and blended geometrically. The plasticizer was added and blended. The blend was then charged to the barrel of Melt Flow Rate apparatus and extruded. The extrudate was cut into appropriate size and packed in polyethylene lined Al foil, heat sealed and sterilized by gamma radiation.

### Conclusion

Eye is a very sensitive part of human body which needs to be handled very carefully to protect its integrity. The nasolacrimal drainage, less contact time, small contact area and many other factors makes the ocular drug delivery very challenging. Hence, in past two decades, the research focused on the development of prolong and controlled drug delivery system to improve the drug resident time and reduces the wastage of drug. thus, enhances the drug absorption and finally the bioavailability. The novel strategies including the ocular inserts, biodegradable polymeric devices, nanocarrier system and collagen shield also concern about improving the patient compliance by reducing the dosing frequency which also decreases the side effects of drug.

# Bibliography


1. Achouri, D., et al., Recent advances in ocular drug delivery. Drug Dev Ind Pharm, 2013. 39(11): p. 1599-617.

2. Ali, J., et al., Colloidal drug delivery system: amplify the ocular delivery. Drug Deliv, 2016. 23(3): p. 710-26.

3. Baranowski, P., et al., Ophthalmic drug dosage forms: characterisation and research methods. ScientificWorldJournal, 2014. 2014: p. 861904.

4. Barar, J., et al., Advanced drug delivery and targeting technologies for the ocular diseases. Bioimpacts, 2016. 6(1): p. 49-67.

5. Basaran, E. and Y. Yazan, Ocular application of chitosan. Expert Opin Drug Deliv, 2012. 9(6): p. 701-12.

6. Del Amo, E.M., et al., Pharmacokinetic aspects of retinal drug delivery. Prog Retin Eye Res, 2017. 57: p. 134-185.

7. Fangueiro, J.F., et al., Ocular Drug Delivery - New Strategies for Targeting Anterior and Posterior Segments of the Eye. Curr Pharm Des, 2016. 22(9): p. 1135-46.

8. Goyal, G., et al., Current nanotechnological strategies for treating glaucoma. Crit Rev Ther Drug Carrier Syst, 2014. 31(5): p. 365-405.

9. Janagam, D.R., L. Wu, and T.L. Lowe, Nanoparticles for drug delivery to the anterior segment of the eye. Adv Drug Deliv Rev, 2017. 122: p. 31-64.

10. Kang-Mieler, J.J., et al., Extended ocular drug delivery systems for the anterior and posterior segments: biomaterial options and applications. Expert Opin Drug Deliv, 2017. 14(5): p. 611-620.

11. Kaur, I.P. and M. Kanwar, Ocular preparations: the formulation approach. Drug Dev Ind Pharm, 2002. 28(5): p. 473-93.

12. Kels, B.D., A. Grzybowski, and J.M. Grant-Kels, Human ocular anatomy. Clin Dermatol, 2015. 33(2): p. 140-6.

13. Ludwig, A., The use of mucoadhesive polymers in ocular drug delivery. Advanced Drug Delivery Reviews, 2005. 57(11): p. 1595-1639.

14. Mandal, A., et al., Polymeric micelles for ocular drug delivery: From structural frameworks to recent preclinical studies. J Control Release, 2017. 248: p. 96-116.

15. Maulvi, F.A., T.G. Soni, and D.O. Shah, A review on therapeutic contact lenses for ocular drug delivery. Drug Deliv, 2016. 23(8): p. 3017-3026.

16. Moisseiev, E. and A. Loewenstein, Drug Delivery to the Posterior Segment of the Eye. Dev Ophthalmol, 2017. 58: p. 87-101.

17. Sharma, O.P., V. Patel, and T. Mehta, Nanocrystal for ocular drug delivery: hope or hype. Drug Deliv Transl Res, 2016. 6(4): p. 399-413.

18.  Tashakori-Sabzevar, F. and S.A. Mohajeri, Development of ocular drug delivery systems using molecularly imprinted soft contact lenses. Drug Dev Ind Pharm, 2015. 41(5): p. 703-13.

19.  Wadhwa, S., et al., Chitosan and its role in ocular therapeutics. Mini Rev Med Chem, 2009. 9(14): p. 1639-47.

20.  Wadhwa, S., et al., Nanocarriers in ocular drug delivery: an update review. Curr Pharm Des, 2009. 15(23): p. 2724-50.

21.  Yellepeddi, V.K. and S. Palakurthi, Recent Advances in Topical Ocular Drug Delivery. J Ocul Pharmacol Ther, 2016. 32(2): p. 67-82.

# Exercise

## A. Multiple Choice Questions

1.  Which of the following statements is correct?
    (a)  The cornea consists of only one membrane, the epithelium,
    (b)  The cornea consists of only one membrane, the endothelium,
    (c)  The cornea consists of only one membrane, stroma.
    (d)  The cornea consists of three layers- epithelium, stroma and endothelium.

2.  According to the result of histological studies
    (a)  The choroidal thickness is about 200 µm at birth.
    (b)  The choroidal thickness is about 100 µm at birth.
    (c)  The choroidal thickness is about 90 µm at birth.
    (d)  The choroidal thickness is about 80 µm at birth.

3.  According to the result of histological studies
    (a)  The choroidal thickness does not change with age
    (b)  The choroidal thickness decreases with increasing age
    (c)  The choroidal thickness increases with age
    (d)  The choroidal thickness remains constant from birth to old age.

4.  The limitation of absorption of drug in the eye is
    (a)  Drainage from eye              (b)  Lacrimation
    (c)  Conjunctival absorption        (d)  All of the above

5.  The rate of permeation through the corneal membrane in cul-de-sac depends
    (a)  Only on lipophilicity and solubility of the drug,
    (b)  Only on the molecular size and shape of the drug,
    (c)  Only on the charge and degree of ionization of the drug
    (d)  All of the above

6. The stability of a drug in an ophthalmic product depends
   (a) Chemical nature of the drug substance in solution or suspension, product pH, method of preparation (particularly temperature exposure), solution additives, and type of packaging.
   (b) pH of the product, method of preparation (particularly temperature exposure), solution additives, and type of packaging.
   (c) Method of preparation (particularly temperature exposure), solution additives, and type of packaging.
   (d) Solution additives, and type of packaging.

7. Which of the following statements is correct?
   (a) The most common inactive ingredient is the product's vehicle.
   (b) The most common inactive ingredient is the viscosity enhancer.
   (c) The most common inactive ingredient is the buffer solution.
   (d) The most common inactive ingredient is the preservative.

8. Which of the following statements is correct?
   (a) The osmotic pressure of the aqueous intraocular fluid is slightly higher than tears measuring about 505 mOsm.
   (b) The osmotic pressure of the aqueous intraocular fluid is slightly higher than tears measuring about 405 mOsm.
   (c) The osmotic pressure of the aqueous intraocular fluid is slightly higher than tears measuring about 305 mOsm.
   (d) The osmotic pressure of the aqueous intraocular fluid is slightly higher than tears measuring about 205 mOsm.

9. Which of the following statements is correct?
   (a) The viscosity imparting substances are used at concentrations that produce viscosities in the range of about 500 to 700cps.
   (b) The viscosity imparting substances are used at concentrations that produce viscosities in the range of about 200 to 500cps.
   (c) The viscosity imparting substances are used at concentrations that produce viscosities in the range of about 300 to 600cps.
   (d) The viscosity imparting substances are used at concentrations that produce viscosities in the range of about 5 to 100cps.

10. Which of the following statements is correct?
   (a) Either water in oil or oil in water emulsions is termed as compound base.
   (b) Only water in oil emulsion is termed as compound base
   (c) Only oil in water emulsion is termed as compound base.
   (d) White petrolatum and lanolin base is termed as compound base.

11. Which of the following statements is correct?
    (a) The excellent biocompatibility and safety of collagen shields are due to its chemical characteristics.
    (b) The excellent biocompatibility and safety of collagen shields are due to its physical characteristics.
    (c) The excellent biocompatibility and safety of collagen shields are due to its biological characteristics.
    (d) The extent of biocompatibility and safety of collagen shields are not satisfactory.

12. Which of the following statements is correct?
    (a) Ocular iontophoresis offers a drug delivery system that is fast, painless and safe; and in most cases, it results in the delivery of a high concentration of the drug to a specific site.
    (b) Ocular iontophoresis offers a drug delivery system that is fast, but painful; and in most cases, it results in the delivery of a high concentration of the drug to a specific site.
    (c) Ocular iontophoresis offers a drug delivery system that is fast, painless and unsafe; and in most cases, it results in the delivery of a high concentration of the drug to a specific site.
    (d) Ocular iontophoresis offers a drug delivery system that is fast, painless and safe; and in most cases, it results in the delivery of a low concentration of the drug to a specific site.

13. Which of the following statements is correct?
    (a) Ocuserts are not felt by the patients as an extraneous body in the eye.
    (b) Patients are not oversensitive to ocuserts as an extraneous body in the eye.
    (c) Ocuserts provide better patients' compliance compared to all ophthalmic preparations.
    (d) Ocuserts are felt by the (often oversensitive) patients as an extraneous body in the eye.

14. Preservative used in ocusert may lead to
    (a) Better patients' compliance      (b)   Sensitivity reaction
    (c) No sensitivity reaction           (d)   Easy insertion

15. Which of the following statements is correct?
    (a) Ocusert may interfere with the vision.
    (b) Ocusert does not have any effect on the vision.
    (c) Ocusert improves the vision.
    (d) Ocusert is not affected on rubbing the eyes.

16. Which of the following statements is correct?
    (a) Ocusert is easy to place in the eye.
    (b) The ocusert remains in the eye in liquid state
    (c) Ocusert fails to deliver accurate dose of a drug.
    (d) Ocusert reduces the frequency of dosing.

17. Which of the following statements is correct?
    (a) The inserts are placed in the upper fornix and less frequently, in the lower fornix.
    (b) The inserts are placed in the upper fornix, even not on the cornea.
    (c) The inserts are placed in the lower fornix and less frequently, in the upper fornix or on the cornea.
    (d) The inserts are placed in the upper fornix only.

18. Which of the following statements is correct?
    (a) Hydrogels are two-dimensional, hydrophilic, polymeric networks capable of imbibing large amount of water or biological fluids.
    (b) Hydrogels are three-dimensional, hydrophilic, polymeric networks capable of imbibing large amount of water or biological fluids.
    (c) Hydrogels are three-dimensional, hydrophobic, polymeric networks capable of imbibing large amount of water or biological fluids.
    (d) Hydrogels are three-dimensional, hydrophobic, polymeric networks capable of imbibing large amount of water.

19. Which of the following statements is correct?
    (a) The hydrogel can be made responsive by pH, temperature, electric field, solvent, external stress, and light only.
    (b) The hydrogel can be made responsive by only electric field, ionic strength, solvent, external stress, light only.
    (c) The hydrogel cannot be made responsive by pH, temperature, electric field, ionic strength, salt type, solvent, external stress, light, or a combination of these.
    (d) The hydrogel can be made responsive by pH, temperature, electric field, ionic strength, salt type, solvent, external stress, light, or a combination of these.

20. Which of the following statements is correct?
    (a) Liposomes are more stable than niosomes.
    (b) Liposomes are less stable than niosomes.
    (c) Liposomes and niosomes are equally stable.
    (d) Liposomes are made of carbohydrate for which they are more stable than niosomes.

## B. Short Questions

1. What are the advantages and disadvantages of ocular drug delivery system?
2. Explain in brief about eye-drops.
3. Write a note on the semisolid-state ocular dosage form.
4. Write down the advantages and disadvantages of ocusert.
5. What are corneal shield and artificial tear inserts?
6. Write a note on ocusert.

## C. Long Questions

1. Discuss briefly the structure of eye.
2. Explain in brief the intraocular barriers and how can these be overcome?
3. Discuss briefly the studies to be conducted before development of an ophthalmic product.
4. Write a note on the solid-state ocular dosage forms.
5. Discuss on the novel formulations to overcome intraocular barriers.
6. Discuss briefly about the excipients used in ophthalmic preparations.
7. Discuss briefly the various techniques used to manufacture ocusert

## CHAPTER 11

# Intrauterine Drug Delivery Systems

*Introduction, advantages and disadvantages, development of intra uterine devices (IUDs) and applications.*

## Introduction

An intrauterine device (IUD) usually is a small, flexible plastic frame. It often has copper wire or copper sleeves on it. It is inserted into a woman's uterus through her vagina. Almost all brands of IUDs have two strings, or threads, tied to them. The strings hang through the opening of the cervix into the vagina. A provider can remove the IUD by pulling gently on the strings with forceps. The intrauterine device (IUD) is a long-term birth control method. Unlike IUDs that were used in the 1970s, present-day IUDs are small, safe, and highly effective. An Intrauterine Device (IUD) is a small piece of plastic that is inserted by a clinician into the uterus to prevent pregnancy. It is approximately 1½ inches (3cm) in length. There are several different types of IUDs. The most common IUD is T-shaped and coated with copper. This can be left in the uterus for 2-5 years. Another type of IUD contains a hormone (progestin) but it needs to be replaced once a year.

Attached to the IUD are two plastic threads or strings that hang down through the cervix into the vagina (fig. 11.1). The cervix is the opening to the uterus. The threads or strings do not hang outside the body. The IUD can also be used as an emergency method of birth control. If an IUD is inserted within 7 days after unprotected vaginal sex it may prevent a pregnancy. An intrauterine device (IUD) is a small T-shaped plastic device that is placed in the uterus to prevent pregnancy. A plastic string is attached to the end to ensure correct placement and for removal.

IUDs are an easily reversible form of birth control, and they can be easily removed. However, an IUD should only be removed by a medical professional. An IUD, or intrauterine device, is a small contraceptive device made of flexible plastic. It's inserted into the uterus, where it provides highly effective long-term contraception. Two IUDs are currently available in the United States: The Copper T 380A (called Para Gard), which is wrapped in fine copper wire and lasts for ten years before it needs to be replaced. Many providers recommend the progestin IUD for women who suffer from extremely heavy, prolonged, or painful menstruation because it tends to lighten their periods or even suppress them altogether. And because they lose less blood, women using this IUD are less likely to develop iron-deficiency anaemia, a condition that can cause fatigue and other symptoms. Some studies have found that women with copper IUDs tend to have a lower risk of endometrial cancer. And some experts suspect that the progestin IUD has the same effect, since that's the case for progestin-only contraceptives like the mini-pill and the shot.

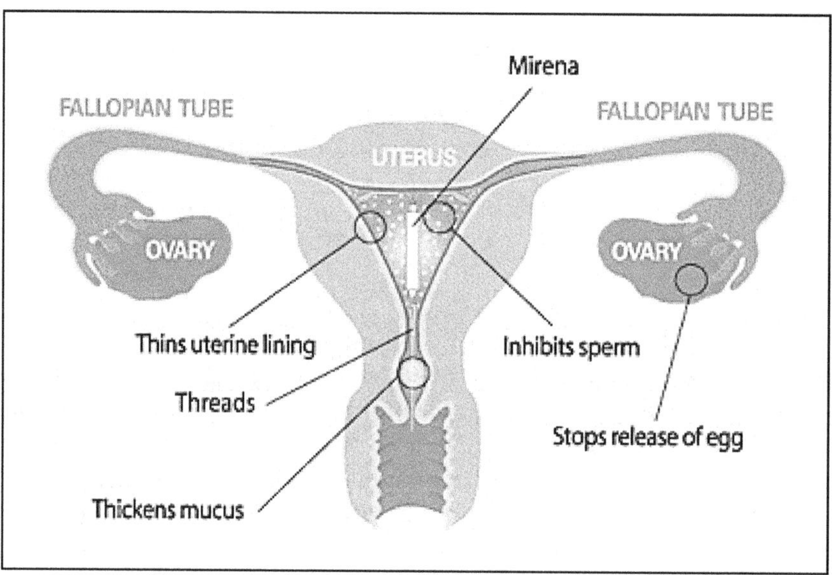


**Fig. 11.1:** Intra-uterine device

Intrauterine devices can be used as emergency contraception to prevent pregnancy up to 5 days after unprotected sexual intercourse, or sexual intercourse during which the primary contraception is believed to have failed (e.g. a condom was used, but it broke). Insertion of a copper-T IUD as emergency contraception is more than 99% effective, making it more effective than emergency contraceptive pills. The IUD is the worlds most widely used safe and effective method of reversible birth control, currently used by nearly 160 million women. An Intrauterine Device (IUD) is a small object that is inserted through the cervix and placed in the uterus to prevent pregnancy. A small string hangs down from the IUD into the upper part of the vagina.

The IUD is not noticeable during intercourse. IUDs can last 1-10 years. They affect the movements of eggs and sperm to prevent fertilization. They also change the lining of the uterus and prevent implantation. IUDs are 99.2-99.9% effective as birth control. They do not protect against sexually transmitted infections, including HIV/AIDS. The IUD is 98% effective in preventing pregnancy.

## Types of IUDS

1. **First Generation IUDs: Plastic Devices:** IUD technology has come a long way since the first plastic IUDs appeared on the scene. The first of the so-called "first generation" IUDs, represented by the "Margulies spiral", was introduced in 1960. After many experiments, Dr Jack Lippes invented the double-S Loop (the Lippes Loop) in 1962 (9).

It was made from polyethylene, with barium sulphate added for visibility under X-rays, and was available in four sizes, from A to D. This IUD was the first to have a nylon thread attached to the lowest part of the device; this made it easier to remove, and it was also possible to verify by simple vaginal examination that the IUD was in the uterine cavity. It became the standard inert device; all the major studies on the IUD were made using this device. Due to its particular shape (trapezoid) (fig. 11.2), the Lippes Loop fits the relaxed uterine cavity snugly. The Lippes Loop was to become extremely popular and, of all the first-generation IUDs, had the greatest worldwide impact.

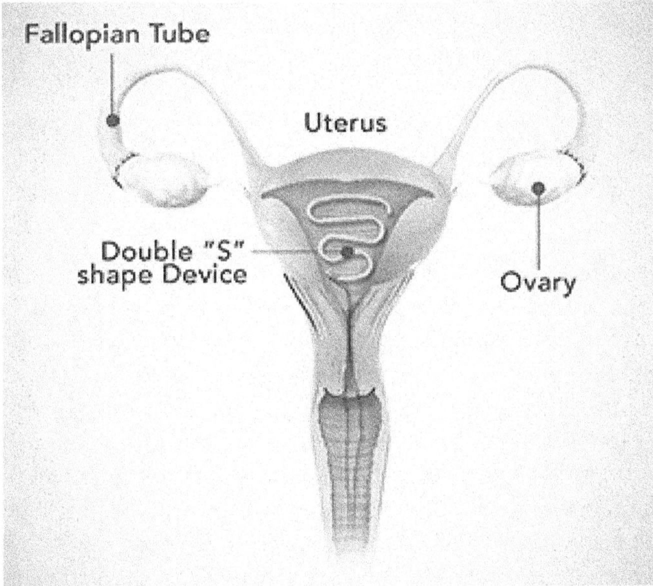


**Fig. 11.2:** Lippes Loop

In subsequent years, resourceful investigators produced scores of original, and sometimes peculiarly shaped, plastic IUDs. One of these was the Dalkon Shield (fig. 11.3), developed by Dr Hugh Davis, and released in 1971. The Dalkon Shield was a plastic device which looked like a round bug with one large eye and five legs on each side. It had a unique tail: not a single filament, but many fibres wound together and enclosed in a sheath. Because of the Dalkon Shield's unique shape made it difficult to remove, a multifilament string was used (instead of the usual stiff monofilament polyethylene thread) to provide increased tensile strength during removal. The multifilament tail string, unique to the Dalkon Shield, was most probably responsible for the facilitated ascent of bacteria from the vagina upward into the uterine cavity, causing pelvic infections. Shortly after its release, reports of septic abortion and other infections reached to a serious level.

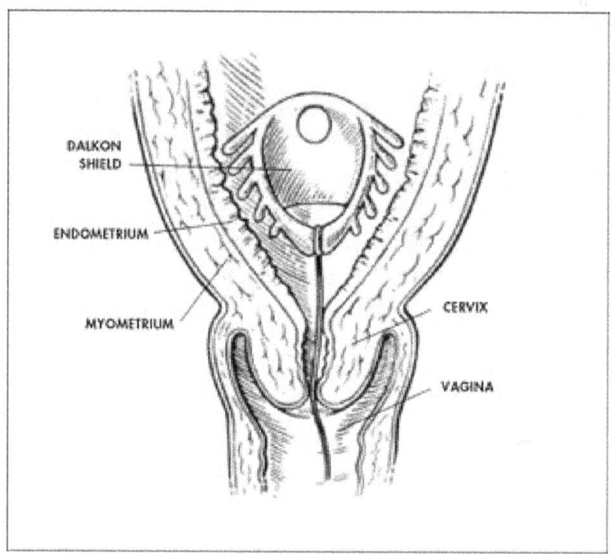


**Fig. 11.3:** Dalkon Shield

2. **Second generation IUDs: Copper IUDs:** Towards the end of the 1960's, it was discovered that adding copper to the plastic produced an IUD that was more effective in preventing pregnancy and less frequently caused bleeding problems. The development of the first copper-bearing IUD (Cu-IUD) was announced in 1969 by Dr Jaime Zipper and Dr Howard Tatum. Dr Tatum invented the plastic T–IUD and Dr Zipper investigated the device clinically. It is the most commonly used type of IUD. It can be left in the body for up to 10 years. It can be removed at any time if a woman wishes to become pregnant or if she does not want to use it anymore. The arms of this IUD contain some copper, which is slowly released into the uterus. The copper prevents sperm from making their way through the uterus into the tubes and prevents fertilization. If fertilization does occur, the copper prevents the fertilized egg from implanting on the wall of the uterus.

3. **Third Generation IUDs: Steroid Mediated Device:** In the late 1960s, Dr Antonio Scommegna, having demonstrated the uterine effects of progesterone, postulated that the endometrial atrophy elicited by the natural steroid hormone would be useful in preventing implantation and reducing menstrual bleeding. He developed a hormone releasing device and showed that it is as effective in preventing pregnancy as the copper-bearing IUD. Dr Scommegna devised a T-shaped device (fig. 11.4a), consisting of a permeable polymer membrane which releases

progesterone at a predictable, controlled rate of 65 mg per 24 h over the period of a year. Unfortunately, this IUD did not gain wide popularity on account of its short (1-year) effective lifespan. The levonorgestrel IUS is a T-shaped polyethylene device with a steroid reservoir around the vertical stem (fig. 11.4b). The cylindrical reservoir contains a mixture of silicone (polydimethylsiloxane) and 52 mg levonorgestrel, a progestin widely used in implants, oral contraceptives, and vaginal rings. This allows a steady, local release of 20 µg levonorgestrel per day through the rate-limiting surface membrane. The reservoir is covered by a silicone membrane, and the frame contains barium sulphate, which makes it radiopaque. A monofilament removal thread is attached to a loop at the end of the vertical stem. The introduction of LNG-IUS has brought a significant change in the side effects in IUD users, with a dramatic reduction in blood loss and the number of days of bleeding per cycle. However, during the first months of use, bleeding can be erratic or even heavy at times, with more than 30% of users experiencing prolonged bleeding of more than 8 days duration. The LNG IUS is licensed for 5 years' use. Many studies, reporting more than 12,000 women/years of use, have confirmed the excellent efficacy of the LNG IUS, with Pearl indices of 0–0.3. There is no statistically significant difference between the efficacy of the LNG IUS and CuT380 at 7 years. A European multicentre trial showed an incidence of ectopic pregnancy of only 0.02 per 100 women-years, representing an 80-90 % reduction in risk compared with women not using contraception. Approximately 20% of conceptions with the LNG IUS are ectopic; the possibility of ectopic pregnancy should therefore not be ignored in a woman with an LNG IUS *in situ*. Expulsion rates have been found to be similar to those with other framed devices.

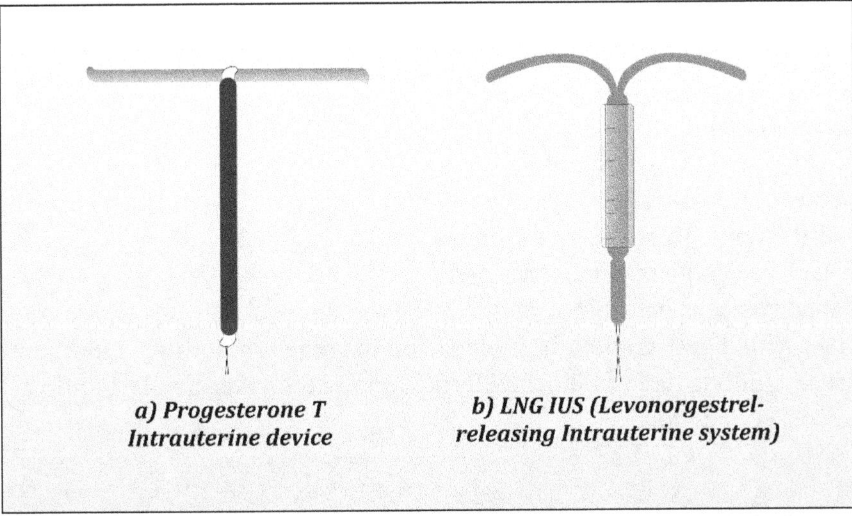


**Fig. 11.4:** Steroid mediated IUDs.

## Risk/Side Effects

Every woman is different and IUDs are not recommended for all women. Due to the risk of serious health problems, women with the following conditions should not use IUDs:

- ➢ Recent or repeated pelvic infection
- ➢ Known or suspected pregnancy
- ➢ Severe cervicitis
- ➢ Salpingitis
- ➢ Malignant lesions in the genital tract
- ➢ Unexplained vaginal bleeding
- ➢ HIV/AIDS
- ➢ History of ectopic pregnancy
- ➢ History of Toxic Shock Syndrome
- ➢ Physical inability to check IUD

IUDs are not recommended for women who are at risk for PID, have lower immune response, abnormal pap smear, heart disease, anaemia, a history of severe menstrual cramping and heavy flow, a history of ectopic pregnancy, or previous problems with an IUD. Copper IUDs are not recommended for women with Wilson's disease or allergies to copper.

- ➢ Women with a history of breast cancer cannot use the Mirena IUD.
- ➢ Women with diabetes should be monitored carefully if they use the Mirena IUD.
- ➢ Breastfeeding women should be aware the synthetic hormone in the Mirena IUD is excreted in breast milk.

## Advantages

- ➢ Prolonged release,
- ➢ Minimal systemic side effects,
- ➢ An increase in bioavailability,
- ➢ Use of less total drug than an oral dose,
- ➢ First-pass metabolism can be avoided,
- ➢ Self-medication is possible.
- ➢ Contact with digestive fluid is avoided and degradation of drug is minimized3.
- ➢ Nausea, vomiting, emesis induced through oral administration is avoided.
- ➢ Quick onset of action.

## Disadvantages

- ➢ Gender specificity,
- ➢ Patient incompliance,

➢ Only a few drugs are administered by this route,
➢ Variability in drug absorption related with menstrual cycle, menopause and pregnancy,
➢ Influence with sexual intercourse.
➢ Personal hygiene.
➢ Some drugs are sensitive at vaginal pH

## Development of Intrauterine Devices (IUDs) and Applications

Several new intrauterine devices (IUDs) are under development or in the early marketing phase. These new devices contain various modifications designed to improve patient continuation and physician satisfaction. Modifications include those designed to facilitate easier insertion and removal, to decrease the rates of accidental expulsion, and reduce complaints of pain or bleeding (responsible for 30 % to 50 % of discontinuations). Devices are being designed to address these issues by modifying IUD size, shape, and flexibility. Some devices are under development or have recently been introduced. These devices include:

1. **CuSafe 300:** This device was developed specifically to decrease the incidence of unwanted side effects such as bleeding, pain and expulsion. The plastic frame of the device is smaller and more flexible than most other framed devices. Both ends of the device's transverse arms curve inwards to reduce uterine tissue irritation. The side arms are thinner than the central stem, allowing easier insertion by a simple push-in technique, and are bent back on themselves in order to reduce trauma to the endometrium. In addition, its monofilament tail is welded into the shaft, instead of knotted, to reduce ectocervical abrasion. This design facilitates easier and less painful insertion and removal, but the curved, "fundal-seeking" arms also resist expulsion. The device bears 300 mm copper on its central stem. The CuSafe 300 is a T-shaped copper IUD with flexible, uniquely shaped arms. It carries a recommended lifespan of 5 years.

   Early studies were encouraging. In a non-comparative study in over 1000 women, 80% of them nulliparous, the 1-year pregnancy and expulsion rates were both 0.6 per 100. Removals for bleeding and pain were also low, at 4.2 and 1.5 per 100, respectively. However, a randomised trial, comparing the device to the TCu380A in 600 nulliparous and parous women, apparently produced a higher pregnancy rate which was not significant, and a significantly higher expulsion rate for the Cu-Safe than the TCu380A. In the study comparing CuSafe and TCu380A IUDs, removals for pain and bleeding occurred significantly less frequently among CuSafe IUD users. On the other hand, the study found that the CuSafe had higher, although statistically nonsignificant, rates of pregnancy and expulsion.

2. **Fincoid-350L** The Fincoid-350, is also designed to resist accidental expulsion. The IUD has a plastic skeleton comprised of two parts: curved horizontal arms, and a copper-coated vertical stem. The horizontal arms lock into a groove on the vertical

stem. The resulting movable joint easily constricts and expands with uterine contractions, adjusting to variations in uterine size and shape. The Fincoid-350 comes in two sizes: standard and short. Studies indicate continuation rates of 90% for the Fincoid-350 device. A study of 792 women found a pregnancy rate of 0.6%, an expulsion rate of 3.7%, and a rate of removal for pain or bleeding of 2.6 %. Another study of 90 women found a higher failure rate of 2.8 %.

3. **GyneFix®:** To minimize failure and side effects of intrauterine devices (IUDs), especially abnormal bleeding, pain, partial and complete expulsion, and other complications due to disharmony, the "frameless" intrauterine system (IUS) was developed. Total elimination of the frame would create perfect harmony and reduce the surface area of the foreign body. However, to retain the IUS in the uterine cavity, the device should be fixed to the uterine wall. This approach seemed a logical and practical way to obtain a significant improvement in IUD performance. This "frameless" IUD consists of six 5 mm copper sleeves with an effective copper surface area of 330 mm, fixed on a length of semi-rigid suture thread. The knot at the upper extremity of the device is anchored (implanted) in the myometrium of the uterine fundus. This device was originally called the Cu-Fix 390, then later the FlexiGard 330 (identical to GyneFix in all but insertion instrument). The device has under-gone 10 years of testing and several modifications to its insertion and anchoring mechanisms. The upper and lower copper sleeves are crimped onto the suture thread to prevent slippage. The proximal end of the suture contains a knot that is insertede1 cm into the fundal myometrium to anchor the device into the uterine muscle. Variations of the device for postpartum use include a larger knot and a cone shaped biodegradable tip that help anchor it securely.

4. **Intracervical fixing device (ICFD):** The intracervical fixing device (ICFD) differs substantially in both construction and placement from other IUDs . The device consists of a rod-shaped, copper-coated polyethylene frame that is about 4 cm long, with a 5 mm projection at the distal end. Through this projection, the ICFD is anchored (fixed) to the inner cervical wall using a modified tenaculum. Removal is facilitated by grasping the stem with sponge forceps. Investigators believe the ICFD's anchoring mechanism could be improved, however, and new fixing techniques are being studied. Better anchoring mechanisms could help to prevent expulsions. One potential advantage of the device is that the insertion procedure is not blind. In addition, because of the intracervical location, the device is less likely to be associated with spotting, bleeding and pain.

5. **Sof-T:** The Sof-T is a copper IUD with a unique shape to enhance effectiveness. The device has soft, flexible knobs, or occlusion bodies, on each end of its flexible transverse arms. These knobs theoretically block the entrances into the fallopian tubes. The insertion procedure for the Sof-T is similar to that for currently available copper IUDs. Ultrasound must be used, however, to ensure exact placement of the device. The device's potential ability to occlude the fallopian tubes could, in theory, reduce the incidence of tubal infection and ectopic pregnancy; however, comparative trials have yet to be performed.

6. **Multiload Mark II:** The Multiload Mark II is an updated version of the original Multiload 375 (ML 375). The original device has a record of dependability, with low patient cessation rates due to pregnancy, expulsion or bleeding and pain. The ML 375 has been associated with problematic insertions, however, because its arms do not fit into the inserter; the arms are open during insertion, making placement more difficult. Developers hope the Multiload Mark II will overcome these insertion limitations. Like its prototype, the Multiload Mark II has a 375 mm copper-coated shaft; however, it has shorter, more flexible arms that allow the device to be folded completely into its inserter. As a result, the new inserter's diameter is smaller than the original model. In addition, the inserter has three other improvements: its design prevents the IUD from getting pushed beyond the inserter; it can function as a uterine sound; and it has a single-handed expulsion action. These innovations may help limit the risk of uterine perforation.

## Conclusion

The latest IUDs are innovative form of contraception which removes the disadvantages of the older contraception techniques and also offers some other health benefits. These are once for a longer time device which eliminates the need of daily contraceptive pills or any other methods very few side effects. However, some severe contradictions, infection, hormonal imbalance were also reported but in case of any harm it can be easily removed. The progestin IUD can also regularize the menstrual cycle and other hormonal irregularities. At the same time, the copper IUD and progestin IUD can also reduce the risk of endometrial cancer. These are not recommended if the women are already having any STD or any other infection.

## Bibliography


1. Bahamondes, L., M. Valeria Bahamondes, and L.P. Shulman, Non-contraceptive benefits of hormonal and intrauterine reversible contraceptive methods. Hum Reprod Update, 2015. 21(5): p. 640-51.

2. Batur, P., L.N. Kransdorf, and P.M. Casey, Emergency Contraception. Mayo Clin Proc, 2016. 91(6): p. 802-7.

3. Berry-Bibee, E.N., et al., The safety of intrauterine devices in breastfeeding women: a systematic review. Contraception, 2016. 94(6): p. 725-738.

4. Chai, W., et al., Vesical transmigration of an intrauterine contraceptive device: A rare case report and literature review. Medicine (Baltimore), 2017. 96(40): p. e8236.

5.    Fok, W.K. and P.D. Blumenthal, Update on emergency contraception. Curr Opin Obstet Gynecol, 2016. 28(6): p. 522-529.

6.    Hsia, J.K. and M.D. Creinin, Intrauterine Contraception. Semin Reprod Med, 2016. 34(3): p. 175-82.

7.    Hubacher, D. and D.A. Grimes, Noncontraceptive health benefits of intrauterine devices: a systematic review. Obstet Gynecol Surv, 2002. 57(2): p. 120-8.

8.    Jatlaoui, T.C., H.E.M. Riley, and K.M. Curtis, The safety of intrauterine devices among young women: a systematic review. Contraception, 2017. 95(1): p. 17-39.

9.    Johnson, M.J. and K.W. Morgan, Intrauterine contraception benefits extend beyond birth control. Nurse Pract, 2005. 30(2): p. 50-5.

10.    Kallat, A., et al., [Intrauterine device: about a rare complication and literature review]. Pan Afr Med J, 2017. 27: p. 193.

11.    Lethaby, A., et al., Progesterone or progestogen-releasing intrauterine systems for heavy menstrual bleeding. Cochrane Database Syst Rev, 2015(4): p. Cd002126.

12.    Lopez, L.M., et al., Immediate postpartum insertion of intrauterine device for contraception. Cochrane Database Syst Rev, 2015(6): p. Cd003036.

13.    Lopez, L.M., et al., Interventions for pain with intrauterine device insertion. Cochrane Database Syst Rev, 2015(7): p. Cd007373.

14.    Matthews, L.R., L. O'Dwyer, and E. O'Neill, Intrauterine Device Insertion Failure After Misoprostol Administration: A Systematic Review. Obstet Gynecol, 2016. 128(5): p. 1084-1091.

15.    Ortiz, M.E. and H.B. Croxatto, Copper-T intrauterine device and levonorgestrel intrauterine system: biological bases of their mechanism of action. Contraception, 2007. 75(6 Suppl): p. S16-30.

16.    Pagano, H.P., et al., Safety of hormonal contraception and intrauterine devices among women with depressive and bipolar disorders: a systematic review. Contraception, 2016. 94(6): p. 641-649.

17.    Patil, E. and P.H. Bednarek, Immediate Intrauterine Device Insertion Following Surgical Abortion. Obstet Gynecol Clin North Am, 2015. 42(4): p. 583-91.

18.    Salma, U., et al., Efficacy of intrauterine device in the treatment of intrauterine adhesions. Biomed Res Int, 2014. 2014: p. 589296.

19.    Schwarz, E.B., R. Hess, and J. Trussell, Contraception for cancer survivors. J Gen Intern Med, 2009. 24 Suppl 2: p. S401-6.

20.    Sivin, I. and I. Batar, State-of-the-art of non-hormonal methods of contraception: III. Intrauterine devices. Eur J Contracept Reprod Health Care, 2010. 15(2): p. 96-112.

21.    Sonalkar, S. and N. Kapp, Intrauterine device insertion in the postpartum period: a systematic review. Eur J Contracept Reprod Health Care, 2015. 20(1): p. 4-18.

22. Stephen Searle, E., The intrauterine device and the intrauterine system. Best Pract Res Clin Obstet Gynaecol, 2014. 28(6): p. 807-24.

23. van Os, W.A., The intrauterine device and its dynamics. Adv Contracept, 1999. 15(2): p. 119-32.

24. Whaley, N.S. and A.E. Burke, Intrauterine contraception. Womens Health (Lond), 2015. 11(6): p. 759-67.

25. Zapata, L.B., et al., Intrauterine device use among women with ovarian cancer: a systematic review. Contraception, 2010. 82(1): p. 38-40.

26. Zapata, L.B., et al., Medications to ease intrauterine device insertion: a systematic review. Contraception, 2016. 94(6): p. 739-759.


# Exercise

## A. Multiple Choice Questions

1. An intrauterine device (IUD) are administered through
   (a) Injectables
   (b) Skin
   (c) Vagina
   (d) Mouth

2. An IUD should only be removed by a
   (a) Pharmacist
   (b) Dentist
   (c) Physiotherapist
   (d) Medical professional

3. The "first generation" IUDs was introduced in
   (a) 1960    (b) 1946    (c) 1981    (d) 1978

4. Dalkon Shield was developed by
   (a) Hugh Davis
   (b) Sergei Yudin
   (c) Vladimir Yourkevitch
   (d) Vladimir Zworykin

5. Copper IUDs are not recommended for women with
   (a) Pott's Spine
   (b) Blood Sugar
   (c) Wilson's disease
   (d) Alzheimer disease

6. The CuSafe 300 is a T-shaped copper IUD has a lifespan of
   (a) 1 Year    (b) Six months    (c) 10 Years    (d) 5 Years

7. What is the success rate of an IUD for birth control
   (a) 10 %    (b) 50 %    (c) 80 %    (d) 99 %

8. The IUD is a method of
   (a) Chance
   (b) Repetitive surgeries
   (c) Long-acting reversible contraception (LARC)
   (d) Invasion

9. Conditions which may indicate to use an IUD are
    (a) you might already be pregnant
    (b) have an untreated sexually transmitted infection or pelvic infection
    (c) have problems with your uterus or cervix
    (d) people with a healthy uterus
10. Removal of IUDs is a
    (a) Painful                    (b)    Simple and easy
    (c) Difficult and complex      (d)    Required major surgery

## B. Short Questions

1. What is IUDs?
2. Write a brief note on efficacy of IUDs?
3. Who can use IUDs?
4. Write the advantages and disadvantages of IUDs?
5. What are the health risks involved with the use of IUDs?

## C. Long Questions

1. What do you mean by IUDs? Explain its different types in detail.
2. Explain in detail the working of CuSafe 300.
3. Explain in details about the various generation of the IUDs.

# Answers

## CHAPTER 1

| | | | | |
|---|---|---|---|---|
| 1. (b) | 2. (a) | 3. (b) | 4. (d) | 5. (c) |
| 6. (a) | 7. (b) | 8. (c) | 9. (d) | 10. (a) |
| 11. (d) | 12. (a) | 13. (b) | 14. (d) | 15. (c) |
| 16. (a) | 17. (b) | 18. (c) | 19. (d) | 20. (a) |

## CHAPTER 2

| | | | | |
|---|---|---|---|---|
| 1. (d) | 2. (d) | 3. (b) | 4. (a) | 5. (c) |
| 6. (a) | 7. (b) | 8. (a) | 9. (c) | 10. (b) |
| 11. (b) | 12. (a) | 13. (c) | 14. (d) | 15. (b) |
| 16. (d) | 17. (d) | 18. (d) | 19. (a) | 20. (d) |

## CHAPTER 3

| | | | | |
|---|---|---|---|---|
| 1. (c) | 2. (b) | 3. (d) | 4. (a) | 5. (b) |
| 6. (a) | 7. (d) | 8. (c) | 9. (b) | 10. (a) |
| 11. (c) | 12. (a) | 13. (d) | 14. (c) | 15. (a) |
| 16. (b) | 17. (d) | 18. (b) | 19. (a) | 20. (d) |

## CHAPTER 4

| | | | | |
|---|---|---|---|---|
| 1. (a) | 2. (c) | 3. (d) | 4. (b) | 5. (a) |
| 6. (d) | 7. (d) | 8. (a) | 9. (c) | 10. (b) |
| 11. (a) | 12. (c) | 13. (b) | 14. (d) | 15. (a) |
| 16. (a) | 17. (c) | 18. (d) | 19. (b) | 20. (a) |

## CHAPTER 5

| | | | | |
|---|---|---|---|---|
| 1. (b) | 2. (a) | 3. (c) | 4. (d) | 5. (a) |
| 6. (d) | 7. (a) | 8. (d) | 9. (a) | 10. (d) |
| 11. (b) | 12. (d) | 13. (a) | 14. (d) | 15. (c) |
| 16. (c) | 17. (b) | 18. (d) | 19. (a) | 20. (b) |

## CHAPTER 6

| | | | | |
|---|---|---|---|---|
| 1. (b) | 2. (d) | 3. (a) | 4. (c) | 5. (b) |
| 6. (b) | 7. (a) | 8. (b) | 9. (a) | 10. (b) |
| 11. (c) | 12. (c) | 13. (a) | 14. (b) | 15. (c) |
| 16. (d) | 17. (b) | 18. (d) | 19. (d) | 20. (b) |

## CHAPTER 7

| | | | | |
|---|---|---|---|---|
| 1. (c) | 2. (d) | 3. (a) | 4. (b) | 5. (c) |
| 6. (a) | 7. (b) | 8. (c) | 9. (a) | 10. (d) |
| 11. (b) | 12. (a) | 13. (d) | 14. (d) | 15. (a) |
| 16. (b) | 17. (c) | 18. (b) | 19. (a) | 20. (d) |

## CHAPTER 8

| | | | | |
|---|---|---|---|---|
| 1. (b) | 2. (d) | 3. (a) | 4. (c) | 5. (b) |
| 6. (a) | 7. (d) | 8. (c) | 9. (b) | 10. (a) |
| 11. (c) | 12. (d) | 13. (d) | 14. (a) | 15. (d) |
| 16. (b) | 17. (c) | 18. (a) | 19. (b) | 20. (c) |

## CHAPTER 9

| | | | | |
|---|---|---|---|---|
| 1. (a) | 2. (d) | 3. (b) | 4. (c) | 5. (d) |
| 6. (a) | 7. (c) | 8. (b) | 9. (d) | 10. (a) |
| 11. (c) | 12. (b) | 13. (a) | 14. (d) | 15. (c) |
| 16. (a) | 17. (b) | 18. (c) | 19. (d) | 20. (a) |

# CHAPTER 10

| 1. (d) | 2. (a) | 3. (b) | 4. (d) | 5. (d) |
| 6. (a) | 7. (b) | 8. (c) | 9. (d) | 10. (a) |
| 11. (c) | 12. (a) | 13. (d) | 14. (b) | 15. (a) |
| 16. (d) | 17. (c) | 18. (b) | 19. (d) | 20. (b) |

# CHAPTER 11

| 1. (c) | 2. (d) | 3. (a) | 4. (a) | 5. (c) |
| 6. (d) | 7. (d) | 8. (c) | 9. (d) | 10. (b) |

# Index

## C

Polyethylene glycol 11, 119, 139, 179, 203
Polylactic acid 151, 155, 203
Polymer chain branching 45
Polymer matrix/drug reservoir 180-181
Polymer properties 118, 216
Polymeric matrix 50, 143, 147
Polymers 37-38, 40, 43, 48, 239,
Polysaccharides 37, 96, 123, 164, 206
Polystyrene 66, 74, 95, 208, 272
Polystyrene sulfonic acid resin 272
Positive displacement pumps 152, 154
Posterior segment 259, 265, 280
Pourability of the suspension 64
Powders 63, 218, 232
Precorneal cavity 262
Preparation of different types of gels 64
Preparation of individual
matrix solution 188
Pressure sensitive adhesive (PSA) 181, 183
Pressurised metered dose inhalers 219, 231
Principle involved in transdermal
penetration 171
Principles of bioadhession/
mucoadhesion 107
Processes used to prepare
controlled-release formulations 15
Processing rate 45
Prodrugs 276
Progestasert IUD 137
Progestin 138, 287
Progestin IUD 288, 295
Prolonged action dosage form 4
Properties of polymers 42, 46, 47, 79,
96, 118
Protective function 166
Protein backbones 240
Pulmonary drug delivery 217, 219
Punching of laminated roll/
making unit dose 189

## Q

Quantum dots 241, 246
Quick adherence 203

## R

Race 175, 177
Radiation barrier 166, 167
Rationale of Controlled Drug Delivery 4
Receptor targeting 3, 35
Receptor-mediated adhesion 203, 214
Regional variation 175, 176
Release liner 54, 181, 184, 195,
Reservoir effect of horny layer 175, 176
Reservoir systems 11, 35, 49, 53, 72
Reservoir type 9, 12, 57, 151
Residence time 6, 58, 121, 146, 168, 197,
218, 231, 244, 279
Residual volume 223
Reticuloendothelial system 238
Retina 260, 265
Riboflavin 21
Rigidization of coating 88,
Robustness 226
Route of administration 7, 21, 35, 51, 145,
158, 197, 217, 229, 260
Rubber or elastomer 41

## S

Saliva 106, 115, 118, 127
Saliva and mucous 118
Sclemm's canal 262
Sclera 260, 264 278
Sebum and surface material 168, 170, 194
Second generation iuds 290
Selection of drug candidates for controlled
release dosage form 7
Selection of implant material 149
Self-aggregation 242
Self-protecting mechanism 202
Semipermeable membrane 137, 147, 207
Semi-synthetic polymer 39
Short residence time 121, 218, 231
Side groups of polymer side chain 44
Single layer floating tablet
/hydrodynamically balanced system 202
Site-specific targeting 3
Skin appendages 165, 169, 196